Protein Misfolding Disorders: A Trip into the ER

Editor: Claudio Hetz

CONTENTS

FOREWORD

Secretory cells require an expanded endoplasmic reticulum (ER) to carry out their task. Efficient protein folding inevitably leads to the accumulation of misfolded proteins as well, a normal byproduct of the protein maturation process. Hence, specialized secretory activity is accompanied by constant ER stress, constituting a threat to the life of a cell. Adaptation to the stress of protein misfolding is accomplished by the activation of a complex signaling pathway known as the unfolded protein response (UPR). Genetic manipulation of the UPR supports the notion that components of the pathway are essential to sustain the function of secretory cells such as B lymphocytes and pancreatic exocrine and endocrine cells.

Emerging evidence suggests that the occurrence of ER stress influences diseases ranging from cancer to autoimmunity and diabetes. Perturbation in organelle function has also been observed in many neurological disorders related to protein misfolding and aggregation. Most neurodegenerative disorders share a common neuropathology, primarily featuring the presence of abnormal protein aggregates containing specific misfolded proteins. These diseases include pathological conditions such as amyotrophic lateral sclerosis (ALS), Alzheimer's Disease (AD), Parkinson's Disease (PD), Prion-related Disorders (PrD), Huntington's Disease (HD), and others.

In this informative E-Book, Claudio Hetz has brought together experts in the UPR to provide an overview of the emerging role of ER stress and protein misfolding in different physiological and pathological conditions. Several chapters focus on the role of the UPR in specific diseases such as diabetes, cancer, and neurodegeneration; other chapters discuss biochemical and genetic mechanisms underpinning the UPR, autophagy and the ubiquitin-proteasome system. Auhors include Amy Lee, an expert in chaperone biology and cancer; Randal Kaufman, a pioneer in identifying the components of the UPR; Claudio Soto, Hidenori Hichijo, and Takashi Momoi, experts in neurodegeneration and protein misfolding, and many others. An important focus of the book is considering the potential therapeutic benefits of targeting ER stress pathways in the context of human disease. Readers interested in understanding how a cell handles protein folding stress and the consequences of dysregulation of this process for human disease will find this book invaluable.

Laurie H. Glimcher, *M.D.*
Irene Heinz Given
Professor of Immunology,
Harvard School of Public Health
Professor of Medicine,
Harvard Medical School

PREFACE

The functional and structural integration between different subcellular compartments is essential for the proper function of a cell. At each organelle, different molecular sentinels permanently sense stressful cellular conditions and initiate complex responses that aim either to adapt to the new conditions restoring homeostasis, or to induce cell suicide to eliminate the damaged cell. One particular organelle, the endoplasmic reticulum (ER), had merged as a main subcellular compartment affected in diverse pathological conditions as diverse as cancer, diabetes, and brain disorders. The ER has important roles in physiology including regulating and executing many post-translational modifications of proteins, ensuring their proper folding and facilitating formation of functional protein complexes. The ER is also the place where the biosynthesis of steroids, cholesterol, and other lipids occurs, playing a crucial role in organelle biogenesis and signaling through the generation of lipid second messengers. The ER is well-known as a major calcium store in the cells and thus constitutes a signaling organelle that modulates many cellular processes including proliferation, cell death and differentiation via calcium release.

A number of physiological and pathological conditions alter the protein folding status at the ER, leading to the accumulation of unfolded or misfolded proteins in the ER lumen, a cellular condition referred as "ER stress". ER stress triggers a complex adaptive reaction known as the unfolded protein response (UPR), which aims the restoration of the homeostasis of this organelle. Activation of the UPR affects the expression of proteins involved in nearly every aspect of the secretory pathway, including protein entry into the ER, folding, glycosylation, ER-associated degradation (ERAD), ER biogenesis, lipid metabolism and vesicular trafficking. The UPR restores the folding capacity to decrease unfolded protein load. Different physiological conditions can induce the UPR by increasing the demand of protein synthesis/secretion or by the generation of excessive misfolded proteins as described for B lymphocytes and pancreatic ☐ cells. Also, abnormal metabolic conditions, such as glucose deprivation can trigger the UPR. Components of the ER stress pathway have been shown to be an important factor for tumor survival and growth due to an adaptation to hypoxia conditions. In addition, in different neurodegenerative conditions associated with protein misfolding (including Huntington's disease, Alzheimer's, Prion-related disorders, amyotrophic lateral sclerosis and others), an irreversible alteration of ER homeostasis has been proposed to be a critical mediator of neuronal dysfunction.

In this book we put together many specialized chapters discussing the emerging role of ER stress and protein misfolding in diverse pathologies. Dr. Fumico Urano from UMASS gives a comprehensive summary of the experimental data supporting the role of the UPR in diabetes. Crucial mediators in the alleviation of the stress in the ER are protein chaperones and foldases of the Glucose Regulated Protein (GRPs) family. Amy Lee, one of the pioneers in the study of GRPs in apoptosis and ER stress, presents an overview of the multiple functional roles of this family of proteins in cancer. Randal Kaufman, a recognized pioneer in the field, prepared a detailed analysis of the function and interconnection between different UPR signaling pathways.

Accumulation of abnormal protein aggregates composed of misfolded proteins is a common denominator in many neurological disorders. Diferent specialist in diverse neurological disorders, including Drs. Julie Atkin, Hidenori Hichijo, Takashi Momoi, Othman Ghribi, Nibaldo Inestrosa, Claudio Soto, and myself, discuss recent evidences suggesting the involvement of ER stress and other signaling pathways in protein misfolding disorders affecting the nervous system and the possible therapeutic benefits of targeting the UPR. As the reader will conclude from this selected group of chapters, pharmacological targeting of different components of the UPR/ER stress pathway may have therapeutic application for the treatment of many pathological conditions, such as diabetes, cancer and neurological disorders.

Claudio Hetz, *PhD*
Director Laboratory Cellular Stress and Biomedicine
Institute of Biomedical Sciences,
University of Chile,
Santiago, Chile.
and Adjunct Professor
Harvard School of Public Health,
Boston, USA

CONTRIBUTORS

Claudio Hetz	Institute of Biomedical Sciences, University of Chile. Independencia 1027, Santiago, Chile, P.O.BOX 70086
Randal J. Kaufman	Howard Hughes Medical Institute, University of Michigan Medical Center, Ann Arbor, MI 48109-0650 USA
Amy S. Lee	USC/Norris Comprehensive Cancer Center, University of Southern California Keck School of Medicine, Los Angeles, California 90089, USA
J.D. Atkin	Howard Florey Institute, University of Melbourne, Parkville, Victoria 3010, Australia
Fumihiko Urano	University of Massachusetts Medical School, Worcester, MA 01605, USA
Takashi Momoi	Divisions of Development and Differentiation, Department of Human Inherited Metabolic Disease, National Institute of Neuroscience, 4-1-1 Ogawahigashi-machi, Kodaira, Tokyo 187-8502, Japan
Hidenori Ichijo	Cell Signaling, Graduate School of Pharmaceutical Sciences, The University of Tokyo, 7-3-1 Hongo, Bunkyo-ku, Tokyo 113-0033, Japan
Nibaldo C. Inestrosa	Centro de Envejecimiento y Regeneración (CARE), Facultad de Ciencias Biológicas, Pontificia Universidad Católica de Chile, Santiago, Chile
Othman Ghribi	Department of Pharmacology, Physiology and Therapeutics, University of North Dakota School of Medicine, Grand Forks, ND, 58202, USA
Claudio Soto	Protein Misfolding Disorders Laboratory, George and Cynthia Mitchell Center for Neurodegenerative Diseases, Dept of Neurology, University of Texas Medical School at Houston, USA
J. Paul Taylor	Department of Developmental Neurobiology, St. Jude Children's Research Hospital, 262 Danny Thomas Place, Memphis, TN 38120 USA
Danny Galleguillos	FONDAP Center for Molecular Studies of the Cell, University of Chile, Santiago, Chile, Faculty of Medicine, Independencia 1027, Santiago, Chile

Vicente Valenzuela	FONDAP Center for Molecular Studies of the Cell, University of Chile, Santiago, Chile, Faculty of Medicine, Independencia 1027, Santiago, Chile
Pamela Valdés	FONDAP Center for Molecular Studies of the Cell, University of Chile, Santiago, Chile, Faculty of Medicine, Independencia 1027, Santiago, Chile
Alexis Martínez	FONDAP Center for Molecular Studies of the Cell, University of Chile, Santiago, Chile, Faculty of Medicine, Independencia 1027, Santiago, Chile
Soledad Matus	FONDAP Center for Molecular Studies of the Cell, University of Chile, Santiago, Chile, Faculty of Medicine, Independencia 1027, Santiago, Chile
Melissa Nassif	FONDAP Center for Molecular Studies of the Cell, University of Chile, Santiago, Chile, Faculty of Medicine, Independencia 1027, Santiago, Chile
Mauricio Torres	FONDAP Center for Molecular Studies of the Cell, University of Chile, Santiago, Chile, Faculty of Medicine, Independencia 1027, Santiago, Chile
Gabriela Martínez	FONDAP Center for Molecular Studies of the Cell, University of Chile, Santiago, Chile, Faculty of Medicine, Independencia 1027, Santiago, Chile
Sung Hoon Back	Howard Hughes Medical Institute, University of Michigan Medical Center, Ann Arbor, MI 48109-0650 USA
Justin R. Hassler	Howard Hughes Medical Institute, University of Michigan Medical Center, Ann Arbor, MI 48109-0650 USA
Risheng Ye	University of Southern California Keck School of Medicine, Los Angeles, California 90089, USA
Yi Zhang	University of Southern California Keck School of Medicine, Los Angeles, California 90089, USA
Sonya G. Fonseca	University of Massachusetts Medical School, Worcester, MA 01605, USA
A.K. Walker	Howard Florey Institute, University of Melbourne, Parkville, Victoria 3010, Australia

| B.J. Turner | Howard Florey Institute, University of Melbourne, Parkville, Victoria 3010, Australia |

| Eriko Fujita | Divisions of Development and Differentiation, Department of Human Inherited Metabolic Disease, National Institute of Neuroscience, 4-1-1 Ogawahigashi-machi, Kodaira, Tokyo 187-8502, Japan |

| Hideki Nishitoh | Graduate School of Pharmaceutical Sciences, The University of Tokyo, Tokyo 113-0033, Japan |

| Hisae Kadowaki | Graduate School of Pharmaceutical Sciences, The University of Tokyo, Tokyo 113-0033, Japan |

| Kohsuke Takeda | Graduate School of Pharmaceutical Sciences, The University of Tokyo, Tokyo 113-0033, Japan |

| Catalina Grabowski | Centro de Envejecimiento y Regeneración (CARE), Facultad de Ciencias Biológicas, Pontificia Universidad Católica de Chile, Santiago, Chile |

| Macarena Arrázola | Centro de Envejecimiento y Regeneración (CARE), Facultad de Ciencias Biológicas, Pontificia Universidad Católica de Chile, Santiago, Chile |

| Lorena Varela-Nallar | Centro de Envejecimiento y Regeneración (CARE), Facultad de Ciencias Biológicas, Pontificia Universidad Católica de Chile, Santiago, Chile |

| Enrique M. Toledo | Centro de Envejecimiento y Regeneración (CARE), Facultad de Ciencias Biológicas, Pontificia Universidad Católica de Chile, Santiago, Chile |

| Abhisek Mukherjee | Protein Misfolding Disorders Laboratory, George and Cynthia Mitchell Center for Neurodegenerative Diseases, Dept of Neurology, University of Texas Medical School at Houston,USA |

| Natalia B. Nedelsky | Department of Developmental Neurobiology, St. Jude Children's Research Hospital, 262 Danny Thomas Place, Memphis, TN 38120 USA |

CHAPTER 1

Targeting Endoplasmic Reticulum Stress Pathways to Treat Neurological Disorders Associated with Protein Misfolding

Danny Galleguillos, Soledad Matus, Vicente Valenzuela, Pamela Valdés, Alexis Martínez, Melissa Nassif, Mauricio Torres, Gabriela Martínez and Claudio Hetz

Program of Cellular and Molecular Biology, Institute of Biomedical Sciences, Faculty of Medicine, NEMO Millennium Nucleus, and The FONDAP Center for Molecular Studies of the Cell, University of Chile, Santiago, Chile.

Address correspondence to: Dr. Claudio Hetz, Institute of Biomedical Sciences, University of Chile. Independencia 1027, Santiago, Chile, P.O.BOX 70086, Phone: 56-2-9786506 E-mail: chetz@med.uchile.cl, Website: http://www.annabolteus.com/HetzLab/ Index.html

Abstract: Amyotrophic lateral sclerosis, Alzheimer's Disease, Parkinson's Disease, Prion-related Disorders, Huntington's Disease and several other neurodegenerative disorders share a common neuropathology, primarily featuring the presence of abnormal protein inclusions containing specific misfolded proteins. Recent evidence indicates that alteration in organelle function is a common pathological feature of protein misfolding disorders. The endoplasmic reticulum (ER) is an essential compartment for protein folding, maturation, and secretion. Signs of ER stress have been extensively described in most experimental models of neurological disorders and more recently in the brains of human patients affected with neurodegenerative conditions. ER stress is caused by functional disturbances, which result in the accumulation of unfolded/misfolded proteins at the ER lumen. To cope with ER stress, cells activate an integrated signaling response termed the Unfolded Protein Response (UPR), which aims to reestablish homeostasis through transcriptional upregulation of genes involved in protein folding, quality control and degradation pathways. Small molecules with chaperone-like activity have been shown to alleviate ER stress and decrease protein misfolding in experimental disease settings. In this chapter we overview the role of ER stress in pathological conditions such as protein misfolding disorders and spinal cord injury, and discuss possible pharmacological strategies to target the UPR with therapeutic benefits.

1. INTRODUCTION

Most neurodegenerative disorders share a common neuropathology, primarily featuring the presence of abnormal protein aggregates containing specific misfolded proteins. These diseases are now classified as Protein Misfolding Disorders and include pathological conditions such as Amyotrophic lateral sclerosis (ALS), Alzheimer's Disease (AD), Parkinson's Disease (PD), Prion-related Disorders (PrD), Huntington's Disease (HD), and many others [1-4]. Disease-related misfolded proteins alter essential cellular functions that lead to neurological impairment and, in many cases cellular death. General alterations include synapse abnormalities, alteration in axonal transport, redox changes, proteasome dysfunction, and cytoskeleton disorganization. Increasing evidence indicates that organelle stress is an important pathological target in neurodegeneration. In brain disorders, special attention has been given in the last years to perturbations of a particular subcellular organelle, the endoplasmic reticulum

(ER). The ER is a specialized subcellular compartment essential for the folding of proteins destined to the secretory pathway. In most protein misfolding disorders, upregulation of ER stress markers is commonly observed linked to the activation of an adaptive reaction known as the Unfolded Protein Response (UPR). The UPR aims to reestablish homeostasis by augmenting the cells capacity to produce properly folded proteins. In doing so, activation of the UPR affects expression of proteins involved in nearly every aspect of the secretory pathway, including protein entry into the ER, folding, ER-associated degradation (ERAD), as well as other adaptive responses such as autophagy. Under chronic or irreversible ER damage the UPR will ultimately initiate apoptosis to eliminate injured cells. Although ER stress is observed in neurological disorders, the actual contribution of the pathway to the disease progression remains speculative and most available data is either correlative or based on *in vitro* evidence. This chapter focuses on recent findings correlating the activation of the UPR in pathological conditions affecting the nervous system and the possible use of pharmacological and gene therapy strategies to target this pathway aiming for therapeutic benefits.

2. UNFOLDED PROTEIN RESPONSE: MACHINERY AND OUTCOMES

The primary function of the ER is to facilitate protein folding and secretion. A complex system of protein chaperones is employed to catalyze the efficient folding of proteins and prevent their abnormal aggregation. This organelle is responsible for executing and regulating many posttranslational modifications, ensuring proper protein function and facilitating the formation of functional protein complexes. The ER also serves as the major calcium store, and also plays an essential role in the biosynthesis of steroids, cholesterol, and other lipids, controlling organelle biogenesis and signaling. A number of stress conditions can interfere with its function and therefore lead to abnormal protein folding in the ER lumen. Accumulation of unfolded and/or misfolded proteins causes an imbalance between the synthesis of new proteins and the ER's ability to process this newly synthesized proteins, resulting in failure of the ER to cope with excessive protein load, a condition termed 'ER stress' [5]. As a result, cells activate an integrated signaling cascade, the UPR, to avert ER stress, Fig. (1). Activation of the UPR results in attenuation of the rate of protein synthesis, upregulation of genes encoding chaperones, foldases and proteins related to maturation or involved in the retro-translocation and degradation of ER-generated misfolded proteins by the proteasome. This response is initiated to minimize accumulation and aggregation of misfolded proteins by increasing the functional capacity of the ER to facilitate folding and to degrade abnormal proteins [6, 7].

There are three main ER resident transmembrane signaling proteins that act as stress sensors to initiate different UPR signaling cascades: double-stranded RNA-activated protein kinase (PKR)-like endoplasmic reticulum kinase (PERK), activating transcription factor 6 (ATF6) α and β, and inositol requiring kinase 1 (IRE1) α and β. Each of these stress sensors transduces information of the protein folding status at the ER lumen to the nucleus by controlling expression of specific transcription factors. Thus, PERK, ATF6, and IRE1α operate in concert to ensure adaptation to protein folding stress (reviewed in [8]).

Activation of PERK is mediated by its oligomerization and autophosphorylation, leading to the phosphorylation and inhibition of eukaryotic translation initiation factor 2α (eIF2α) [9]. Alternatively, eIF2α phosphoryla-tion augments the specific translation of ATF4, a UPR transcription factor essential for the upregulation of many UPR genes such as CHOP and Grp78/BiP. Activated ATF6 translocates from the ER to the Golgi Apparatus where it is proteolytically processed, releasing its cytosolic domain which is then translocated to the nucleus to function as an activating transcription factor. This cleaved form of ATF6 upregulates several ER chaperones [10-12].

IRE1α and its downstream target X-Box-binding protein 1 (XBP-1) initiate the third adaptive response. IRE1α is a Serine/Threonine protein kinase and endoribonuclease that, upon activation initiates the unconventional splicing of the mRNA encoding the transcription factor XBP-1 [13-15]. A 26 nucleotide intron of XBP-1 mRNA is removed by activated IRE1α, resulting in an alternative splice form which shifts the mRNA reading frame. This mRNA maturation event promotes the translation of a stable protein, XBP-1s, which is targeted to the nucleus and upon binding to its response elements in the DNA acts as a potent transcriptional activator that controls the upregulation of a subset of UPR-related genes. Through this process IRE1α transduces survival signals into the nucleus to increase the folding capacity of the ER, therefore alleviating stress. In addition, activated IRE1α binds the adaptor protein TRAF2, leading to the activation of several signaling pathways including ERK, JNK and NF-kB [6]. The signaling activity of IRE1α is modulated by the formation of a protein complex termed the *UPRosome* (reviewed in [8, 16]), which is controlled by the binding of different accessory proteins including some members of the BCL-2 protein family and other components [16, 17].

3. PROTEIN MISFOLDING IN THE NERVOUS SYSTEM

As previously mentioned, a common feature of many neurodegenerative diseases is the accumulation and deposition of misfolded proteins that affects neural function and viability [1-4].

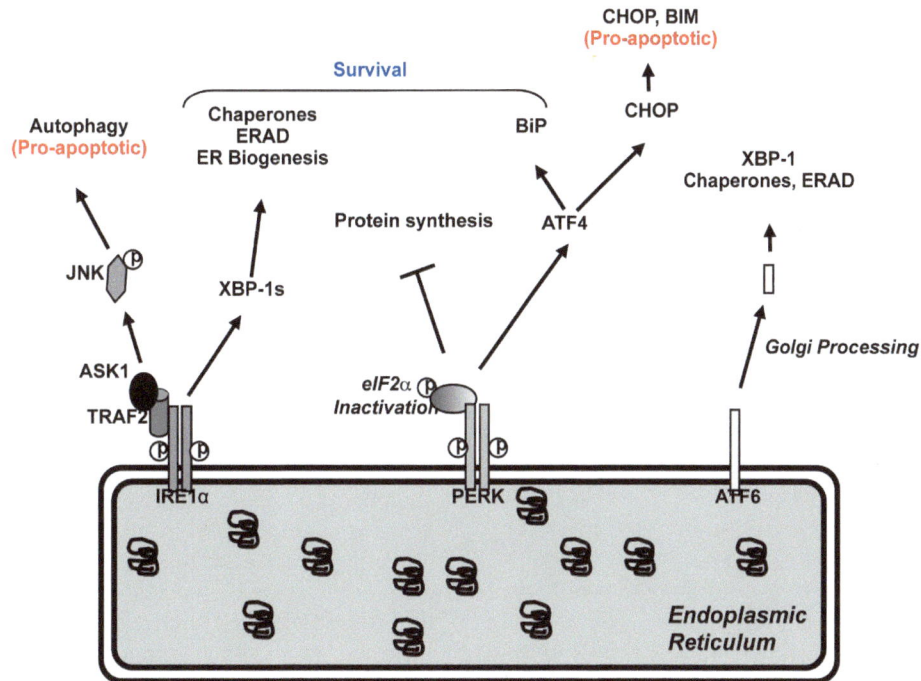

Fig. (1): The unfolded protein response. Accumulation of misfolded protein inside the endoplasmic reticulum (ER) lumen triggers a stress response known as the unfolded protein response (UPR). In cells undergoing ER stress, IRE1 autophosphorylation leads to the activation of its endoribonuclease activity. This activity mediates the processing of the mRNA encoding *XBP-1*, which is a transcription factor that upregulates many essential UPR genes involved in folding, organelle biogenesis, and protein quality control. Alternatively, activation of PERK increases the translation of *ATF4*, a transcription factor that induces the expression of genes such as CHOP that function in amino acid metabolism, antioxidant response, and apoptosis. A third UPR pathway is initiated by ATF6, a type II ER transmembrane protein encoding a bZIP transcriptional factor on its cytosolic domain and localized in the ER in unstressed cells. Upon ER stress induction, ATF6 is processed, increasing the expression of some ER chaperones.

Experimental evidence using mouse models of neurodegeration indicate that several mutations associated with hereditary forms of disease activate various components of the UPR, implying impaired ER function. More importantly, increased expression of ER stress markers has been observed in post-mortem brain tissues and cell culture models of many protein conformational disorders, including PD [18-20], ALS [21, 22], AD [23] and Creutzfeldt-Jacob's disease (CJD) [24, 25]. The expected functional significance of ER stress in the disease process is proposed to be both a protective component during early UPR responses and more deleterious during prolonged or chronic stress due to the irreversible disturbance of ER homeostasis (reviewed in [26, 27]). In the following sections we discuss specific evidence linking ER stress to neurodegeneration in four diseases (ALS, HD, PD and PrD) and also discuss therapeutic strategies that have been tested to target ER stress responses. In addition, recent experimental evidence linking ER stress with Spinal Cord Injury (SCI) conditions is presented.

3.1. Huntington's Disease

HD is an autosomal dominant neurodegenerative disorder characterized by progressive cognitive impairment, neuropsychiatric symptoms, and chorea. A mutation encoding an abnormal expansion of CAG-encoded polyglutamine - poly(Q)- repeats within the Huntingtin protein causes HD. Age of onset depends on the severity of the mutation, usually resulting in symptoms beginning in the fourth or fifth decade of life. Patients typically decline over a 15-20 year period until complications lead to death, as there is no effective treatment for the selective neuronal loss affecting the frontal lobe, striatum, and basal ganglia[28]. The general population exhibits an average of 18 poly(Q) repeats, yet expansions exceeding 35 repeats will almost always result in disease. Increasing numbers of repeats cause the age of onset to decrease, and individuals with more than 60 repeats will develop disease before the age of twenty [29].

The primary histopathological feature observed in HD is the co-localization of Huntingtin positive-aggregates with ubiquitin [30]. In many cases, the formation of intracellular Huntingtin inclusions precede cell death [31-33], and neurotoxicity is also plausible when considering the array of other proteins found within such aggregates [34, 35]. Changes in the subcellular localization of Huntingtin-interacting proteins may also contribute to the pathology [35].

Although the mechanism of expanded poly(Q) pathogenesis is still highly controversial, it is well established that neurotoxicity is provoked by a dominant gain of function. Neuronal apoptosis in HD is proposed to be mediated by several different mechanisms, including mitochondrial dysfunction, altered axonal transport, and proteasome dysfunction, to name a few of them (reviewed in [36]). Recent data also suggests that pro-apoptotic pathways originating from the ER may contribute to HD neurodegeneration. Mutant Huntingtin aggregates impair the function of the ubiquitin-proteasome system [36], resulting in ER stress through general accumulation of abnormally folded proteins, poisoning the cell with abnormal folding intermediates or immature proteins [37].

Recent attempts to understand the function of wild type Huntingtin demonstrated that inhibition of its expression significantly alters ER morphogenesis, network patterning [38] and alters post-Golgi trafficking [39, 40]. In addition, mutant Huntingtin perturbs ER calcium homeos-tasis [41], and the experimental targeting of poly(Q) peptides to the ER decreases aggregation [42]. Thus, increasing evidence suggests that mutant Huntingtin may exert its neurotoxic effect by directly altering ER function. However, the actual involvement of ER stress-related pathways in the disease remains speculative.

The accumulation of mutant poly(Q) inclusions triggers activation of UPR stress sensors IRE1α and PERK *in vitro*, resulting in upregulation of downstream targets [43]. Many groups have shown that ER stress partially mediates toxicity caused by mutant HD associated with activation of JNK, ASK1 and caspase-12 processing, an ER located caspase [44]. ASK1 deficient neurons have been shown to be protected from poly(Q)$_{79}$ toxicity [45]. One of primary roles of the UPR is to regulate the upregulation of a diverse set of chaperones, and many reports have shown that mutant Huntingtin aggregation can be diminished by the expression of cytosolic chaperones such as Hsp70 and Hsp40 [33, 46].

Evidence is beginning to emerge indicating that clearance pathways responsible for elimination of poly(Q) aggregates are closely regulated by the ER through UPR stress sensors such as PERK/eIF2α. PERK controls the expression of the autophagy-related gene ATG12, increasing lysosomal-mediated degradation of mutant Huntingtin [43]. Thus, the UPR and ER stress pathways may affect the accumulation of mutant Huntingtin in the cell. Autophagy is a "large-scale" cellular degradation process for proteins and damaged organelles [47]. Autophagy is divided in three subtypes, including macroauto-phagy, microautophagy, and chaperone-mediated autophagy. This review will focus on macroauto-phagy, hereafter referred to as autophagy. During autophagy, double membrane vesicles termed autophagosomes are formed, sequestering cytosolic proteins and/or organelles as cargoes. Autophagosomes then fuse with lysosomes, and their intracellular components are degraded to ultimately result in macromolecule recycling.

The therapeutic effects of targeting the UPR were recently demonstrated in models of diabetes where ER stress mediates insulin resistance [48]. The authors employed chemical chaperones, including 4-phenyl butyric acid (4-PBA) and trimethylamine N-oxide dihydrate (TMAO), which are a group of low molecular weight compounds known to stabilize protein conformation and improve ER folding capacity (reviewed in [49]). Likewise, endogenous bile acid derivates, such as TUDCA, also modulate ER function [50]. Remarkably, a positive effect of TUDCA administration was demonstrated on different models of Huntington's disease [51], reducing striatal-neuron apoptosis and the size of intranuclear Huntingtin inclusions. Locomotor and sensorimotor deficits were significantly improved in HD animal models upon treatment [51]. The chemical chaperone 4-PBA also significantly extended survival, improved motor performance, and delayed the neuropathological features in the R6/2 transgenic mouse model of HD [52]. The impact these drugs have on ER stress in HD transgenic mouse models remains to be determined.

The ability of chemical chaperones to alleviate ER stress *in vitro* demonstrates the feasibility of targeting organelle function for therapeutic achievements. Accumulating evidence indicates a constant homeostatic cross-talk between the UPR and autophagy [53]. In this line, activation of autophagy with rapamycin, which targets the mTOR pathway, has the capacity to increase the survival of HD animal models and recover motor performance. Autophagy occurs at basal levels in most tissues [54-56], yet activation preferentially occurs mainly under two different stress conditions: during starvation it acts to promote survival, and in times when misfolded proteins or damaged organelles are present it acts to clear out the cell of altered intracellular components. The therapeutic effects of rapamycin in HD models were associated with a decrease in Huntingtin aggregate size, indicating that pharmacological strategies aiming to increase autophagy-mediated clearance of protein aggregates may be clinically effective [57]. A relatively new drug, trehalose, was recently shown to act both as a chemical chaperone and an autophagy activator, decreasing the aggregation of mutant Huntingtin and α–synuclein *in vitro* [58]. The same group recently performed a small-molecule screen in yeast which identified novel small-molecule modulators of mammalian autophagy based on their ability to modulate the cytostatic effects of rapamycin [59]. Three enhancers induced autophagy independently of rapamycin in mammalian cells, facilitating the clearance of mutant Huntingtin and Parkinson's related α-synuclein[A53T]. These autophagy enhancers, which seem to act either independently or downstream of rapamycin, attenuated mutant Huntingtin-fragment toxicity in Huntington's disease *in vitro* models as well as in *D. melanogaster* [59], reinforcing the therapeutic potential of the clearance of mutant protein aggregates identified in neurodegenerative conditions.

3.2. Amyotrophic Lateral Sclerosis

ALS, also known as Lou Gehrig's disease, is a progressive and deadly adult-onset motor neuron disease characterized by muscle weakness, spasticity, atrophy, paralysis and premature death. The pathological hallmark of ALS is the selective degeneration of motoneurons in the spinal ventral horn, most brainstem nuclei and the cerebral cortex. Average onset occurs around age 50, with an incidence estimated at 1-2 per 100,000 individuals, males being more frequently affected than females. The majority of ALS patients lack a defined hereditary genetic component (sporadic ALS), while approximately 10% of cases are hereditary (familial ALS). Over 100 mutations affecting the gene encoding Superoxide Dismutase-1 (SOD1) has been associated with hereditary ALS. These mutations trigger the misfolding and abnormal aggregation of SOD1, which leads to neurotoxicity. Overexpression of

human fALS-linked SOD1 mutations in transgenic mice recapitulates essential features of the human pathology, provoking age-dependent protein aggregation, paralysis and motor neuron degeneration (see general reviews in [60, 61]).

The primary mechanism by which mutations in SOD1 contribute to progressive motoneuron loss in fALS remains unknown, but it has been proposed that neuronal loss is mediated by mitochondrial dysfunction, altered axonal transport, and non-neuronal components (reviewed in [60, 61]). Recent data also suggests that stress responses originating from the ER may contribute to ALS [62], Fig. (**2**). Activation of the UPR was recently described in post-mortem samples from sALS patients [21, 22], and Golgi ultrastructural abnormalities are a common hallmark of sALS (reviewed in [63]). Similarly, ER stress responses are observed in transgenic rodents expressing different fALS-related SOD1 mutations [64-71] and biochemical and histological studies revealed that a fraction of mutant SOD1 accumulates inside the ER and Golgi *in vivo*, where it forms insoluble high molecular weight species [66, 68, 69, Urushitani, 2008 #120, 72]. A direct interaction between mutant SOD1 and the ER chaperones Grp78/BiP and PDI was observed in microsomal fractions of spinal cord extracts [66, 68]. Significantly, a proteomic analysis of spinal cord tissue from SOD1[G93A] transgenic mice revealed that two UPR targets, PDI and Grp58, are among the most induced proteins in this ALS model [68]. Moreover, involvement of pro-apoptotic BIM and PUMA, both essential for ER stress-induced apoptosis [73, 74], in motoneuron loss and disease progression has recently been described in mouse models of fALS [71, 75]. Another gene mutation related to fALS in the ALS8 gene (synaptobrevin-associated protein B - VAMPB), was shown to result in cytoplasmic inclusions, ubiquitination, and UPR activation [76]. Moreover, VAMPB was found to interact with ATF6, attenuating its activity [77]. Finally, expression of mutant VAMPB or reduction of VAMPB by short hairpin RNA in primary neurons causes Golgi dispersion and cell death [78]. These results support the proposal of a broad ER-stress involvement in ALS disease. Although a strong correlation between ER stress, SOD1 aggregation and ALS progression has been described the actual role of the UPR in the disease process has not been addressed directly.

Several pieces of evidence suggest that chronic or irreversible ER stress may play an important role in motoneuron loss in ALS. Many groups have

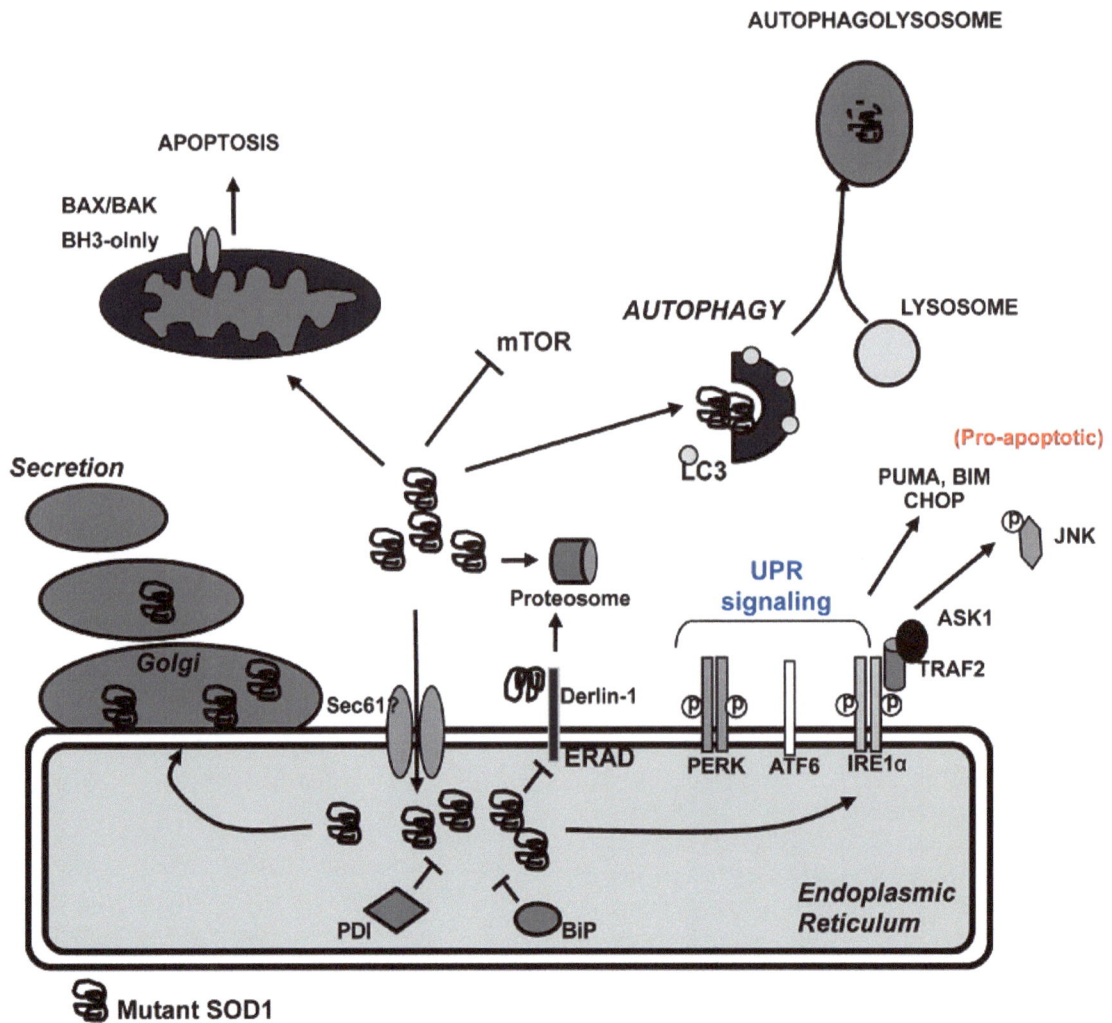

Fig. (2): Mutant SOD1 pathway in fALS. Mutant SOD1 forms abnormal protein aggregates that are found in the cytosol, ER, mitochondria, and Golgi apparatus. In the ER mutant, SOD1 interacts with ER chaperons and presumably activates UPR stress sensors. In the cytosol, mutant SOD1 generates ERAD impairment through its interaction with Derlin-1, and the protein aggregates activate autophagy via mTOR dependent and independent pathways. In Golgi the mutant protein interacts with chromogranins (CgA/CgB), which could mediate its secretion.

described upregulation of ER stress related pro-apoptotic factors in the spinal cord of late stage disease animals, including GADD153/ CHOP and pro-caspase-12 processing [64, 67, 68, 70, 71]. In addition, ER stress inducible BCL-2 pro-apoptotic genes such as BIM and PUMA are upregulated in symptomatic mutant SOD1 transgenic mice [71, 75]. More importantly, genetic deletion of BIM or PUMA delays ALS disease onset, possibly due to a significant decrease of apoptosis in motoneurons. This data is in agreement with the fact that BAX deficient or BCL-2 transgenic mice exhibit an increased life span due to augmented motoneuron survival [79-81]. A novel pathogenic mechanism of mutant SOD1-induced ER stress was described, in which mutant SOD1 protein specifically interacts with Derlin-1, a component of the ERAD machinery, resulting in impaired ERAD and ER-

stress-dependent activation of IRE1α-TRAF2-ASK1 pathway, resulting in motor neuron death [82].

In support of the role of ER stress on ALS, salubrinal, a small molecule described as an ER stress inhibitor [79], was shown to suppress aggregation of mutant SOD1 as well as SOD1-induced apoptotic cell death in Neuro2A cells [80]. Salubrinal selectively engages the translational control branch of the UPR by inducing eIF2α phosphorylation without affecting the transcription-dependent component of the UPR [79]. However, it remains to be shown that this protective effect is due to the delay of aggregate formation or inhibition of downstream ER stress responses caused by mutant SOD1 oligomers.

Neuroprotective therapies that target specific molecular mechanisms in ALS mice, including expression of anti-apoptotic genes and growth factors through viral-mediated gene therapy, have potential to delay onset and slow progression of disease. In addition, targeting of mutant SOD1 with small interfering RNA and lentiviral vectors has therapeutic potential in animal models of ALS [83], and small molecules have also been shown to have therapeutic benefits [84-86]. 4-PBA was recently shown to decrease motoneuron apoptosis in SOD1 transgenic mice, improving motor performance and life span. However, the effects of 4-PBA as a chemical chaperone were not evaluated [87]. How cells manage to accumulate mutant SOD1 is still an open question. Kabuta and colleagues reported that activation of autophagy reduces SOD1^{G93A} mediated toxicity and overall protein levels in a neuroblastoma cell line, proposing that the contribution of autophagy to mutant SOD1 degradation was comparable to that of proteasome pathway [88]. Increased levels of LC3 processing and inhibition of mTOR were observed in SOD1^{G93A} transgenic mice [89], possibly inferring that autophagy has a relevant role as a mechanism to eliminate SOD1 aggregates. However, the authors did not provide further evidence to clarify if the altered number of LC3-possitive autopohagosomes was due to increased autophagy or to decreased lysosomal fusion/ degradative activity.

Based on these outcomes, therapeutic benefits of targeting autophagy are becoming more attractive for treatment of ALS. In a recent work, the use of lithium, a recognized compound for treatment of depression and bipolar disorder, delayed the progression of the disease in human ALS patients [90]. Lithium treatment significantly delayed cell death of spinal cord neurons in SOD1^{G93A} transgenic mice, improving motor performance and extending life span. Interestingly, lithium produced a marked regression of SOD1 aggregates, decreased levels of ubiquitinated proteins, and increased the number of autophagosomes. In a mTOR-independent manner, lithium acts as a positive modulator of autophagy by blocking inositol-3-phosphate (IP$_3$) activity [91], possibly explaining its protective effect in ALS. Clinical trials are now underway to test the efficacy of treating ALS with lithium, preliminarily, slower disease progression has been observed in lithium treated patients in comparison with control individuals. While these trials are still preliminary, it is encouraging that evidence gained from fALS mouse models is translatable to treatment of the

disease in sALS human patients. Large clinical trials are now required to establish the safety and efficacy of treating with lithium and other autophagy initiating therapeutics to reduce the progression of ALS.

Recent data indicates that other pathological conditions affecting the spinal cord trigger ER stress. Spinal cord injury (SCI) is an alteration of the spinal cord function that considerably affects the patient's life quality due to a partial or complete loss of mobility. SCI can be produced by mechanical trauma, ischemia, tumor action or development-related disease. The injury itself produces a myelophaty or damage to the white matter or myelinated fiber tracts that carry sensory and motor information to and from the brain. These events occur immediately after injury, producing ischemia, blood-brain barrier rupture and the consequent release of cytokines, neurotransmitters and free radicals, triggering in the long-term apoptosis. Contusion-injured studies in rats have shown an increase in caspases activation as fast as one hour post-injury [92].

Ischemia-induced SCI induces ER stress in rodents, associated with the upregulation of different UPR markers including Grp78, CHOP and the XBP-1 mRNA splicing [93, 94]. These results suggest that ER stress responses may be a relevant factor associated with SCI and motoneuron dysfunction.

3.3. Prion-related Disorders

PrDs, also known as transmissible spongiform encephalopathies (TSEs), are fatal neurodegenerative disorders characterized by spongiform degeneration of the brain accompanied by accumulations of a misfolded and partially protease-resistant form of the prion protein (PrP^{Sc} or PrP^{RES}) [95]. Etiologically, TSEs can be classified as sporadic, infectious, or autosomal dominant inherited forms, affecting both humans and other mammals. In humans, PrDs include classic CJD, new variant CJD (Gerstmann-Sträussler-Scheinker syndrome), fatal familial insomnia and kuru. Prion diseases in other mammals include bovine spongiform encephalopathy, commonly known as mad cow disease, chronic wasting disease in elk and deer, and scrapie in sheep and goats [96]. This group of diseases generally presents a long incubation period followed by rapid progression to death shortly after the first clinical signs appear. Although clinical symptoms and progression vary among PrD, they commonly include progressive dementia and ataxia as a result of extensive neuronal death due to reactive astrocytosis and activated microglia during neuro-inflammation [97].

The most widely accepted "protein-only" hypothesis postulates that infectious prion pathogenicity results from a conformational change of normal cellular prion protein (PrP^C) from its primarily α-helical structure to an insoluble β sheet

conformation (PrP^{Sc}), initiated by a direct interaction between the two PrP forms. No amino acid sequence or posttranslational modification differences have been detected between normal host PrP^C and its pathological form, PrP^{Sc} [98]. Like other membrane proteins, PrP^C undergoes post translational processing in the ER and Golgi. Then, it localizes to cholesterol-rich lipid rafts, where it is anchored to the outer surface of the plasma membrane with a glycosyl phosphatidyl inositol (GPI) anchor [99], Fig. (**3**). Despite the

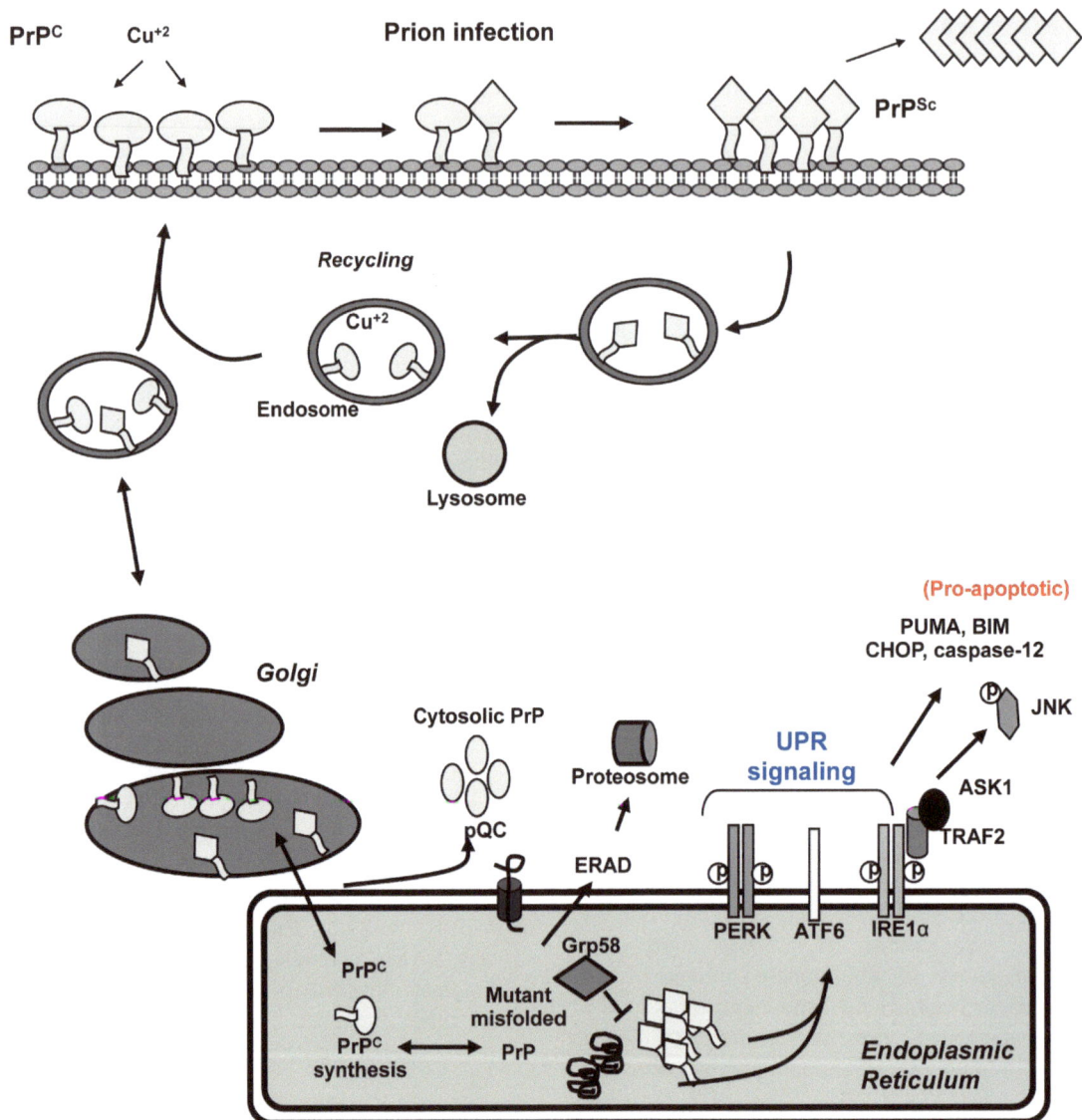

Fig. (3): Pathways involved in the neurotoxicity of the prion protein. Cellular prion protein (PrP^C) is a GPI-anchored plasma-membrane glycoprotein that is synthesized and processed in the ER and Golgi apparatus. The mature form is carried to cell surface and is usually associated with detergent-resistant membrane subdomains (lipid rafts). Scrapie infection triggers PrP^{Sc} generation at the plasma membrane and early endocytic vesicles. In familial TSE-associated mutant PrP^C molecules, spontaneous folding abnormalities can occur in the ER. During synthesis, misfolded PrP^C can be subject to the ER-associated degradation pathway (ERAD). PrP^{Sc} may trigger ER stress that is negatively regulated by different components of the UPR including Grp58 and many other chaperones. Chronic ER stress also leads to activation of a "pre-emptive" quality control system (pQC) resulting in cytosolic accumulation of PrP and neurotoxicity.

vast body of research, the physiological role of PrP^C is still under debate [100].

Apoptosis has been described in the brains of patients affected by CJD and Fatal Familial Insomnia, as well as scrapie-infected hamsters, mice and sheep (reviewed in [101]). Several *in vitro* and *in vivo* models for PrD have been developed to understand the molecular basis of neuronal dysfunction in infectious and inherited forms of PrD [102-105]. However, the exact mechanism by which Prion misfolding affects neuronal function is not well understood. Several groups have shown an engagement of ER stress responses in PrD models, where XBP-1 splicing [106] and the activation of stress signaling pathways linked to ER stress, such as JNK and ERK, are observed in scrapie-infected mice [106, 107]. In both human CJD patients and mouse models, the upregulation of UPR-responsive chaperones such as Grp78/BiP, Grp94, and Grp58 is observed in the brain [24, 108, 109]. In addition, a proteomic analysis of post-mortem CJD brain samples demonstrated that the disulfide isomerase Grp58 was highly expressed in the cerebellum of human patients affected with sporadic CJD [25]. *In vitro* studies using Neuro2a neuroblastoma cells demonstrated that inhibition of Grp58 expression using RNA interference leads to a significant enhancement of PrP^{Sc} toxicity. Conversely, overexpression of Grp58 protects cells from PrP^{Sc} toxicity and decreases the rate of caspase-12 activation, suggesting that ER stress is an early protective cellular response to prion replication, acting as a neuroprotective mechanism against prion neurotoxicity [110]. Recent evidence indicates that the activation of UPR components such as IRE1α, XBP-1 and others determines the rate of PrP^C aggregation *in vitro* under stress conditions [111, 112] and in yeast models [113], suggesting that the UPR has an active role in preventing neurodegeneration. We recently described conditions in which ER stress facilitates *in vitro* conversion of PrP^C into PrP^{Sc} due to partial misfolding of PrP^C [111], which was reverted by activation of UPR components such as XBP-1, ATF4 and ATF6. In addition, scrapie infected neuroblastoma cells are more sensitive to ER stress mediated apoptosis [24]. Because PrP^{Sc} induces ER stress, it seems that a vicious cycle exists in which alterations of ER physiology cause PrP^C to be more susceptible to conversion into PrP^{Res}, therefore causing additional ER stress. This most likely explains the rapid progression of the disease.

Other studies concerning the pathogenic mechanisms of prion diseases demonstrate that normal expression of PrP^C is necessary to generate neuronal damage. Early experiments demonstrate that brain regions knocked out for the PrP^C were resistant to degeneration caused by PrP^{Sc} [114]. More recently, selective postnatal knockout of PrP^C in neurons halted and even reversed the damage caused by either pre-existing PrP^{Sc} or newly generated PrP^{Sc} [115, 116]. These observations suggest that neurotoxic molecules are actively generated from newly synthesized PrP^C possibly through a conformational change, and that accumulation of PrP^{Sc} might not be directly responsible for neurodegeneration. At least three models can explain this requirement for PrP^C expression: first, the conversion of PrP^C to PrP^{Sc} might generate neurotoxic intermediate species that requires PrP^C expression for its continuous formation (as proposed by Collinge [96]). A second possibility is that PrP^{Sc} interacts with PrP^C, triggering a signal transduction pathway that alters cellular metabolism inducing neurodegeneration (reviewed in [117]). The third possibility was described recently by Rane and colleagues, suggesting that neurodegeneration in prion diseases might be dependent on chronic ER stress produced by PrP^{Sc} accumulation, leading to persistent activation of a "preemptive" quality control system (pQC) that aborts the RE translocation of PrP leading to cytosolic accumulation of PrP, resulting in neurotoxicity [109].

Despite the fact that chronic ER stress has been extensively described in neurodegenerative conditions linked to protein misfolding and aggregation, the role of the UPR in the central nervous system had not been studied directly. To address this question, we recently described the generation of a brain specific XBP-1 conditional knockout strain (XBP-1$^{Nes-/-}$) and assessed the function of XBP-1 prion pathogenesis [106]. To our surprise, the activation of stress responses triggered by prion replication, such as Grp58 and PDI induction, caspase-12 processing, JNK and ERK phosphorylation, were not influenced by XBP-1 deficiency, their activation remaining unaltered during the disease process. Neither prion aggregation, neuronal loss nor animal survival were affected. These findings imply that this highly conserved arm of the UPR may not contribute to the occurrence or pathology of neurodegenerative conditions associated with Prion misfolding, despite predictions that such diseases are related to

ER stress. Since the UPR is not restricted to the IRE1α/XBP-1 pathway in mammals, an activation of other UPR pathways may possibly compensate for XBP-1 deficiency in our prion model. The contribution of ATF6 and PERK to prion pathogenesis remains to be determined using genetic manipulation *in vivo*.

Similarly, Steele *et al* recently described that caspase-12 knockout mice are normally susceptible to prion infection and pathogenesis despite a clear activation of the UPR in their model [107]. Pro-apoptotic BH3-only proteins such as BIM and PUMA are induced in two different models of scrapie, suggesting that other ER stress related pro-apoptotic pathways might modulate neuronal loss in infectious Prion-related disorders [106, 118]. However, neither BAX deletion or BCL-2 overexpression affect infectious prion pathogenesis, suggesting that apoptosis is not essential for disease progression, and that it may be a downstream effect of neuronal dysfunction [118].

Based on several *in vitro* and animal studies, different categories of drugs have been suggested as candidates for treatment of prion disease [119, 120]. Therapeutic interventions in human have included the use of antiviral drugs (acyclovir, amantadine, vidarabine), antimalarial (quinacrina), antifungal (amphotericin), anticoa-gulant (pentosan polysulfate), anticonvulsant (levetiracetam, topiramate, phenytoin) and analgesic drugs (flupirtine), together with antioxidants, vitamins and biologic response modifiers including interferon [121]. However, despite a marked *in vitro* "anti-prion" activity of some drugs tested, including quinacrina, a transient benefit or no effect on clinical symptoms is observed. Moreover, these trials did not appear to stop disease progression because no significant differences in survival following treatments were reported [121].

Chemical chaperones have been employed to reduce PrP^C to PrP^{Sc} conversion in mouse neuroblastoma cells. Exposure to compounds with chemical chaperone activity, including glycerol, TMAO and dimethylsulfoxide (DMSO), can influence PrP folding, stabilizing PrP^C and preventing prion replication [122]. Anilino-naphtalene compounds, which are used to label amyloid deposits, inhibit the aggregation of a PrP neurotoxic peptide, also binding to PrP^{Sc} [123]. Doxycycline, a semi-synthetic tetracyc-line, also showed an anti-prion activity, reverting the effects of PrP^{Sc} in a cellular model [124]. Since doxycycline is already approved for use in humans,

future clinical trials are required to establish the efficacy of treating patients affected with TSEs. Trehalose, a disaccharide approved by the FDA, showed to reduce the size of PrP^{Sc} aggregates and modifies their subcellular localization, promoting cellular resistance to oxidative damage in prion infected cells, suggesting the use of trehalose as a potential therapeutic agent [125]. The discovery of novel chemical chaperones with low toxicity and higher permeability to the blood-brain barrier could lead to promising methods for treating this devastating disease. Autophagic vesicles are also observed in the brain of patients affected with PrD [126]. The role of autophagy in the progression of prion diseases is unknown, but the potential to promote clearance of misfolded protein aggregates may be a promising therapeutic approach [120].

Beta-sheet breakers constitute a new class of drugs that were originally designed to specifically bind AD amyloid-beta peptide and block or reverse the abnormal conformational change [127, 128]. The effects of a 13-residue beta-sheet breaker peptide (iPrP13) were shown to be effective in reverting PrP^{Sc} to a biochemical and structural state similar to that of PrP^C [128]. More importantly, treatment of PrP^{Sc} with iPrP13 delayed the appearance of clinical symptoms and decreased infectivity by 90-95% in mice with experimental scrapie [128]. These peptides or their derivatives provide a useful tool to study the role of PrP conformation and may represent a novel therapeutic approach for prion-related disorders.

3.4. Parkinson Disease and α-Synucleinopathies

PD is the second most common neurodegenerative disease affecting near 2% of the population over 65 years old [129]. It is a slowly progressing neurodegenerative disorder with no clear etiology recognized only by its clinical symptoms (bradykinesia, resting tremor, rigidity, postural instability, and periods of freezing) resulting of an extensive dopaminergic neuron death in the Substancia Nigra pars compacta (SNpc) in the ventral mesencephalon with a concomitant decrease of the dopamine content in the Striatum. Most of the cases are idiopatic but mutations in a few genes accounting for 2-3% of the cases have been associated to the disease, been the most common affected gene in familial PD LRRK2 (Dardarin) a kinase linked to several intracellular transduction pathways and Parkin, the most common early onset PD associated gene. One of the most studied genes related to PD is α-synuclein [130]. One of the pathological hallmarks of the disorder is the presence of Lewy Bodies (LBs) intracytoplasmic inclusions of a variety of proteins, but mainly composed of fibrillar aggregated and misfolded α-synuclein protein. This intracellular aggregate is not exclusive of PD, Dementia with Lewy Bodies (DLB) and other α-synucleinopathies also present these spherical masses. Mutations in this gene have been identified in rare families with dominant PD, indicating that aggregation of this protein in LBs is probably a crucial step in the

molecular pathogenesis of the disorder. Despite this, the mechanism involved in dopaminergic neuron loss in PD remains speculative.

Several evidences implicate the participation of the UPR in the disease process. A recent study demonstrated that the earliest defect following α-synuclein accumulation includes the impairment in the degradation of selective ERAD substrates, producing a block in ER to Golgi vesicular trafficking with concomitant UPR activation [131], resulting in growth arrest and cell death, Fig. (**4**).

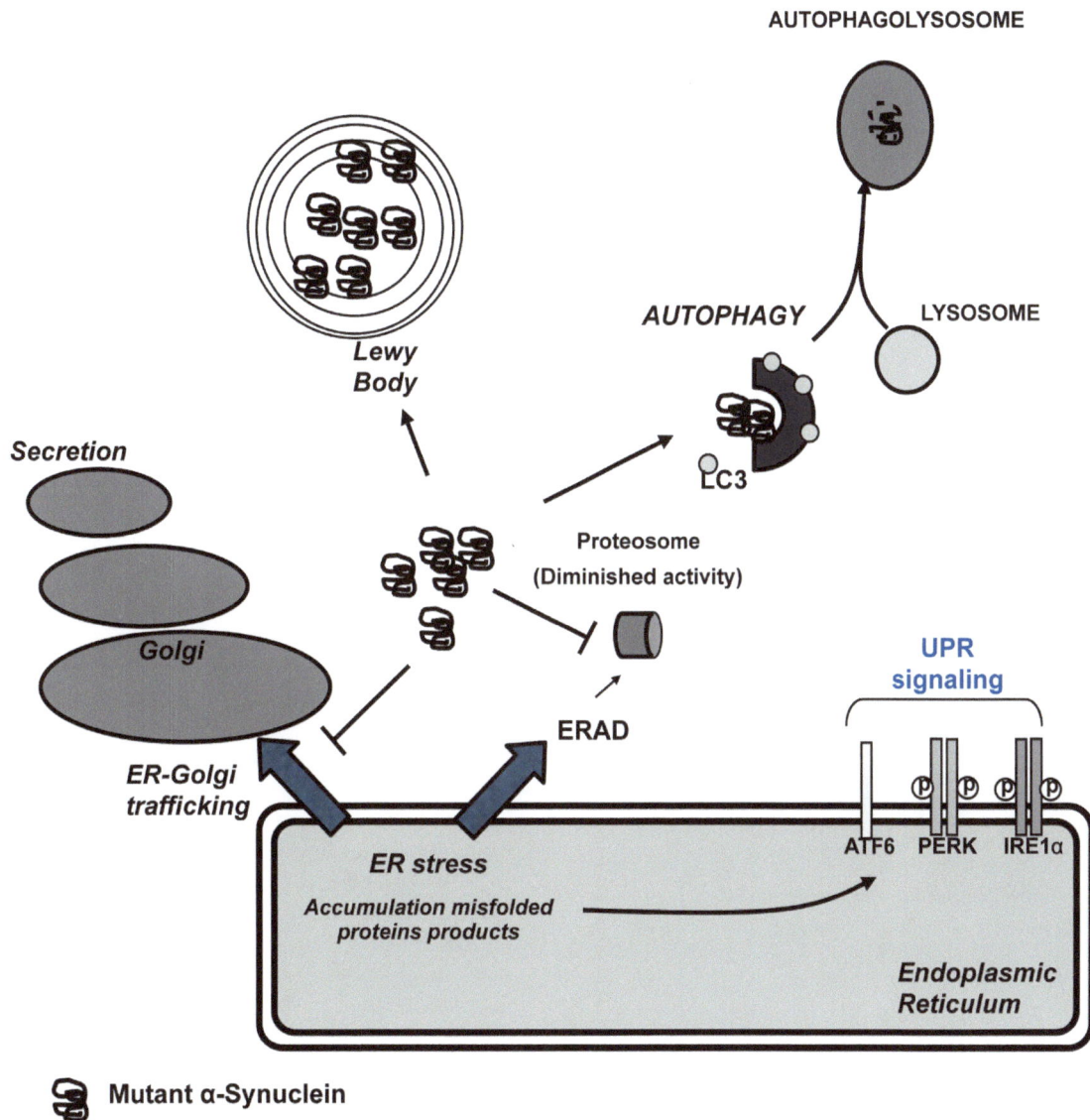

Fig. (4): UPR activation in Parkinson's Disease. α-Synuclein plays a predominant role in PD. During the pathogenesis of the disease α-Synuclein accumulates inside Lewy Bodies. It also induces a block in ER to Golgi trafficking concomitant with the impairment of the ERAD, without affecting proteasome function. Mutant α-Synuclein also induces ER stress by an unknown mechanism, leading to UPR activation and mitochondrial dysfunction. *In vivo* different markers of the UPR activation have been detected in brain tissue of human patients. This is also observed in toxicological models of the disease (6OHDA, MPTP).

Among mutations in α-synuclein, the A53T variant (α-Syn^{A53T}) shows more severe effects in the disease. Forced expression of α-Syn^{A53T} in PC12 cells induces ER stress and mitochondrial dysfunction resulting in neuronal cell death [132]. The decrease of the proteasome activity, increasing levels of cytosolic cytochrome c and the activation of caspase 9 and caspase 3 has been implicated in the toxic process.

Toxicological models resembling sporadic PD also suggest an involvement of ER stress in the pathology. Two independent gene expression profile analysis on dopaminergic neuron models revealed a striking increase in different transcripts associated with the UPR [133, 134]. In these *in vitro* models, the treatment with 6-hydroxidopamine (6-OHDA) reveals the induction of ER stress genes, ER stress, and increase of UPR markers, such as BiP, CHOP, and ATF4. More importantly, activation of the UPR was recently described in post-mortem tissue from sporadic PD human cases [18]. Immunoreactivity for the UPR activation markers activated PERK and phosphorylated eIF2α is detected in neuromelanin containing dopaminergic neurons in the Substantia Nigra of PD cases. In addition, phospho-PERK immunoreactivity is co-localized with increased α-synuclein expression in dopaminergic neurons

The hypothesis that ER dysfunction plays an important role in the development of PD is not only supported by the α-synuclein associated cases. Mutations in Parkin has been associated with ER-induced cell death, which results in recessive juvenile PD. Parkin mutations reduce or abolish its E3-ligase activity, a crucial part of the cellular machinery that tags proteins with ubiquitin, targeting them for the degradation by the proteasome. Consequently, these Parkin mutations results in an impairment to deal with some toxic substrates that accumulates inside the cell. A wide spectrum of oxidative stress-inducers such as rotenone, MPTP, 6-OHDA, paraquat, nitric oxide and iron, in addition to dopamine, alters the Parkin solubility and results in its aggregation. The diminished capacity of the cell to cope with intracellular aggregates would indirectly induce ER stress, activating the UPR [135, 136].

Trehalose has been assayed *in vitro* as a therapeutic approach to decrease the neurotoxicity of α-synuclein [58]. Whereas some of the protective effects may be explained by its chemical chaperone activity, its actions are largely unknown. A novel function of trehalose was reported in the α-synuclein model, acting as an mTOR-independent autophagy activator. Trehalose-induced autophagy enhanced the clearance of autophagy substrates such as α-Syn^{A30P} and α-Syn^{A53T} mutants. Furthermore, trehalose and mTOR inhibition by rapamycin together exerted an additive effect on the clearance of these aggregates due to increased autophagic activity. Trehalose also protects cells against subsequent pro-apoptotic insults via the mitochondrial pathway. The dual protective properties of trehalose and the combinatorial strategy with rapamycin may be relevant for the treatment of PD [58]. The role of the UPR and autophagy in PD *in vivo* remains to be determined.

4. CONCLUDING REMARKS

The UPR is an essential pathway that controls adaptive processes to stress, which results in global changes of ER function including ERAD, ER/Golgi biogenesis, protein folding, translocation into the ER, and autophagy [137]. Essential UPR transcription factors such as XBP-1, ATF4 and ATF6 enforce changes in cellular structure and function consistent with the requirements of the UPR to maintain proper function of professional secretory cells, but the exact role of the UPR in the CNS is mostly unknown. A genetic link is observed between an XBP-1 promoter polymorphism and the occurrence of bipolar disorders [138], schizophrenia [139] and certain personality types in the Japanese population [140]. As discussed here, extensive studies indicate a strong association between accumulation of misfolded proteins and ER stress induction in several important neurodegenerative conditions [26, 117]. Direct evidence indicating that perturbation of ER function could result in neurodegeneration came from the characterization of the Woozy mutant mouse, where disruption of a BiP co-chaperone triggers neuronal dysfunction associated with spontaneous protein aggregation in the brain [141]. Similarly, recent reports indicate that autophagy is critical for the maintenance of neuronal homoeostasis and has a role in the basal elimination of misfolded, ubiquitinated proteins. Brain specific knockout animals for essential autophagic-related genes develop spontaneous neurodegeneration with pathological features similar to AD and PD [54, 55]. These data suggest that the continuous clearance of cellular proteins in the brain through basal autophagy is required to prevent abnormal accumulation, therefore acting as a neuro-protective mechanism. However, most of the evidence supporting the involvement of ER stress in neurodegeneration is correlative, and manipulation of the UPR *in vivo* was required to define the actual contribution of the pathway to the disease process.

Strong correlations have been described between the misfolding and aggregation of an underlying protein and the occurrence of ER stress in neurodegenerative conditions. Additionally, increasing reports describe activation of the UPR in human post-mortem samples from patients affected with diverse types of protein misfolding disorders, suggesting a role as a general cellular response to neurodegeneration. Despite this evidence, little causal relationship is available to link the UPR and ER stress to neurological disorders *in vivo*. Predictions for the role of ER stress in disease processes are not obvious because activation of the UPR may decrease neurodegeneration by increasing folding, protein quality control and autophagy. However, extensive or chronic ER stress may result in irreversible neuronal damage and apoptosis. Promising results have been obtained with pharmacological strategies to target ER stress in a disease context. Small molecules, including chemical chaperones and autophagy activators, have been shown to have protective effects against neurodegeneration in certain disease models *in vivo*, decreasing protein misfolding and aggregation. Genetic manipulation of UPR components *in vivo* will ultimately identify the role of these processes in neurodegeneration.

5. ACKNOWLEDGMENTS

This work was supported by: Millennium Nucleus NEMO, FONDECYT N° 1070444, FONDAP grant N° 15010006, High Q Foundation, Michael J. Fox Foundation for Parkinson's Research, The Muscular Dystrophy Association (CH), FONDECYT N° 3085017 (SM), and CONICYT Ph.D fellowship (MN and MT).

6. REFERENCES

1. Kopito, R. R., Ron, D. Conformational disease. Nat Cell Biol, 2000; 2(11): E207-209.
2. Rao, R. V., Bredesen, D. E. Misfolded proteins, endoplasmic reticulum stress and neurodegeneration. Curr Opin Cell Biol, 2004; 16(6): 653-662.
3. Selkoe, D. J. Folding proteins in fatal ways. Nature, 2003; 426(6968): 900-904.
4. Taylor, J. P., Hardy, J., Fischbeck, K. H. Toxic proteins in neurodegenerative disease. Science, 2002; 296(5575): 1991-1995.
5. Ron, D., Walter, P. Signal integration in the endoplasmic reticulum unfolded protein response. Nat Rev Mol Cell Biol, 2007; 8(7): 519-529.
6. Schroder, M., Kaufman, R. J. The mammalian unfolded protein response. Annu Rev Biochem, 2005; 74(739-789.
7. Hetz, C. A., Torres, V., Quest, A. F. Beyond apoptosis: nonapoptotic cell death in physiology and disease. Biochem Cell Biol, 2005; 83(5): 579-588.
8. Hetz, C., Glimcher, L. XBP-1 and the UPRosome: Mastering secretory cell function. Curr Immunol Rev, 2008; In Press.
9. Harding, H. P., Zhang, Y., Ron, D. Protein translation and folding are coupled by an endoplasmic-reticulum-resident kinase. Nature, 1999; 397(6716): 271-274.
10. Chen, X., Shen, J., Prywes, R. The luminal domain of ATF6 senses endoplasmic reticulum (ER) stress and causes translocation of ATF6 from the ER to the Golgi. J Biol Chem, 2002; 277(15): 13045-13052.
11. Haze, K., Yoshida, H., Yanagi, H., Yura, T., Mori, K. Mammalian transcription factor ATF6 is synthesized as a transmembrane protein and activated by proteolysis in response to endoplasmic reticulum stress. Mol Biol Cell, 1999; 10(11): 3787-3799.
12. Ye, J., Rawson, R. B., Komuro, R., Chen, X., Dave, U. P., Prywes, R., Brown, M. S., Goldstein, J. L. ER stress induces cleavage of membrane-bound ATF6 by the same proteases that process SREBPs. Mol Cell, 2000; 6(6): 1355-1364.
13. Lee, K., Tirasophon, W., Shen, X., Michalak, M., Prywes, R., Okada, T., Yoshida, H., Mori, K., Kaufman, R. J. IRE1-mediated unconventional mRNA splicing and S2P-mediated ATF6 cleavage merge to regulate XBP1 in signaling the unfolded protein response. Genes Dev, 2002; 16(4): 452-466.
14. Calfon, M., Zeng, H., Urano, F., Till, J. H., Hubbard, S. R., Harding, H. P., Clark, S. G., Ron, D. IRE1 couples endoplasmic reticulum load to secretory capacity by processing the XBP-1 mRNA. Nature, 2002; 415(6867): 92-96.
15. Yoshida, H., Matsui, T., Yamamoto, A., Okada, T., Mori, K. XBP1 mRNA is induced by ATF6 and spliced by IRE1 in response to ER stress to produce a highly active transcription factor. Cell, 2001; 107(7): 881-891.
16. Hetz, C., Glimcher, L. The daily job of night killers: alternative roles of the BCL-2 family in organelle physiology. Trends Cell Biol, 2008; 18(1): 38-44.
17. Hetz, C., Bernasconi, P., Fisher, J., Lee, A. H., Bassik, M. C., Antonsson, B., Brandt, G. S., Iwakoshi, N. N., Schinzel, A., Glimcher, L. H., Korsmeyer, S. J. Proapoptotic BAX and BAK modulate the unfolded protein response by a direct interaction with IRE1alpha. Science, 2006; 312(5773): 572-576.
18. Hoozemans, J. J., van Haastert, E. S., Eikelenboom, P., de Vos, R. A., Rozemuller, J. M., Scheper, W. Activation of the unfolded protein response in Parkinson's disease. Biochem Biophys Res Commun, 2007; 354(3): 707-711.
19. Uehara, T., Nakamura, T., Yao, D., Shi, Z. Q., Gu, Z., Ma, Y., Masliah, E., Nomura, Y., Lipton, S. A. S-nitrosylated protein-disulphide isomerase links protein misfolding to neurodegeneration. Nature, 2006; 441(7092): 513-517.
20. Conn, K. J., Gao, W., McKee, A., Lan, M. S., Ullman, M. D., Eisenhauer, P. B., Fine, R. E., Wells, J. M. Identification of the protein disulfide isomerase family member PDIp in experimental Parkinson's disease and Lewy body pathology. Brain Res, 2004; 1022(1-2): 164-172.

21.   Ilieva, E. V., Ayala, V., Jove, M., Dalfo, E., Cacabelos, D., Povedano, M., Bellmunt, M. J., Ferrer, I., Pamplona, R., Portero-Otin, M. Oxidative and endoplasmic reticulum stress interplay in sporadic amyotrophic lateral sclerosis. Brain, 2007; 130(Pt 12): 3111-3123.

22.   Atkin, J. D., Farg, M. A., Walker, A. K., McLean, C., Tomas, D., Horne, M. K. Endoplasmic reticulum stress and induction of the unfolded protein response in human sporadic amyotrophic lateral sclerosis. Neurobiol Dis, 2008; 30(3): 400-407.

23.   Unterberger, U., Hoftberger, R., Gelpi, E., Flicker, H., Budka, H., Voigtlander, T. Endoplasmic reticulum stress features are prominent in Alzheimer disease but not in prion diseases in vivo. J Neuropathol Exp Neurol, 2006; 65(4): 348-357.

24.   Hetz, C., Russelakis-Carneiro, M., Maundrell, K., Castilla, J., Soto, C. Caspase-12 and endoplasmic reticulum stress mediate neurotoxicity of pathological prion protein. Embo J, 2003; 22(20): 5435-5445.

25.   Yoo, B. C., Krapfenbauer, K., Cairns, N., Belay, G., Bajo, M., Lubec, G. Overexpressed protein disulfide isomerase in brains of patients with sporadic Creutzfeldt-Jakob disease. Neurosci Lett, 2002; 334(3): 196-200.

26.   Lindholm, D., Wootz, H., Korhonen, L. ER stress and neurodegenerative diseases. Cell Death Differ, 2006; 13(3): 385-392.

27.   Matus, S., Lisbona, F., Torres, M., Leon, C., Thielen, P., Hetz, C. The stress rheostat: an interplay between the unfolded protein response (UPR) and autophagy in neurodegeneration. Curr Mol Med, 2008; 8(3): 157-172.

28.   A novel gene containing a trinucleotide repeat that is expanded and unstable on Huntington's disease chromosomes. The Huntington's Disease Collaborative Research Group. Cell, 1993; 72(6): 971-983.

29.   Kremer, B., Goldberg, P., Andrew, S. E., Theilmann, J., Telenius, H., Zeisler, J., Squitieri, F., Lin, B., Bassett, A., Almqvist, E., et al. A worldwide study of the Huntington's disease mutation. The sensitivity and specificity of measuring CAG repeats. N Engl J Med, 1994; 330(20): 1401-1406.

30.   Rubinsztein, D. C. Lessons from animal models of Huntington's disease. Trends Genet, 2002; 18(4): 202-209.

31.   Hackam, A. S., Singaraja, R., Wellington, C. L., Metzler, M., McCutcheon, K., Zhang, T., Kalchman, M., Hayden, M. R. The influence of huntingtin protein size on nuclear localization and cellular toxicity. J Cell Biol, 1998; 141(5): 1097-1105.

32.   Lunkes, A., Mandel, J. L. A cellular model that recapitulates major pathogenic steps of Huntington's disease. Hum Mol Genet, 1998; 7(9): 1355-1361.

33.   Wyttenbach, A., Carmichael, J., Swartz, J., Furlong, R. A., Narain, Y., Rankin, J., Rubinsztein, D. C. Effects of heat shock, heat shock protein 40 (HDJ-2), and proteasome inhibition on protein aggregation in cellular models of Huntington's disease. Proc Natl Acad Sci U S A, 2000; 97(6): 2898-2903.

34.   Nucifora, F. C., Jr., Sasaki, M., Peters, M. F., Huang, H., Cooper, J. K., Yamada, M., Takahashi, H., Tsuji, S., Troncoso, J., Dawson, V. L., Dawson, T. M., Ross, C. A. Interference by huntingtin and atrophin-1 with cbp-mediated transcription leading to cellular toxicity. Science, 2001; 291(5512): 2423-2428.

35.   Ravikumar, B., Rubinsztein, D. C. Role of autophagy in the clearance of mutant huntingtin: a step towards therapy? Mol Aspects Med, 2006; 27(5-6): 520-527.

36.   Momoi, T. Conformational diseases and ER stress-mediated cell death: apoptotic cell death and autophagic cell death. Curr Mol Med, 2006; 6(1): 111-118.

37.   Kopito, R. R. Aggresomes, inclusion bodies and protein aggregation. Trends Cell Biol, 2000; 10(12): 524-530.

38.   Omi, K., Hachiya, N. S., Tokunaga, K., Kaneko, K. siRNA-mediated inhibition of endogenous Huntingtin disease gene expression induces an aberrant configuration of the ER network in vitro. Biochem Biophys Res Commun, 2005; 338(2): 1229-1235.

39.   Strehlow, A. N., Li, J. Z., Myers, R. M. Wild-type huntingtin participates in protein trafficking between the Golgi and the extracellular space. Hum Mol Genet, 2007; 16(4): 391-409.

40.   del Toro, D., Canals, J. M., Gines, S., Kojima, M., Egea, G., Alberch, J. Mutant huntingtin impairs the post-Golgi trafficking of brain-derived neurotrophic factor but not its Val66Met polymorphism. J Neurosci, 2006; 26(49): 12748-12757.

41.   Rockabrand, E., Slepko, N., Pantalone, A., Nukala, V. N., Kazantsev, A., Marsh, J. L., Sullivan, P. G., Steffan, J. S., Sensi, S. L., Thompson, L. M. The first 17 amino acids of Huntingtin modulate its sub-cellular localization, aggregation and effects on calcium homeostasis. Hum Mol Genet, 2007; 16(1): 61-77.

42.   Rousseau, E., Dehay, B., Ben-Haiem, L., Trottier, Y., Morange, M., Bertolotti, A. Targeting expression of expanded polyglutamine proteins to the endoplasmic reticulum or mitochondria prevents their aggregation. Proc Natl Acad Sci U S A, 2004; 101(26): 9648-9653.

43.   Kouroku, Y., Fujita, E., Tanida, I., Ueno, T., Isoai, A., Kumagai, H., Ogawa, S., Kaufman, R. J., Kominami, E., Momoi, T. ER stress (PERK/eIF2alpha phosphorylation) mediates the polyglutamine-induced LC3 conversion, an essential step for autophagy formation. Cell Death Differ, 2007; 14(2): 230-239.

44.   Nakagawa, T., Zhu, H., Morishima, N., Li, E., Xu, J., Yankner, B. A., Yuan, J. Caspase-12 mediates endoplasmic-reticulum-specific apoptosis and cytotoxicity by amyloid-beta. Nature, 2000; 403(6765): 98-103.

45.   Nishitoh, H., Matsuzawa, A., Tobiume, K., Saegusa, K., Takeda, K., Inoue, K., Hori, S., Kakizuka, A., Ichijo, H. ASK1 is essential for endoplasmic reticulum stress-induced neuronal cell death triggered by expanded polyglutamine repeats. Genes Dev, 2002; 16(11): 1345-1355.

46.   Jana, N. R., Tanaka, M., Wang, G., Nukina, N. Polyglutamine length-dependent interaction of Hsp40 and Hsp70 family chaperones with truncated N-terminal huntingtin: their role in suppression of aggregation and cellular toxicity. Hum Mol Genet, 2000; 9(13): 2009-2018.

47.   Maiuri, M. C., Zalckvar, E., Kimchi, A., Kroemer, G. Self-eating and self-killing: crosstalk between autophagy and apoptosis. Nat Rev Mol Cell Biol, 2007; 8(9): 741-752.

48.   Ozcan, U., Yilmaz, E., Ozcan, L., Furuhashi, M., Vaillancourt, E., Smith, R. O., Gorgun, C. Z., Hotamisligil, G. S. Chemical chaperones reduce ER stress and restore glucose homeostasis in a mouse model of type 2 diabetes. Science, 2006; 313(5790): 1137-1140.

49.   Welch, W. J., Brown, C. R. Influence of molecular and chemical chaperones on protein folding. Cell Stress Chaperones, 1996; 1(2): 109-115.

50.   Xie, Q., Khaoustov, V. I., Chung, C. C., Sohn, J., Krishnan, B., Lewis, D. E., Yoffe, B. Effect of

tauroursodeoxycholic acid on endoplasmic reticulum stress-induced caspase-12 activation. Hepatology, 2002; 36(3): 592-601.

51. Keene, C. D., Rodrigues, C. M., Eich, T., Chhabra, M. S., Steer, C. J., Low, W. C. Tauroursodeoxycholic acid, a bile acid, is neuroprotective in a transgenic animal model of Huntington's disease. Proc Natl Acad Sci U S A, 2002; 99(16): 10671-10676.

52. Gardian, G., Browne, S. E., Choi, D. K., Klivenyi, P., Gregorio, J., Kubilus, J. K., Ryu, H., Langley, B., Ratan, R. R., Ferrante, R. J., Beal, M. F. Neuroprotective effects of phenylbutyrate in the N171-82Q transgenic mouse model of Huntington's disease. J Biol Chem, 2005; 280(1): 556-563.

53. Hoyer-Hansen, M., Jaattela, M. Connecting endoplasmic reticulum stress to autophagy by unfolded protein response and calcium. Cell Death Differ, 2007; 14(9): 1576-1582.

54. Komatsu, M., Waguri, S., Chiba, T., Murata, S., Iwata, J., Tanida, I., Ueno, T., Koike, M., Uchiyama, Y., Kominami, E., Tanaka, K. Loss of autophagy in the central nervous system causes neurodegeneration in mice. Nature, 2006; 441(7095): 880-884.

55. Hara, T., Nakamura, K., Matsui, M., Yamamoto, A., Nakahara, Y., Suzuki-Migishima, R., Yokoyama, M., Mishima, K., Saito, I., Okano, H., Mizushima, N. Suppression of basal autophagy in neural cells causes neurodegenerative disease in mice. Nature, 2006; 441(7095): 885-889.

56. Ravikumar, B., Rubinsztein, D. C. Can autophagy protect against neurodegeneration caused by aggregate-prone proteins? Neuroreport, 2004; 15(16): 2443-2445.

57. Floto, R. A., Sarkar, S., Perlstein, E. O., Kampmann, B., Schreiber, S. L., Rubinsztein, D. C. Small molecule enhancers of rapamycin-induced TOR inhibition promote autophagy, reduce toxicity in Huntington's disease models and enhance killing of mycobacteria by macrophages. Autophagy, 2007; 3(6): 620-622.

58. Sarkar, S., Davies, J. E., Huang, Z., Tunnacliffe, A., Rubinsztein, D. C. Trehalose, a novel mTOR-independent autophagy enhancer, accelerates the clearance of mutant huntingtin and alpha-synuclein. J Biol Chem, 2007; 282(8): 5641-5652.

59. Sarkar, S., Perlstein, E. O., Imarisio, S., Pineau, S., Cordenier, A., Maglathlin, R. L., Webster, J. A., Lewis, T. A., O'Kane, C. J., Schreiber, S. L., Rubinsztein, D. C. Small molecules enhance autophagy and reduce toxicity in Huntington's disease models. Nat Chem Biol, 2007; 3(6): 331-338.

60. Boillee, S., Vande Velde, C., Cleveland, D. W. ALS: a disease of motor neurons and their nonneuronal neighbors. Neuron, 2006; 52(1): 39-59.

61. Pasinelli, P., Brown, R. H. Molecular biology of amyotrophic lateral sclerosis: insights from genetics. Nat Rev Neurosci, 2006; 7(9): 710-723.

62. Turner, B. J., Atkin, J. D. ER stress and UPR in familial amyotrophic lateral sclerosis. Curr Mol Med, 2006; 6(1): 79-86.

63. Gonatas, N. K., Stieber, A., Gonatas, J. O. Fragmentation of the Golgi apparatus in neurodegenerative diseases and cell death. J Neurol Sci, 2006; 246(1-2): 21-30.

64. Vlug, A. S., Teuling, E., Haasdijk, E. D., French, P., Hoogenraad, C. C., Jaarsma, D. ATF3 expression precedes death of spinal motoneurons in amyotrophic lateral sclerosis-SOD1 transgenic mice and correlates with c-Jun phosphorylation, CHOP expression, somato-dendritic ubiquitination and Golgi fragmentation. Eur J Neurosci, 2005; 22(8): 1881-1894.

65. Nagata, T., Ilieva, H., Murakami, T., Shiote, M., Narai, H., Ohta, Y., Hayashi, T., Shoji, M., Abe, K. Increased ER stress during motor neuron degeneration in a transgenic mouse model of amyotrophic lateral sclerosis. Neurol Res, 2007; 29(8): 767-771.

66. Kikuchi, H., Almer, G., Yamashita, S., Guegan, C., Nagai, M., Xu, Z., Sosunov, A. A., McKhann, G. M., 2nd, Przedborski, S. Spinal cord endoplasmic reticulum stress associated with a microsomal accumulation of mutant superoxide dismutase-1 in an ALS model. Proc Natl Acad Sci U S A, 2006; 103(15): 6025-6030.

67. Wootz, H., Hansson, I., Korhonen, L., Napankangas, U., Lindholm, D. Caspase-12 cleavage and increased oxidative stress during motoneuron degeneration in transgenic mouse model of ALS. Biochem Biophys Res Commun, 2004; 322(1): 281-286.

68. Atkin, J. D., Farg, M. A., Turner, B. J., Tomas, D., Lysaght, J. A., Nunan, J., Rembach, A., Nagley, P., Beart, P. M., Cheema, S. S., Horne, M. K. Induction of the unfolded protein response in familial amyotrophic lateral sclerosis and association of protein-disulfide isomerase with superoxide dismutase 1. J Biol Chem, 2006; 281(40): 30152-30165.

69. Urushitani, M., Sik, A., Sakurai, T., Nukina, N., Takahashi, R., Julien, J. P. Chromogranin-mediated secretion of mutant superoxide dismutase proteins linked to amyotrophic lateral sclerosis. Nat Neurosci, 2006; 9(1): 108-118.

70. Wootz, H., Hansson, I., Korhonen, L., Lindholm, D. XIAP decreases caspase-12 cleavage and calpain activity in spinal cord of ALS transgenic mice. Exp Cell Res, 2006; 312(10): 1890-1898.

71. Kieran, D., Woods, I., Villunger, A., Strasser, A., Prehn, J. H. Deletion of the BH3-only protein puma protects motoneurons from ER stress-induced apoptosis and delays motoneuron loss in ALS mice. Proc Natl Acad Sci U S A, 2007; 104(51): 20606-20611.

72. Urushitani, M., Ezzi, S. A., Matsuo, A., Tooyama, I., Julien, J. P. The endoplasmic reticulum-Golgi pathway is a target for translocation and aggregation of mutant superoxide dismutase linked to ALS. Faseb J, 2008; 22(7): 2476-2487.

73. Morishima, N., Nakanishi, K., Tsuchiya, K., Shibata, T., Seiwa, E. Translocation of Bim to the endoplasmic reticulum (ER) mediates ER stress signaling for activation of caspase-12 during ER stress-induced apoptosis. J Biol Chem, 2004; 279(48): 50375-50381.

74. Puthalakath, H., O'Reilly, L. A., Gunn, P., Lee, L., Kelly, P. N., Huntington, N. D., Hughes, P. D., Michalak, E. M., McKimm-Breschkin, J., Motoyama, N., Gotoh, T., Akira, S., Bouillet, P., Strasser, A. ER stress triggers apoptosis by activating BH3-only protein Bim. Cell, 2007; 129(7): 1337-1349.

75. Hetz, C., Thielen, P., Fisher, J., Pasinelli, P., Brown, R. H., Korsmeyer, S., Glimcher, L. The proapoptotic BCL-2 family member BIM mediates motoneuron loss in a model of amyotrophic lateral sclerosis. Cell Death Differ, 2007; 14(7): 1386-1389.

76. Tsuda, H., Han, S. M., Yang, Y., Tong, C., Lin, Y. Q., Mohan, K., Haueter, C., Zoghbi, A., Harati, Y., Kwan, J., Miller, M. A., Bellen, H. J. The amyotrophic lateral sclerosis 8 protein VAPB is cleaved, secreted, and acts as a ligand for Eph receptors. Cell, 2008; 133(6): 963-977.

77. Gkogkas, C., Middleton, S., Kremer, A. M., Wardrope, C., Hannah, M., Gillingwater, T. H., Skehel, P. VAPB interacts with and modulates the activity of ATF6. Hum Mol Genet, 2008; 17(11): 1517-1526.

78. Teuling, E., Ahmed, S., Haasdijk, E., Demmers, J., Steinmetz, M. O., Akhmanova, A., Jaarsma, D., Hoogenraad, C. C. Motor neuron disease-associated mutant vesicle-associated membrane protein-associated protein (VAP) B recruits wild-type VAPs into endoplasmic reticulum-derived tubular aggregates. J Neurosci, 2007; 27(36): 9801-9815.

79. Boyce, M., Bryant, K. F., Jousse, C., Long, K., Harding, H. P., Scheuner, D., Kaufman, R. J., Ma, D., Coen, D. M., Ron, D., Yuan, J. A selective inhibitor of eIF2alpha dephosphorylation protects cells from ER stress. Science, 2005; 307(5711): 935-939.

80. Oh, Y. K., Shin, K. S., Yuan, J., Kang, S. J. Superoxide dismutase 1 mutants related to amyotrophic lateral sclerosis induce endoplasmic stress in neuro2a cells. J Neurochem, 2008; 104(4): 993-1005.

81. Ohta, Y., Kamiya, T., Nagai, M., Nagata, T., Morimoto, N., Miyazaki, K., Murakami, T., Kurata, T., Takehisa, Y., Ikeda, Y., Asoh, S., Ohta, S., Abe, K. Therapeutic benefits of intrathecal protein therapy in a mouse model of amyotrophic lateral sclerosis. J Neurosci Res, 2008; 86(13): 3028-3037.

82. Nishitoh, H., Kadowaki, H., Nagai, A., Maruyama, T., Yokota, T., Fukutomi, H., Noguchi, T., Matsuzawa, A., Takeda, K., Ichijo, H. ALS-linked mutant SOD1 induces ER stress- and ASK1-dependent motor neuron death by targeting Derlin-1. Genes Dev, 2008; 22(11): 1451-1464.

83. Raoul, C., Abbas-Terki, T., Bensadoun, J. C., Guillot, S., Haase, G., Szulc, J., Henderson, C. E., Aebischer, P. Lentiviral-mediated silencing of SOD1 through RNA interference retards disease onset and progression in a mouse model of ALS. Nat Med, 2005; 11(4): 423-428.

84. Azzouz, M., Hottinger, A., Paterna, J. C., Zurn, A. D., Aebischer, P., Bueler, H. Increased motoneuron survival and improved neuromuscular function in transgenic ALS mice after intraspinal injection of an adeno-associated virus encoding Bcl-2. Hum Mol Genet, 2000; 9(5): 803-811.

85. Kirik, D., Bjorklund, A. Modeling CNS neurodegeneration by overexpression of disease-causing proteins using viral vectors. Trends Neurosci, 2003; 26(7): 386-392.

86. Azzouz, M., Kingsman, S. M., Mazarakis, N. D. Lentiviral vectors for treating and modeling human CNS disorders. J Gene Med, 2004; 6(9): 951-962.

87. Petri, S., Kiaei, M., Kipiani, K., Chen, J., Calingasan, N. Y., Crow, J. P., Beal, M. F. Additive neuroprotective effects of a histone deacetylase inhibitor and a catalytic antioxidant in a transgenic mouse model of amyotrophic lateral sclerosis. Neurobiol Dis, 2006; 22(1): 40-49.

88. Kabuta, T., Suzuki, Y., Wada, K. Degradation of amyotrophic lateral sclerosis-linked mutant Cu,Zn-superoxide dismutase proteins by macroautophagy and the proteasome. J Biol Chem, 2006; 281(41): 30524-30533.

89. Morimoto, N., Nagai, M., Ohta, Y., Miyazaki, K., Kurata, T., Morimoto, M., Murakami, T., Takehisa, Y., Ikeda, Y., Kamiya, T., Abe, K. Increased autophagy in transgenic mice with a G93A mutant SOD1 gene. Brain Res, 2007; 1167(112-117.

90. Fornai, F., Longone, P., Cafaro, L., Kastsiuchenka, O., Ferrucci, M., Manca, M. L., Lazzeri, G., Spalloni, A., Bellio, N., Lenzi, P., Modugno, N., Siciliano, G., Isidoro, C., Murri, L., Ruggieri, S., Paparelli, A. Lithium delays progression of amyotrophic lateral sclerosis. Proc Natl Acad Sci U S A, 2008; 105(6): 2052-2057.

91. Sarkar, S., Floto, R. A., Berger, Z., Imarisio, S., Cordenier, A., Pasco, M., Cook, L. J., Rubinsztein, D. C. Lithium induces autophagy by inhibiting inositol monophosphatase. J Cell Biol, 2005; 170(7): 1101-1111.

92. Springer, J. E., Azbill, R. D., Knapp, P. E. Activation of the caspase-3 apoptotic cascade in traumatic spinal cord injury. Nat Med, 1999; 5(8): 943-946.

93. Penas, C., Guzman, M. S., Verdu, E., Fores, J., Navarro, X., Casas, C. Spinal cord injury induces endoplasmic reticulum stress with different cell-type dependent response. J Neurochem, 2007; 102(4): 1242-1255.

94. Yamauchi, T., Sakurai, M., Abe, K., Matsumiya, G., Sawa, Y. Impact of the endoplasmic reticulum stress response in spinal cord after transient ischemia. Brain Res, 2007; 1169(24-33.

95. Prusiner, S. B. Prions. Proc Natl Acad Sci U S A, 1998; 95(23): 13363-13383.

96. Collinge, J. Prion diseases of humans and animals: their causes and molecular basis. Annu Rev Neurosci, 2001; 24(519-550.

97. Budka, H., Aguzzi, A., Brown, P., Brucher, J. M., Bugiani, O., Gullotta, F., Haltia, M., Hauw, J. J., Ironside, J. W., Jellinger, K., *et al.* Neuropathological diagnostic criteria for Creutzfeldt-Jakob disease (CJD) and other human spongiform encephalopathies (prion diseases). Brain Pathol, 1995; 5(4): 459-466.

98. Pan, K. M., Baldwin, M., Nguyen, J., Gasset, M., Serban, A., Groth, D., Mehlhorn, I., Huang, Z., Fletterick, R. J., Cohen, F. E., *et al.* Conversion of alpha-helices into beta-sheets features in the formation of the scrapie prion proteins. Proc Natl Acad Sci U S A, 1993; 90(23): 10962-10966.

99. Vey, M., Pilkuhn, S., Wille, H., Nixon, R., DeArmond, S. J., Smart, E. J., Anderson, R. G., Taraboulos, A., Prusiner, S. B. Subcellular colocalization of the cellular and scrapie prion proteins in caveolae-like membranous domains. Proc Natl Acad Sci U S A, 1996; 93(25): 14945-14949.

100. Hetz, C., Maundrell, K., Soto, C. Is loss of function of the prion protein the cause of prion disorders? Trends Mol Med, 2003; 9(6): 237-243.

101. Hetz, C., Soto, C. Protein misfolding and disease: the case of prion disorders. Cell Mol Life Sci, 2003; 60(1): 133-143.

102. Chiesa, R., Drisaldi, B., Quaglio, E., Migheli, A., Piccardo, P., Ghetti, B., Harris, D. A. Accumulation of protease-resistant prion protein (PrP) and apoptosis of cerebellar granule cells in transgenic mice expressing a PrP insertional mutation. Proc Natl Acad Sci U S A, 2000; 97(10): 5574-5579.

103. Ma, J., Wollmann, R., Lindquist, S. Neurotoxicity and neurodegeneration when PrP accumulates in the cytosol. Science, 2002; 298(5599): 1781-1785.

104. Supattapone, S., Bosque, P., Muramoto, T., Wille, H., Aagaard, C., Peretz, D., Nguyen, H. O., Heinrich, C., Torchia, M., Safar, J., Cohen, F. E., DeArmond, S. J., Prusiner, S. B., Scott, M. Prion protein of 106 residues creates an artifical transmission barrier for prion replication in transgenic mice. Cell, 1999; 96(6): 869-878.

105. Supattapone, S., Bouzamondo, E., Ball, H. L., Wille, H., Nguyen, H. O., Cohen, F. E., DeArmond, S. J., Prusiner, S. B., Scott, M. A protease-resistant 61-residue prion peptide causes neurodegeneration in transgenic mice. Mol Cell Biol, 2001; 21(7): 2608-2616.

106. Hetz, C., Lee, A. H., Gonzalez-Romero, D., Thielen, P., Castilla, J., Soto, C., Glimcher, L. H. Unfolded

protein response transcription factor XBP-1 does not influence prion replication or pathogenesis. Proc Natl Acad Sci U S A, 2008; 105(2): 757-762.

107. Steele, A. D., Hetz, C., Yi, C., Jackson, W., Borkowski, A., Yuan, J., Wollmann, R., Lindquist, S. Prion disease in caspase-12 knockout mice. Proc Natl Acad Sci U S A, 2008.

108. Brown, A. R., Rebus, S., McKimmie, C. S., Robertson, K., Williams, A., Fazakerley, J. K. Gene expression profiling of the preclinical scrapie-infected hippocampus. Biochem Biophys Res Commun, 2005; 334(1): 86-95.

109. Rane, N. S., Kang, S. W., Chakrabarti, O., Feigenbaum, L., Hegde, R. S. Reduced translocation of nascent prion protein during ER stress contributes to neurodegeneration. Dev Cell, 2008; 15(3): 359-370.

110. Hetz, C., Russelakis-Carneiro, M., Walchli, S., Carboni, S., Vial-Knecht, E., Maundrell, K., Castilla, J., Soto, C. The disulfide isomerase Grp58 is a protective factor against prion neurotoxicity. J Neurosci, 2005; 25(11): 2793-2802.

111. Hetz, C., Castilla, J., Soto, C. Perturbation of endoplasmic reticulum homeostasis facilitates prion replication. J Biol Chem, 2007; 282(17): 12725-12733.

112. Orsi, A., Fioriti, L., Chiesa, R., Sitia, R. Conditions of endoplasmic reticulum stress favor the accumulation of cytosolic prion protein. J Biol Chem, 2006; 281(41): 30431-30438.

113. Apodaca, J., Kim, I., Rao, H. Cellular tolerance of prion protein PrP in yeast involves proteolysis and the unfolded protein response. Biochem Biophys Res Commun, 2006; 347(1): 319-326.

114. Brandner, S., Isenmann, S., Raeber, A., Fischer, M., Sailer, A., Kobayashi, Y., Marino, S., Weissmann, C., Aguzzi, A. Normal host prion protein necessary for scrapie-induced neurotoxicity. Nature, 1996; 379(6563): 339-343.

115. Mallucci, G., Dickinson, A., Linehan, J., Klohn, P. C., Brandner, S., Collinge, J. Depleting neuronal PrP in prion infection prevents disease and reverses spongiosis. Science, 2003; 302(5646): 871-874.

116. Mallucci, G. R., White, M. D., Farmer, M., Dickinson, A., Khatun, H., Powell, A. D., Brandner, S., Jefferys, J. G., Collinge, J. Targeting cellular prion protein reverses early cognitive deficits and neurophysiological dysfunction in prion-infected mice. Neuron, 2007; 53(3): 325-335.

117. Hetz, C. A., Soto, C. Stressing out the ER: a role of the unfolded protein response in prion-related disorders. Curr Mol Med, 2006; 6(1): 37-43.

118. Steele, A. D., King, O. D., Jackson, W. S., Hetz, C. A., Borkowski, A. W., Thielen, P., Wollmann, R., Lindquist, S. Diminishing apoptosis by deletion of Bax or overexpression of Bcl-2 does not protect against infectious prion toxicity in vivo. J Neurosci, 2007; 27(47): 13022-13027.

119. Kristiansen, M., Messenger, M. J., Klohn, P. C., Brandner, S., Wadsworth, J. D., Collinge, J., Tabrizi, S. J. Disease-related prion protein forms aggresomes in neuronal cells leading to caspase activation and apoptosis. J Biol Chem, 2005; 280(46): 38851-38861.

120. Rubinsztein, D. C., Gestwicki, J. E., Murphy, L. O., Klionsky, D. J. Potential therapeutic applications of autophagy. Nat Rev Drug Discov, 2007; 6(4): 304-312.

121. Korth, C., May, B. C., Cohen, F. E., Prusiner, S. B. Acridine and phenothiazine derivatives as pharmacotherapeutics for prion disease. Proc Natl Acad Sci U S A, 2001; 98(17): 9836-9841.

122. Korth, C., Peters, P. J. Emerging pharmacotherapies for Creutzfeldt-Jakob disease. Arch Neurol, 2006; 63(4): 497-501.

123. Stewart, L. A., Rydzewska, L. H., Keogh, G. F., Knight, R. S. Systematic review of therapeutic interventions in human prion disease. Neurology, 2008; 70(15): 1272-1281.

124. Tatzelt, J., Prusiner, S. B., Welch, W. J. Chemical chaperones interfere with the formation of scrapie prion protein. Embo J, 1996; 15(23): 6363-6373.

125. Beranger, F., Crozet, C., Goldsborough, A., Lehmann, S. Trehalose impairs aggregation of PrPSc molecules and protects prion-infected cells against oxidative damage. Biochem Biophys Res Commun, 2008; 374(1): 44-48.

126. Cordeiro, Y., Lima, L. M., Gomes, M. P., Foguel, D., Silva, J. L. Modulation of prion protein oligomerization, aggregation, and beta-sheet conversion by 4,4'-dianilino-1,1'-binaphthyl-5,5'-sulfonate (bis-ANS). J Biol Chem, 2004; 279(7): 5346-5352.

127. Soto, C. Unfolding the role of protein misfolding in neurodegenerative diseases. Nat Rev Neurosci, 2003; 4(1): 49-60.

128. Soto, C., Kascsak, R. J., Saborio, G. P., Aucouturier, P., Wisniewski, T., Prelli, F., Kascsak, R., Mendez, E., Harris, D. A., Ironside, J., Tagliavini, F., Carp, R. I., Frangione, B. Reversion of prion protein conformational changes by synthetic beta-sheet breaker peptides. Lancet, 2000; 355(9199): 192-197.

129. de Rijk, M. C., Launer, L. J., Berger, K., Breteler, M. M., Dartigues, J. F., Baldereschi, M., Fratiglioni, L., Lobo, A., Martinez-Lage, J., Trenkwalder, C., Hofman, A. Prevalence of Parkinson's disease in Europe: A collaborative study of population-based cohorts. Neurologic Diseases in the Elderly Research Group. Neurology, 2000; 54(11 Suppl 5): S21-23.

130. Klein, C., Lohmann-Hedrich, K. Impact of recent genetic findings in Parkinson's disease. Curr Opin Neurol, 2007; 20(4): 453-464.

131. Cooper, A. A., Gitler, A. D., Cashikar, A., Haynes, C. M., Hill, K. J., Bhullar, B., Liu, K., Xu, K., Strathearn, K. E., Liu, F., Cao, S., Caldwell, K. A., Caldwell, G. A., Marsischky, G., Kolodner, R. D., Labaer, J., Rochet, J. C., Bonini, N. M., Lindquist, S. Alpha-synuclein blocks ER-Golgi traffic and Rab1 rescues neuron loss in Parkinson's models. Science, 2006; 313(5785): 324-328.

132. Smith, W. W., Jiang, H., Pei, Z., Tanaka, Y., Morita, H., Sawa, A., Dawson, V. L., Dawson, T. M., Ross, C. A. Endoplasmic reticulum stress and mitochondrial cell death pathways mediate A53T mutant alpha-synuclein-induced toxicity. Hum Mol Genet, 2005; 14(24): 3801-3811.

133. Ryu, E. J., Harding, H. P., Angelastro, J. M., Vitolo, O. V., Ron, D., Greene, L. A. Endoplasmic reticulum stress and the unfolded protein response in cellular models of Parkinson's disease. J Neurosci, 2002; 22(24): 10690-10698.

134. Holtz, W. A., O'Malley, K. L. Parkinsonian mimetics induce aspects of unfolded protein response in death of dopaminergic neurons. J Biol Chem, 2003; 278(21): 19367-19377.

135. Abou-Sleiman, P. M., Muqit, M. M., Wood, N. W. Expanding insights of mitochondrial dysfunction in Parkinson's disease. Nat Rev Neurosci, 2006; 7(3): 207-219.

136. Wang, H. Q., Takahashi, R. Expanding insights on the involvement of endoplasmic reticulum stress in

Parkinson's disease. Antioxid Redox Signal, 2007; 9(5): 553-561.

137.   Lee, A. H., Iwakoshi, N. N., Glimcher, L. H. XBP-1 regulates a subset of endoplasmic reticulum resident chaperone genes in the unfolded protein response. Mol Cell Biol, 2003; 23(21): 7448-7459.

138.   Kakiuchi, C., Iwamoto, K., Ishiwata, M., Bundo, M., Kasahara, T., Kusumi, I., Tsujita, T., Okazaki, Y., Nanko, S., Kunugi, H., Sasaki, T., Kato, T. Impaired feedback regulation of XBP1 as a genetic risk factor for bipolar disorder. Nat Genet, 2003; 35(2): 171-175.

139.   Chen, W., Duan, S., Zhou, J., Sun, Y., Zheng, Y., Gu, N., Feng, G., He, L. A case-control study provides evidence of association for a functional polymorphism -197C/G in XBP1 to schizophrenia and suggests a sex-dependent effect. Biochem Biophys Res Commun, 2004; 319(3): 866-870.

140.   Kusumi, I., Masui, T., Kakiuchi, C., Suzuki, K., Akimoto, T., Hashimoto, R., Kunugi, H., Kato, T., Koyama, T. Relationship between XBP1 genotype and personality traits assessed by TCI and NEO-FFI. Neurosci Lett, 2005; 391(1-2): 7-10.

141.   Zhao, L., Longo-Guess, C., Harris, B. S., Lee, J. W., Ackerman, S. L. Protein accumulation and neurodegeneration in the woozy mutant mouse is caused by disruption of SIL1, a cochaperone of BiP. Nat Genet, 2005; 37(9): 974-979.

CHAPTER 2

The Unfolded Protein Response in Mammalian Cells

Sung Hoon Back[1], Justin R. Hassler[2] and Randal J. Kaufman[1,2,3]

[1]*Howard Hughes Medical Institute, Departments of* [2]*Biological Chemistry and* [3]*Internal Medicine, University of Michigan Medical Center, Ann Arbor, MI 48109-0650 USA*

Address correspondence to: Dr. Randal J. Kaufman, Howard Hughes Medical Institute, University of Michigan Medical Center, Ann Arbor, MI 48109-0650 USA; Tel: 734-763-9037; Fax. 734-763-9323; Email: kaufmanr@umich.edu

Abstract: The endoplasmic reticulum (ER) is a well-orchestrated factory where secretory and membrane proteins are manufactured, modified and correctly folded prior to trafficking to their final destinations. Conditions that interfere with ER function lead to an evolutionarily conserved cellular stress response termed the unfolded protein response (UPR). The UPR initially transduces signals to re-establish ER homeostasis but with prolonged or acute ER stress these signals undergo a transition that initiate cell death. In this review, we summarize our current understanding of the mammalian UPR and discuss the cell-type and tissue-specific functions of UPR components revealed by studies from genetic mouse models.

1. INTRODUCTION

The endoplasmic reticulum (ER) is a network of interconnected tubules, vesicles, and sacs [1]. The ER is the first station of the secretory pathway and the site of synthesis for proteins resident in the ER or destined for the Golgi compartment, endosomes, lysosomes, the plasma membrane or the extracellular milieu [2]. It also serves as a site of biosynthesis for steroids, cholesterol and other lipids, calcium storage and as a signaling platform between the nucleus and cytosol. [3,4]. Efficient ER function relies on numerous resident quality control factors such as molecular chaperones and folding enzymes, a high level of calcium, and an oxidative environment. Nascent polypeptides that are translocated into the ER lumen undergo post-translational modifications and rounds of folding interactions required for optimal function. Properly folded proteins exit from the ER and progress through the secretory pathway, whereas irreparably unfolded proteins are retro-translocated from the ER and degraded by cytoplasmic proteasomes [5,6]. The flux of nascent polypeptides into the ER is variable because it changes rapidly in response to the physiological state and environmental conditions of the cell. In order to handle this dynamic situation, cells must adjust their ER protein-folding capacity according to their environmental and physiological context, thereby ensuring that the quality of membranous and secreted proteins is maintained with high fidelity. Given the importance of ER function for normal cellular function, it is not surprising that the ER

affects a diverse number of cellular processes such as transcription, translation, cell cycle control, intracellular signaling and programmed cell death. When ER homeostasis is altered, signaling pathways are activated eliciting an adaptive response that is collectively called the unfolded protein response (UPR). The UPR includes expansion of ER size, enhanced folding capacity, reduced protein synthesis through transcriptional or translational controls, and increased clearance of unfolded or misfolded proteins [7-11]. When these mechanisms fail to restore ER homeostasis, numerous death signaling pathways are activated [12-15]. Mammalian UPR signaling pathways are initiated by three transmembrane ER-proximal sensors of unfolded protein: inositol-requiring protein 1 (IRE1), activating transcription factor 6 (ATF6), and PKR-like endoplasmic reticulum kinase (PERK) [10, 16] in all cell types. In addition, recent studies suggest that the ER has several tissue specific auxiliary sensors, although the roles of these tissue specific sensors in ER stress are not fully understood. These three main UPR sensors are integral membrane proteins that sense the unfolded protein load in the ER lumen and transmit this information across the ER membrane to the cytosol. Considerable progress has been made in our understanding of the signaling pathways and physiological significance of the UPR. The goal of this review is to summarize our current insight into these processes in the mammalian UPR and furthermore to discuss the specific functions of the UPR revealed by studies of genetic mouse models at both specific cell and tissue levels.

2. THE THREE BRANCHES OF THE UPR

IRE1

The initial characterization of the UPR was performed in the budding yeast *Saccharomyces cerevisiae* [17,18]. A genetic screen revealed that three proteins are required for signal transduction from the ER to activate gene transcription in the nucleus. The first protein, IRE1, is a type 1 transmembrane Ser/The protein kinase that also has a site-specific endoribonuclease (RNase) activity. The second protein is HAC1, a transcriptional activator that regulates transcription of UPR target genes [19,20]. Finally, Rlg1p (tRNA ligase) joins the 5′ and 3′ ends of *Hac1* mRNA that are produced through cleavage by IRE1 [21,22]. The unconventional cytoplasmic splicing of *Hac1* mRNA is required for accumulation of a more efficiently translated HAC1 transcription factor possessing a C-terminal frame shift which mediates the Baker's yeast UPR transcriptional response.

IRE1 is the most proximal component of the yeast UPR pathway that is evolutionarily conserved in mammals. IRE1 has three functional domains [17,18,22,23]. The amino terminal domain resides in the ER lumen and senses the accumulation of unfolded proteins [17]. When cells are not stressed, IRE1 protein kinase is maintained in an inactive monomeric form through interactions with the protein chaperone Kar2p/BiP [24-27]. Accumulation of misfolded proteins in the ER lumen induces IRE1 dimerization and *trans*-autophosphorylation via the cytoplasmic kinase domain. The activation of oligomerized kinase domains subsequently activates the site-specific carboxy-terminal endoribonuclease domain [23,28,29]. In yeast, the only known substrate for the site-specific RNase activity of IRE1 is *Hac1* mRNA, which encodes a basic leucine zipper (bZIP) transcription factor that binds to the UPR element (UPRE) upstream of responsive genes [19,20]. Unspliced *Hac1* mRNA is constitutively transcribed, but the RNA is not translated due to long-range base-pairing interactions between the *Hac1* 5′ UTR and the intron [30]. Upon activation of the UPR, IRE1-mediated cleavage removes the intron and the exons are tethered together by base pairing then ligated by tRNA ligase Rlg1p. The unconventional splicing of *Hac1* mRNA removes a 252-nucleotide intron and changes the open reading frame so that a short carboxy-terminal activation domain consisting of a 19 amino acid segment (Hac1i) replaces the previous 10 amino acid segment (Hac1u) [31]. Hac1i binds to a DNA

sequence motif termed the unfolded protein response element (UPRE; consensus CAGCGTG) as a dimer in the promoters of ER chaperone genes. In addition to activating the transcription of ER chaperone genes, Hac1i activates the transcription of genes that are involved in ER protein folding and modification, phospholipid biosynthesis, ER-associated protein degradation (ERAD), and vesicular transport in the secretory pathway downstream of the ER [32-34].

Although the UPR was first described in the budding yeast *Saccharomyces cerevisiae* [35], higher eukaryotic cells have also maintained the essential and unique properties of IRE1 signaling. However, higher eukaryotes possess additional sensors and control mechanisms to mediate more diverse responses upon activation of the UPR. Three ER-localized, ubiquitously expressed transmembrane proteins, IRE1, PERK, and ATF6 serve as the UPR's proximal sensors responsible for the ER's folding capacity of newly synthesized proteins by attenuating expression, and degradation of misfolded proteins Fig. (1) [7-11,36-39].

Both human and mouse IRE1α proteins respond to the accumulation of unfolded proteins in the ER, undergo kinase activation and thereby trigger their endoribonuclease activity. Upon activation of the UPR in mammals, unconventional cytoplasmic splicing by IRE1α protein removes a 26-nucleotide intron from the unspliced *Xbp1* mRNA (encoding 267 amino acids), to induce a translational frame-shift producing a fusion protein encoded from two evolutionarily conserved open reading frames (ORFs) Fig. (1). The translation product (XBP1s) from spliced *Xbp1* mRNA is a potent transcriptional activator of 371 amino acids that comprises the original amino-terminal DNA binding domain plus an additional transactivation domain in the carboxy-terminus [40-42]. The spliced XBP1 (XBP1s) induces multiple secretory pathway genes, expands the ER, and increases total protein synthesis [43-45] to enforce cellular structure and function consistent with the requirements during ER stress. Unlike yeast where *Hac1* mRNA is the only known substrate for IRE1's RNase activity, human IRE1α cleaves human CD59 (complement defense 59) although the physiological meaning of this observation is not known [46] Fig. (1). Furthermore, *Ire1α* mRNA itself has also been reported to be cleaved *via* an IRE1α RNase dependent mechanism [47]. In addition, it was recently reported that *Drosophila* IRE1 reduces ER burden by selectively

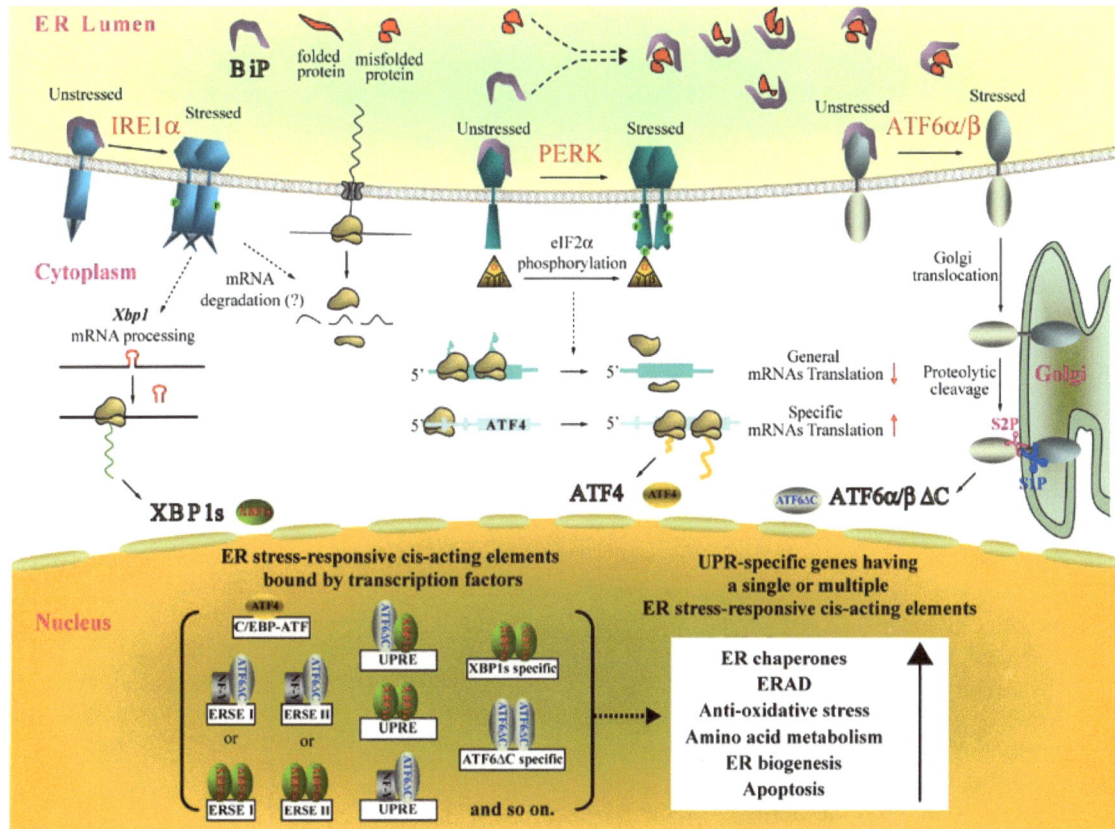

Fig. (1). The unfolded protein response in mammalian cells. Mammalian UPR signaling pathways are initiated by three transmembrane ER-proximal sensors (IRE1, PERK, and ATF6) upon accumulation of unfolded proteins in ER lumen: ER stress causes BiP dissociation from the sensors (IRE1 and PERK) leading to their activation by autophosphorylation and then dimerization or oligomerization. The RNase activity of activated IRE1 initiates *Xbp1* mRNA splicing thereby creating a potent transcriptional activator (XBP1s) and may selectively degrade mRNAs encoding secretory proteins. The kinase activity of activated PERK phosphorylates the α subunit of eIF2 on Ser51, that inhibits translation initiation of general mRNAs but activates translation of some specific genes (such as *Atf4* mRNA). Lastly, ATF6 released from BiP is transported from the ER to the Golgi apparatus, where it is cleaved by Golgi-resident proteases, S1P and S2P to liberate the N-terminal transcription factor domain (ATF6ΔC). The three transcription factors (XBP1s, ATF6ΔC, and ATF4) generated from activation of three UPR sensors localize to nucleus where they bind the promoter regions of UPR-specific genes having single or multiple ER stress-responsive *cis*-acting elements (ERSE1, ERSE II, UPRE, or C/EBP-ATF). The combination of different *cis*-acting elements in the promoter of each gene determines specificity of XBP1s, ATF6ΔC, and ATF4.

cleaving mRNAs encoding secreted proteins during induction of the UPR in fly cells [48].

There are two mammalian IRE1 homologs referred to as IRE1α and IRE1β. IRE1α is expressed in most cells and tissues [49], whereas IRE1β expression is restricted to intestinal epithelial cells [50]. Human IRE1β displays 76% identity to murine IRE1β and 39% identity to human IRE1α [51]. Overexpression of both human and murine IRE1β isolated from colon cDNA library caused apoptotic cell death [50,51], possibly a consequence of expression of the proapoptotic transcription factor CHOP [50] or activation of the JNK pathway [52]. However, the precise mechanism by which IRE1β

overexpression induces cell death is not known. The RNase activity of both human and murine IRE1α to cleave *Xbp1* mRNA has been studied in both *in vivo* and *in vitro* experiments [41,42,53], whereas the RNase activity and RNA substrate specificity of IRE1β are less well understood. In addition, there is no enough evidence that *Xbp1* mRNA is a direct substrate for IRE1β. However, a domain swapping experiment between human IRE1 α and β C-terminal RNase domains suggested that RNase domain of IRE1 determines the functional specificities of these isoforms [54]. Recently, Iqbal J. *et al.* reported that mouse IRE1β inhibited chylomicron production by selectively degrading microsomal triglyceride transfer protein (MTP) mRNA as well as 28S rRNA, however

IRE1β could not induce UPR genes through cleavage of *Xbp1* mRNA [55]. The 28S rRNA cleavage would serve to globally reduce protein synthesis, as characterized for *Drosophila* IRE1 [51]. However, further work is required to understand physiological role of IRE1β RNase activity. Taken together, these findings support an emerging phyisiological role of IRE1-mediated mRNA cleavage as a mode of posttranscriptional regulation to help reduce the accumulation of unfolded proteins by functioning in conjunction with the general translational inhibition mediated by the PERK pathway [56].

Recently the structural analyses of yeast IRE1- and human IRE1α-luminal domain revealed a head-to-head dimerization interface hypothesized to be a consequence of a central groove formed by several α-helices situated around an antiparallel β-sheet [57,58]. The groove present in both yeast IRE1 and human IRE1α crystals shares many features with the peptide-binding domains of major histocompatibility complexes (MHC). For yeast IRE1, it has been proposed that direct binding of unfolded proteins to the deep grooves is required for oligomerization of yeast IRE1 [57]. The proposal was further supported by studies of Kimata Y. *et al.* which suggested that upon ER stress, IRE1 is activated in two steps, in the first step, BiP dissociation from IRE1 leads to cluster formation. In the second step, direct interaction of unfolded proteins with the core stress sensing region (CSSR, aa 112-454 in yeast IRE1) orients the cytosolic effector domains of clustered IRE1 molecules [59]. Although the crystal structures for yeast IRE1- and human IRE1α-luminal domains share significant structural similarity [57,58] the mechanism presented for yeast IRE1 activation may not be applicable to mammalian IRE1α because the crystal structure of the luminal domain of mammalian IRE1α revealed that the MHC-like groove is too narrow for peptide binding and peptide binding to this groove is not required for dimerization. Furthermore, mutations that disrupt the dimerization interface produced IRE1α molecules that failed to either dimerize or activate the UPR upon ER stress [57, 58].

The structural analysis of yeast IRE1 cytosolic domain showed that the domain forms a symetrical dimmer mediated by both kinase-kinase and nuclease-nuclease interactions. In the kinase domain, both N- and C-lobe residues contribute to the dimer interface [60]. Interestingly when leucine 745 (yeast IRE1) [61] or isoleucine 642 (human IRE1α) [7] in the putative ATP/ADP-binding pocket of the kinase domain was mutated to a smaller residue (alanine or glycine) to accommodate binding of a bulky kinase inhibitor 1NM-PP1, remarkably, instead of thwarting the nuclease activity of IRE1, the kinase inhibitor stimulated its activity indicating that the trigger for IRE1's endoribonuclease activity is not phosphorylation *per se,* but rather a conformational change in the kinase domain induced by nucleotide binding and *trans*-autophosphorylation of the kinase activation loop. Although the sequence of events has not been determined NM-PP1 binding with high affinity in the nucleotide-binding cleft of the IRE1 mutant evidently induces the requisite conformational change in the kinase domain without need for phosphorylation of the activation loop. Thus, the structural and mutational analysis to IRE1 cytosolic domain revealed that signal induced trans-autophosphorylation [23,29] of the kinase domain permits unfettered binding of nucleotide (ADP or ATP), which in turn promotes dimerization to compose the ribonuclease active site [7].

Upon activation in response to ER stress, IRE1α performs at least two different functions. First, the endoribonuclease activity of IRE1 cleaves *Xbp1* mRNA, converting it into a potent transcriptional activator. Gene expression analyses were performed by several groups using *Xbp1* null MEFs, *Xbp1*-deficient splenic B cells, or spliced XBP1 overexpressing cells [43,44,62]. Those analyses consistently showed that spliced XBP1 induces a wide spectrum of secretory pathway genes involved in protein folding, translocation of nascent polypeptides, ER-Golgi translocation, ERAD genes, and genes remodeling ER and Golgi structure to restore ER homeostasis and maintain ER quality control in stressed cells. How spliced XBP1 induces several genes will be discussed in the section "**The regulation of gene expression by UPR activation**". Second, recent studies from several laboratories have shown that IRE1α links the UPR to the activation of JNK signaling pathways which we will revisit in the section "**The UPR and cell death**".

PERK

The second ER stress transducer, PERK (EIF2AK3), is a type I transmembrane protein located in the ER, which senses the accumulation of unfolded proteins in the ER lumen [63]. The luminal stress-sensing domain of PERK superficially resembles IRE1, is phylogenetically related, similar in structure and function, and experimentally interchangeable [28, 64]. The cytoplasmic portion of PERK contains a protein kinase domain [63, 65]. In the absence of ER stress, BiP binds to the luminal domain of PERK and keeps it from being activated. In response to ER stress, BiP is released from PERK, and PERK undergoes activating *trans*-autophosphorylation by oligomerization [28,64] Fig. (**1**). Activated PERK phosphorylates at Ser51 on the α-subunit of the heterotrimeric eukaryotic initiation factor 2 (eIF2) [63,65]. The ternary complex of eIF2–GTP–tRNAi^{Met} delivers initiator methionyl tRNA to the 40S ribosomal subunit and is crucial for AUG start-codon selection. Upon 60S ribosomal subunit joining, GTP is hydrolyzed to GDP. To promote another round of initiation, the GDP bound eIF2 requires GTP exchange in a reaction catalyzed by eIF2B. When eIF2α is phosphorylated at Ser51, this exchange reaction is prevented by the sequestration of eIF2B in a complex with eIF2. Because the cellular level of eIF2B is 10 to 20 fold lower than the level of eIF2, very small increases in the degree of eIF2α phosphorylation sequester eIF2 in a complex with eIF2B and reduce the efficiency of AUG codon recognition. As a consequence, translation is changed both quantitatively and qualitatively. The status of eIF2α phosphorylation is controlled by several Ser/Thr protein kinases. To date, four specific eIF2α kinases including PERK have been identified in the mammalian genome [66] (1) the heme-regulated inhibitor kinase (HRI, EIF2AK1) that is expressed in reticulocytes and proposed to coordinate globin polypeptide synthesis with hemin availability in erythroid tissues and also regulated by oxidative stress [67]; (2) the general control of nitrogen metabolism kinase 2 (GCN2, EIF2AK4) which is activated upon nutritional deprivation, UV irradiation, proteasome inhibition, and certain viral infections [68,69]; (3) the dsRNA-activated protein kinase (PKR, EIF2AK2) participates in an anti-viral defense mechanism that is mediated by interferon [70]. Although PERK is mainly responsible for UPR-induced eIF2α phosphorylation, analysis of *Perk*$^{+/+}$ and *Perk*$^{-/-}$ mouse embryo fibroblasts (MEFs) showed that with extended stress conditions, significant eIF2α kinase activity was found even in the *Perk*-null cells [71]. This suggests that the other eIF2α kinases can function during the UPR. However, in double null *Gcn2*$^{-/-}$ *Perk*$^{-/-}$ MEFs the previously observed eIF2α kinase activities were abolished [71]. Cooperativity between the eIF2α kinases PERK and GCN2 was shown to be biologically

important for cell-cycle arrest in response to ER stress [72]. Furthermore, phosphorylation of eIF2α facilitates translational repression of cyclin D, which is central for subsequent arrest in the G1 phase upon the UPR activation [73]. Although deletion of *Perk* alone did not restore cyclin D expression in response to ER stress, the combined deletion of *Perk* and *Gcn2* in MEFs fully abolished eIF2α phosphorylation and restored cyclin D translation [72]. However, recent studies from Raven J.F. *et al.* suggest that PKR and PERK induce the proteosome-dependent degradation of cyclin D *via* a mechanism requiring eIF2α phosphorylation yet in polysome profile experiments showed that the cyclin D message is translated equally well regardless of the state of eIF2α phosphorylation or the inhibition of global protein synthesis [74]. Currently it can be said that the decrease in cyclin D1 during ER stress arrests mammalian cells in G1 but how cyclin D is regulated is not fully understood yet.

Although activated PERK-mediated eIF2α phosphorylation inhibits general mRNA translation initiation, phosphorylation of eIF2α specifically activates translation of some mRNAs encoding several short upstream open reading frames (uORFs) [75,76] Fig. (**1**). Specifically, UPR-mediated activation of PERK stimulates translation of *Atf4* (activating transcription factor 4) mRNA, encoding a basic leucine zipper (bZIP) containing transcription factor that activates a subset of UPR-responsive genes [77, 78]. *Atf4* mRNA contains two uORFs conserved in vertebrates [79]. The second uORF overlaps with the *Atf4* ORF. Mutation of the AUG in uORF1 repressed translation of the *Atf4* ORF and mutation of the AUG in uORF2 derepressed translation of the *Atf4* ORF [79, 80]. Mutational analysis of the *Atf4* mRNA revealed that scanning ribosomes initiate translation efficiently at both uORFs and ribosomes that had translated uORF1 efficiently reinitiate translation at downstream AUGs. During low levels of eIF2α phosphorylation, scanning ribosomes that have translated uORF1 reinitiate at the inhibitory uORF2, which precludes subsequent translation of ATF4. However, high levels of eIF2α phosphorylation reduce formation of eIF2-GTP-tRNAi^{Met} ternary complexes to decrease the probability that ribosomes initiating at uORF1 will acquire these complexes in time to translate the repressive uORF2, but rather will acquire them later to initiate at the *Atf4* AUG. The translated ATF4 induces several genes involved in ER protein folding, ERAD, amino acid biosynthesis and transport function, anti-oxidative stress responses, and apoptosis, such as growth arrest and DNA damage 34 (Gadd34) and CAAT/enhancer-binding protein (C/EBP) homologous protein (*Chop*) [81-84].

eIF2α phosphorylation also activates translation from some internal ribosome entry site elements (IRES) [85]. As part of the adaptive response to nutritional deprivation, cells increase the expression of amino acid biosynthetic and transporter genes. For instance, glucose and/or amino acid limitation increases expression of the Arginine/Lysine Transporter1 gene (*Cat1*) through an increase in *Cat1* mRNA transcription, stability and translation [86]. Phosphorylation of eIF2α during UPR activation, such as glucose deprivation, signals through PERK, whereas, amino acid deprivation signals through GCN2 [75]. Both signaling pathways converge at eIF2 to induce translation of *Cat1* mRNA. The 5'-leader of the *Cat1* mRNA contains an internal ribosome entry site (IRES) with a short uORF. Phosphorylation of eIF2α is required for IRES-dependent translation of *Cat1* mRNA. In the non-translated state, the IRES forms a dormant negative structure in the 5' UTR. Phosphorylation of eIF2α stimulates translation of the uORF to unfold the inhibitory structure and induces a conformational change that activates the IRES. However, the detailed mechanism is presently not known.

Recent studies revealed that NF-E2-related factor 2 (NRF2) is another substrate of PERK kinase activity [87]. NRF2 belongs to the cap 'n' collar (CNC) family of transcription factors, that includes p45/NF-E2, Nrf1, Nrf2, Nrf3, Bach1, and Bach2 [88]. NRF2 activates transcription on the antioxidant response element [(ARE)-(G/C)TGA(C/T)N3GC(A/G)] as a heterodimer with small Maf proteins [89]. Through the ARE, the NRF2-Maf complex controls expression of detoxifying enzymes including NAD(P)H:quinone oxidoreductase 1 (NQO1), hem(e)oxygenase 1 (HO-1), glutathione *S*-transferase (GST), UDP-glucuronosyl transferase and the rate limiting enzyme in glutathione biosynthesis,γ-glutamyl-cysteine sythetase (GCLC) [89]. NRF2 is maintained in an inactive state in the cytosol through interaction with the cytoskeletal anchor protein Kelch like Ech-associated protein 1 (KEAP1) [90]. Upon UPR activation, phosphorylation of NRF2 by PERK dissociates the NRF2-KEAP1 complex, allowing NRF2 to translocate to the nucleus. *Nrf2*-null cells are sensitive to a variety of ER stress conditions, and NRF2 overexpression enhances survival during the

UPR [91]. *Perk-* and *Nrf2*-null cells accumulate reactive oxygen species (ROS) [81,91]. In addition, other studies suggest that defects in the UPR cause the accumulation of ROS in cells [81,92,93]. These data support the notion that PERK phosphorylates multiple substrates to protect cells from oxidative stress.

Translational repression by PERK is a transient response to temporally attenuate protein synthesis in order to permit an efficient response to prolonged ER stress. Two regulatory subunits of protein phosphatase I (PP1), Growth arrest and DNA damage-inducible protein-34) (GADD34) and constitutive repressor of eIF2α phosphory-lation (CREP), have recently been characterized to regulate eIF2α phosphatase activity through their homologous C-terminal domains [94-97]. PP1 dephosphorylates eIF2α and terminates signaling through the PERK-eIF2α pathway. CREP is a constitutive activator of PP1. In contrast, GADD34 is not detected in unstressed cells and is activated transcriptionally during ER stress by ATF4.

ATF6 and ATF6-like Molecules

ATF6 is a type II transmembrane protein that acts as a metazoan-specific ER stress transducer. The luminal domain of ATF6 senses the presence of unfolded proteins [98-100]. The cytoplasmic portion of ATF6 has a DNA-binding domain containing bZIP and transcriptional activation domains. Two homologous proteins, ATF6α and ATF6β/cAMP-response-element-binding protein (CREB)-related protein (CREB-RP)/G13 exist in mammals [98]. Under conditions of ER stress, BiP dissociates from ATF6, and ATF6 is transported from the ER to the Golgi apparatus, where it is cleaved by Golgi-resident proteases, first by S1P (site 1 protease) and then in the intramembrane region by S2P (site 2 protease) to release the N-terminal bZIP transcription factor domain designated ATF6ΔC [101-103] Fig. (**1**). The role of S1P is to reduce the size of the luminal domain to prepare ATF6 to be an optimal S2P substrate [104]. ATF6ΔC enters the nucleus where it activates mainly the transcription of genes encoding ER-localized molecular chaperones and folding enzymes [100,105,106]. Interestingly, it has been shown that the binding and dissociation of BiP is also critical for the activation of ATF6 [102]. The dissociation of BiP from ATF6 appears to be actively triggered upon ER stress rather than resulting from simple competition between ATF6 and unfolded proteins for binding to BiP [107]. In addition, recent research suggests that whereas

IRE1α and PERK are monomers in the unstressed ER, ATF6α occurs as a monomer, dimer, and oligomer in the unstressed ER through the presence of inter- and intramolecular disulfide bridges formed between two conserved cysteine residues (aa 467 and 618) in the luminal domain [108]. ATF6α is reduced in response to ER stress to produce a monomeric ATF6α that transits to the Golgi apparatus where it is cleaved by the sequential actions of S1P and S2P. The reduced monomer ATF6α is a better substrate for S1P than disulfide-bonded oligomeric forms [108]. However the mechanism for the reduction of ATF6α in response to ER stress is unknown.

Recently, several bZIP transcription factors located in the ER and regulated by regulated intramembrane proteolysis (RIP) have been reported. One such transcription factor is the cAMP response element-binding protein H (CREBH) which is expressed in hepatocytes, the pyloric stomach, and small intestine [109]. Pro-inflammatory cytokines IL-6, 1L-1α, and TNFα increase transcription of CREBH to produce an inactive precursor protein that is localized to the ER [110]. On the onset of ER stress, CREBH transits to the Golgi compartment, where it is cleaved by S1P and S2P processing enzymes. However, unlike ATF6, cleaved CREBH does not activate transcription of UPR genes, but rather, induces the transcription of acute-phase response genes [such as C-reactive protein (CRP) and murine serum amyloid P component (SAP)] involved in acute inflammatory responses [110]. These studies identified CREBH as a novel ER-localized transcription factor that has an essential role in induction of innate immune response genes and linked for the first time ER stress to inflammatory responses.

In addition to ATF6 and CREBH, additional similarly-related factors are regulated through ER stress-induced proteolytic processing, although their physiologic significance remains unknown. OASIS (old astrocyte specifically induced substance) is also cleaved by S1P and S2P in response to ER stress in astrocytes and activates the transcription of BiP [111]. BBF2H7 (BBF2 human homolog on chromosome 7) belonging to the OASIS family, is processed by S1P and S2P in response to ER stress [112]. It is noteworthy that BBF2H7 is markedly induced at the translational level during ER stress and has the potential to activate transcription of target genes *via* direct binding to the CRE site. BBF2H7 protein is up-regulated in damaged neurons after ischemia and protects neurons from ER stress-induced cell death.

The spermatid-specific transcription factor, Tisp40 α/β (transcript induced in spermiogenesis), is also cleaved by S1P and S2P and activates the transcription of EDEM [113]. Luman/LZIP/CREB3 can be processed by S1P and S2P to induce expression of *Herpud*-1 during the UPR *via* transactivation of the ER stress response element II (ERSE-II in its promoter [114,115]. CREB4 is also a member of the ER-localized proteins that are regulated by ER stress through cleavage by S1P [116]. The discovery of these numerous RIP-activated proteins raises the question of why cells have evolved multiple ATF6-like molecules in the ER. These ATF6-like molecules might be evolutionarily chosen to respond to specific conditions of ER stress that occur in different tissues to activate tissue-specific expression of genes to resolve ER stress. Further studies are required to elucidate how the trafficking of ATF6-like molecules from the ER to the Golgi apparatus is regulated. In addition, targeted deletion of the gene encoding ATF6-like molecules should identify their significance in the ER-stress signaling pathways.

3. THE REGULATION OF GENE EXPRESSION BY UPR ACTIVATION

Analysis of promoter regions of UPR-inducible genes in mammals identified several ER stress-responsive *cis*-acting elements Fig. (**1**). First, deletion and point mutation analysis of the *BiP*, *Grp94,* and calreticulin (*Crt*) promoters identified the ER stress response element I (ERSE-I) (CCAAT-(N9)-CCACG) [117,118]. Using a yeast one-hybrid screen, Yoshida *et al.* identified two bZIP-containing transcription factors ATF6α and XBP1 that activate transcription from ERSE-I, [118]. Both ATF6ΔC and spliced XBP1 bind to the CCACG region of the ERSE-I while the general transcription factor NF-Y binds to the CCAAT region [100,106]. The ERSE-I is found in the promoters of various UPR targets including transcription factors XBP1 and CHOP, ER chaperones like BiP and GRP94, and ERAD components such as Herpud-1 [62,100,106,119].

Second, the ER stress-responsive *cis*-acting element designated the UPR element (UPRE, TGA<u>CGTGG</u>/A) was identified through affinity selection of oligonucleotides that bind purified ATF6α bZIP proteins [120]. The presence of the CCACG sequence in UPRE (complementary sequence of the underlined sequence identical to the ERSE-I region) suggests that both ATF6ΔC and spliced-XBP1 can bind to the UPRE. Indeed, the UPRE is preferentially bound by XBP1 homodimers without assistance from NF-Y, in contrast to ATF6ΔC that requires NF-Y as a heterodimer to bind ERSE-I [106]. In addition, it seems that ATF6ΔC and XBP1 heterodimerize in ER stressed cells, and these heterodimers have higher binding affinity to the UPRE than the XBP1 homodimer [121]. However, promoters of mammalian genes that require a UPRE have not been identified to date. Acosta-Alvear D. *et al.* recently showed XBP1 can bind several genes containing the UPRE sequence [62].

The third *cis*-acting element was identified in the promoter of the ERAD component Herpud-1 [122]. This promoter contains not only ERSE-I but also a *cis*-acting element different from either ERSE-1 or UPRE [123]. The consensus sequence of this new element, designated ERSE-II, was determined to be ATTGG-N-CCACG by extensive mutational analysis. Evidently, this element contains CCAAT and CCACG as in the case of ERSE-1, although they are separated by a spacer of only one nucleotide and positioned in the opposite orientation compared to ERSE-I. It was also shown that ERSE-II allows the NF-Y–dependent binding of ATF6ΔC , as in the case of ERSE-I, and the NF-Y–independent binding of XBP1, as in the case of the UPRE, and that transcription from ERSE-II is reduced in the absence of XBP1 or ATF6ΔC. Accordingly, the induction of *Herpud-1* mRNA was diminished in the absence of XBP1 or ATF6ΔC [119].

The latest *cis*-acting ER stress responsive element to be discovered was found in the *Chop* promoter [83,124]. The C/EBP homologous protein transcription factor CHOP (GADD153) is one of the UPR targets that is regulated by all three branches of the UPR [83,100,125]. The *Chop* promoter contains both an ERSE-I and an C/EBP-ATF composite site (C/EBP-ATF, TTGCATCA). Deletion and point mutation analysis of either element revealed that both elements are essential for both the basal activity and the ER stress-induction of the *Chop* promoter [125]. The ATF6 and XBP1 transcription factors can bind to ERSE-I

with NF-Y and ATF6 overexpression leads to CHOP induction in cells [100,106]. ATF4 binds to the C/EBP-ATF composite site *in vitro* in an ER stress-dependent manner [83]. Interestingly in *Perk*-null and Ser51Ala *eIF-2α* knock-in cells,

where eIF-2α phosphorylation is blocked during ER stress, the induction of CHOP is completely lost [53,78,126] although the IRE1-XBP1 and ATF6α pathways are still functional. Therefore more studies are required to understand the relative contributions and cross-talk of the three UPR branches in regulating CHOP expression during different cellular stresses.

Recent studies indicate that the three arms of the UPR communicate with each other downstream from the initial independent activation of IRE1, PERK and ATF6 in ER-stressed cells. One good example of cross-talk between the arms of the UPR is the *Herp-1/Herpud-1* promoter. Herpud-1 is an ER localized protein with an N-terminal ubiquitin-like domain [122,127]. The *Herpud-1* promoter has three ER stress-responsive *cis*-acting elements (C/EBP-ATF composite site, ERSE-II, and ERSE-I) [128]. ATF4, induced by the PERK-eIF2α pathway, directly binds to the C/EBP-ATF composite site. However, ATF4 is not essential for Herpud-1 induction during ER stress, but is required for maximal activation [128]. ERSE-II of the *Herpud-1* promoter allows the NF-Y-dependent binding of ATF6 and NF-Y-independent binding of XBP1, and transcription from ERSE-II is reduced in the absence of XBP1 [119]. It was recently shown, using ATF6α-deficient MEFs that ATF6α also contributes to optimal induction of *Herpud-1* through direct binding to both ERSE-II and probably ERSE-1 [121,129]. Thus, all three signaling pathways activated during the mammalian UPR are directly involved in the maximal induction of *Herpud-1* suggesting Herpud-1 is important for the homeostasis of the ER. The biological significance of cross-talk between the arms of the UPR has not yet been carefully examined but it is evident that genes have evolved to utilize different combinations of ER stress-responsive *cis*-acting elements in their promoters to respond to different stresses, and that the cross-talk of the UPR pathways through these *cis*-acting elements helps prevent complete loss of UPR-gene expression when any of the three general ER stress-activated pathways are defective. Additionally, elucidating the developmental roles of each these elements will prove to be an exciting area for future research.

4. THE UPR AND CELL DEATH

Activation of each arm of the UPR initiates adaptive mechanisms to relieve the protein folding defect in the ER. As we described above, this adaptive response includes the rapid phosphorylation of eIF2α by PERK to inhibit general mRNA translation, IRE1α-dependent degradation of a subset of ER-associated mRNAs to help clear the ER membrane of polysome-associated transcripts, and the induction of genes to increase the folding capacity of the ER and remove misfolded proteins from the ER mediated by ATF4, cleaved ATF6, and spliced XBP1. In addition, another mechanism known as preemptive quality control (pQC) also contributes to reduce the burden

of misfolded substrates entering the ER by inhibiting the ER translocation of many, but not all, polypeptides [130]. Thus, the adaptive pathways maintain cellular function and avoid apoptosis during chronic stress. Little is known about how the UPR integrates signals from both adaptive and apoptotic pathways to selectively allow for adaptation or programmed cell death. Rutkowski D.T. *et al.* suggest that when ER stress is mild, survival is favored as a consequence of the intrinsic instabilities of mRNAs and proteins that promote apoptosis compared to the relatively long-lived half-lives of those that facilitate protein folding and adaptation [13,131]. As a consequence, the

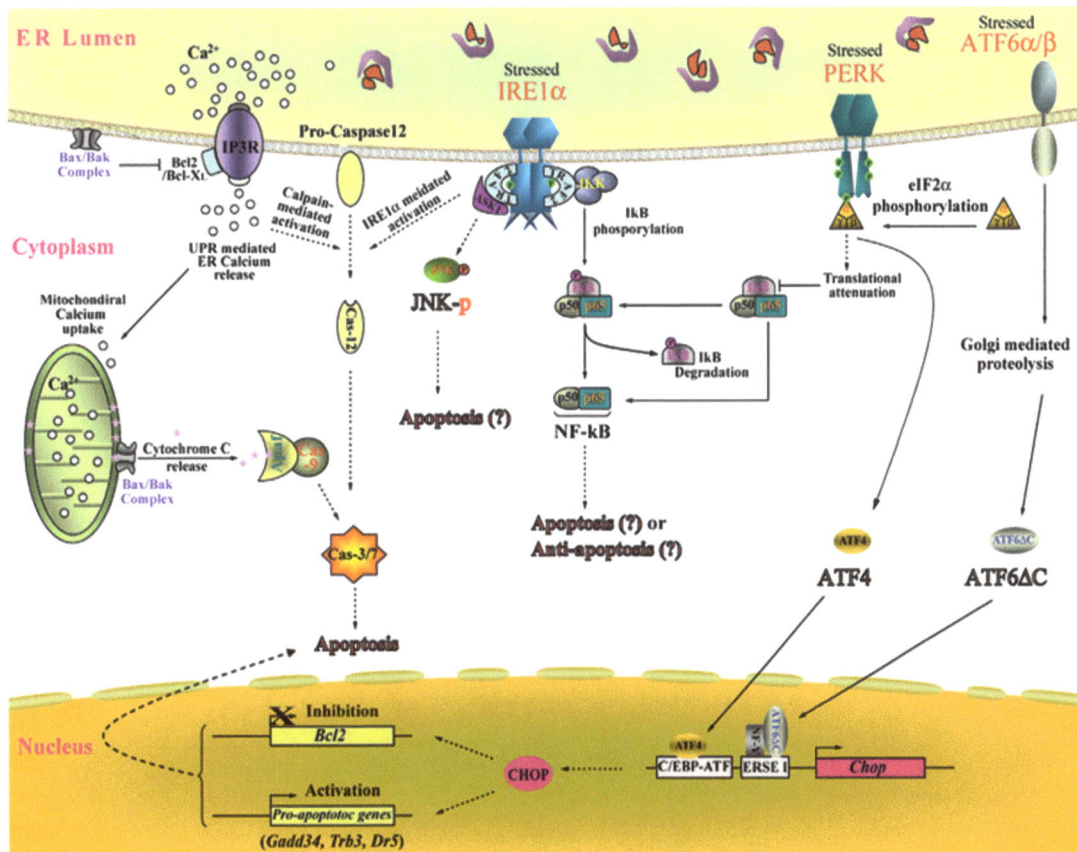

Fig. (2). ER stress-mediated cell death in mammalian cells. ER stress leads to several redundant mitochondria-independent and –dependent apoptotic pathways. Activated IRE1 interacts with the adaptor protein TRAF2, leading to the activation of the JNK and NF-κB pathways. Whether IRE1-TRAF2-dependent JNK and NF-κB pathways protect or sensitize cells to ER stress-induced apoptosis remains controversial. In addition, in response to ER stress, PERK-mediated translational attenuation upregulates NF-κB dependent transcription because IκB has a shorter half-life than NF-κB which is thereby free to translocate to the nucleus. Activated PERK and ATF6ΔC lead to the transcriptional activation of CHOP which induces apoptosis, possibly by inhibiting expression of the antiapoptotic gene *Bcl-2* and/or through regulation of the proapoptotic genes *Gadd34*, *Trb3*, and/or *Dr5*. During ER stress, oligomerized Bax/Bak interacts with InsP₃R in the ER membrane permitting Ca²⁺ efflux into the cytoplasm. Increased cytosolic Ca²⁺ can activate both mitochondria-dependent and -independent caspase cascades. The calcium-dependent protease calpain cleaves and activates the ER-resident procaspase-12 to initiate caspase-dependent apoptosis, although activated IRE1 may also be involved in the activation of procaspase-12 as well. The calcium released from the ER also enters mitochondria to depolarize the inner membrane, promoting cytochrome *c* release and activating APAF (apoptosis protease-activating factor)/procaspase-9–regulated apoptosis.

expression of apoptotic proteins is short-lived as cells adapt to stress. However, if ER stress is severe and chronic, the UPR-mediated efforts to correct the protein-folding defect fail and the apoptotic pathway is preferentially activated over time. Several mechanisms, described below, have been proposed to link the stressed ER to cell death, including direct activation of kinases, transcription factors, caspases, and Bcl-2-family proteins and their modulators. Mitochondrial-dependent and independent cell death pathways trigger apoptosis in response to ER stress Fig. (**2**). In addition, the ER serves as an important compartment where apoptotic signals are generated and integrated to elicit cell death in response to the unbearable accumulation of unfolded proteins, presumably to the advantage of the organism.

IRE1-mediated Cell Death

During ER stress, IRE1α forms a heterooligomeric complex with tumor necrosis factor receptor associated factor 2 (TRAF2) [132] and apoptosis signal-regulating kinase 1 (ASK1) [133] Fig. (**2**). This interaction is abolished by IRE1α kinase-inactivating mutations [132], suggesting that only activated, dimerized, and phosphorylated IRE1α can interact with TRAF2. Studies suggested that this heterotriomeric complex promotes apoptosis through JNK phosphorylation in response to pharmacological induction of ER stress, as it was demonstrated that *Ask1-/-* primary neurons are resistant to ER stress-induced cell death [133]. The kinase pathway initiated by ASK1 leads to JNK-mediated phosphorylation and activation of the proapoptotic protein BIM [134,135], while inhibiting the antiapoptotic protein BCL-2 [136]. During ER stress, the IRE1α-TRAF2 complex simultaneously activates both JNK and NF-κB pathways [132,137,138]. In *Ire1α* or *Traf2*-null MEFs the activation of both JNK and NF-κB is defective or delayed [52,139]. In contrast to ER stress-resistant *Ask1*-null neurons, *Traf2*-null or knockdown cells are more susceptible to apoptosis triggered by ER stress [139]. This susceptibility is at least partially caused by a higher accumulation of reactive oxygen species (ROS) in these deficient cells than wild-type cells when challenged with ER stress. Treatment with the antioxidant *N*-acetyl-L-cysteine (NAC), which abolishes ROS accumulation, protects *Traf2*-null stressed cells from apoptosis [139]. In addition, studies using *Nfκb* p65 subunit knock-out and *Jnk1/2* double knock-out MEFs suggest that TRAF2-mediated activation of NFκB protects from apoptosis by

decreasing ROS levels and regulating JNK activation [139]. However, Hu P. *et al.* showed that blocking of ER stress-induced NFκB activation by over-expression of mutant IκB made cells resistant to ER stress-induced apoptosis [140]. Thus, whether IRE1-TRAF2-dependent JNK and NF-κB pathways protect or sensitize cells to ER stress-induced apoptosis remains controversial.

In addition, three different proteins have been identified to interact with IRE1α including, c-Jun N-terminal inhibitory kinase (JIK), Jun activation domain-binding protein 1 (JAB1) and apoptosis signal-regulating kinase [ASK]1-interacting protein 1 (AIP1) [141-143]. The ability of JIK to bind both IRE1α and TRAF2 was shown by immunoprecipitation and indicates a potential role for JIK in regulating the recruitment of TRAF2 and thus activation of this ER stress-induced MAPK pathway. JAB1 was shown to bind to IRE1α during resting conditions. Mild ER stress enhanced this interaction, whereas strong ER stress diminished it. Thus, JAB1 might regulate the choice between the UPR and apoptosis by association with or dissociation from IRE1α. AIP1 associates with IRE1α to facilitate IRE1α dimerization and interaction with TRAF2 and ASK1 to activate the JNK pathway. Although mild ER stress induces formation of AIP1-IRE1α complex, interaction of IRE1α with AIP1 is independent of the kinase activity of IRE1α. In addition, the ER stress-induced IRE1α-JNK/XBP1 axis is blunted in AIP knockout cells [141].

In summary, IRE1α is involved in the regulation of several pathways when activated by the UPR including XBP1 splicing and the recruitment of TRAF2, and BAK/BAX (discussed below). Understanding how these molecules interact with IRE1α to affect cell survival or death remains unclear.

CHOP-mediated Cell Death

CHOP (GADD153) is a member of the C/EBP family of bZIP transcription factors, and its expression is induced to high levels by ER stress [144]. The *Chop* gene promoter contains both an ERSE and a C/EBP-ATF composite site causing it to be regulated by all of the major inducers of the UPR, including ATF4, ATF6, and XBP1 [83,100,106] Fig. (**2**). *Perk* and *Atf4* knockout cells as well as Ser51Ala *eIF2α* knock-in cells failed to induce *Chop* [78,128,145] whereas, *Ire1α-*, *Xbp1-*, and *Atf6α*-null cells displayed slightly reduced

Chop expression during ER stress [43,121,146], suggesting that the PERK-eIF2α-ATF4 pathway is the main contributor toward ER stress-dependent *Chop* expression.

Overexpression of CHOP represses transcription of the antiapoptotic protein BCL-2, which leads to enhanced oxidant injury and increased apoptosis [147-149] Fig. (**2**). Moreover, *Chop*-null mice are resistant to kidney damage induced by tunicamycin and brain injury resulting from cerebral artery occlusion, further demonstrating a role for CHOP in cell destruction when ER stress is involved [149,150]. Although the precise mechanism by which CHOP mediates apoptosis is unknown, CHOP does activate the transcription of several genes that potentiate apoptosis Fig. (**2**). These include *Gadd34*, endoplasmic reticulum oxidoreductase 1 (*Ero1α*), death receptor 5 (*Dr5*) [151], Tribbles homolog 3 (*Trb3*) [152], and carbonic anhydrase VI [153]. GADD34 is a subunit of protein phosphatase 1 (PP1) which dephosphorylates eIF2α and thus releases the translational block [94]. Expression of GADD34 correlates with apoptosis induced by various signals, and its overexpression can initiate or enhance apoptosis [154]. Therefore both *Chop*-null and *Gadd34*-null cells will have a prolonged reduction in client protein load during ER stress [92]. Furthermore, mice lacking GADD34-directed eIF2α dephosphorylation, like *Chop-null* mice, are resistant to renal toxicity induced by tunicamycin [92]. Moreover, inhibition of eIF2α phosphatases (with salubrinal) was reported to reduce ER stress-induced apoptosis [12], suggesting that reducing protein synthesis during sustained periods of ER stress prevents the initiation of cell death signaling when the UPR is chronically activated. In other words, persistent protein synthesis during periods of ER stress chronically activates the UPR and initiate cell death pathways. *Ero1* encodes an ER oxidoreductase required to maintain PDI in an active state that promotes proper disulfide bond formation during oxidative protein folding in the ER [155]. Increased ERO1 activity creates a hyper-oxidized ER environment that causes an accumulation of ROS in ER stressed cells [92]. In addition, the greater oxidizing environment of the ER is suggested to contribute to the preferred oxidation and inactivation of ER-resident proteins, such as protein disulfide isomerases, thereby contributing to unfolded protein accumulation. *Dr5* encodes a cell-surface death receptor that activates caspase cascades [151]. Thus, CHOP is capable of inducing apoptosis and contributing to cell death through several possible mechanisms in response

to ER stress. However, it is noteworthy that CHOP may not be essential for ER stress-induced cell death of *Perk-null* and Ser51Ala *eIF2α* knock-in cells that fail to significantly induce *Chop* gene expression [78,126].

Caspase-mediated Cell Death

The caspase family (caspases 2, 3, 4, 7, 9, and 12) of proapoptotic cysteine proteases also play a critical role in ER stress-induced apoptosis [156-159]. In rodents, procaspase-12 associates with the activated IRE1α-TRAF2 complex, resulting in proteolytic processing of procaspase-12 [143] Fig. (**2**). Mice lacking caspase-12 display partial resistance to pharmacological inducers of ER stress, such as tunicamycin (inhibitor of N-linked protein glycosylation) and thapsigargin (inhibitor of sarcoplasmic/ endoplasmic reticulum Ca2+ ATPases [SERCAs], which pump Ca2+ into the ER) [160]. However, the mechanisms responsible for proteolysis of procaspase-12 may be indirect, involving calpains activated by Ca2+ released in the vicinity of the ER [161], instead of an induced proximity mechanism where oligomers of IRE1 provide a scaffold for clustering procaspase-12 zymogens. Caspase-3/7 may also activate caspase-12 by translocating from the cytosol to the ER [162]. However, the relevance of caspase-12 to ER-induced apoptosis has been questioned because of the absence of a proteolytically active caspase-12 in most humans [163]. Although human caspase-4 is one of the closest paralogs of rodent caspase-12, the involvement of caspase-4 in ER stress-mediated apoptosis of human cells is still open to question [159]. In addition, data suggest that rodent caspase-12 and human caspase-4 are not required for caspase-dependent ER stress-induced apoptosis, although caspase-9 (a caspase-12 substrate) is clearly involved in the apoptotic pathway [164,165]. Therefore a systematic approach to address caspase involvement in ER stress-induced cell death is needed.

Bcl-2 Family-regulated Cell Death

Bcl-2 family proteins play a central role in regulating apoptosis. These proteins function at the mitochondria to prevent or promote the release of apoptogenic factors such as cytochrome c, AIF, Smac/Diablo, endonuclease G, and Omi [166]. In addition to their mitochondrial localization, some antiapoptotic members of the Bcl-2 family have also been found at the ER and perinuclear membrane regions, suggesting a role of the Bcl-2 family proteins at sites other than mitochondria

[167]. ER stress-induced apoptosis can be inhibited by overexpression of BCL-2 or its homologs [167,168]. Conversely, ER stress itself can upregulate and activate several 'BH3-only' proapoptotic members of the Bcl-2 family, including BIM [169,170], BIK [171,172], and PUMA [173,174]. Therefore, efferent signaling from the stressed ER can engage the Bcl-2 death machinery directly.

Cells with double deletions in the proapoptotic multidomain Bcl-2 family proteins Bax and Bak are remarkably resistant to many forms of apoptosis, including ER stress [175,176], implying that many apoptotic signaling pathways converge on BAX and BAK. In recent reports, ER stress induces cleavage of BID, a member of the BH3 domain only subgroup of BCL-2, at position D59 by caspase-2. The truncated p15 BID (tBID) translocates to mitochondria where it inserts into the mitochondrial outer membrane [177] and induces mitochondrial membrane translocation of BAX permitting reorganization/oligomerization of BAX and BAK to cause the release of cytochrome c from mitochondria to the cytosol [178] Fig. (**2**). Cytosolic cytochrome c binds to Apaf-1 and procaspase 9, resulting in the activation of procaspase 9 which subsequently activates procaspases 3 and 7 ultimately leading to cell death [178]. However, how ER stress activates caspase-2 and whether BAX and BAK activation in the mitochondrial membrane is absolutely dependent on the caspase-2 and BID pathway remains to be clarified.

Several studies have also demonstrated that BAX and BAK regulate ER stress-induced apoptosis [179,180] and it has been shown endogenous BAX and BAK regulate ER stress-induced apoptosis from both the mitochondrial and ER membranes Fig. (**2**). ER stress induces BAX oligomerization on the ER membrane [180]. BAX and BAK are crucial for maintaining the resting level of ER lumenal calcium [179,181], probably through an interaction with the type 1 inositol trisphosphate receptor (InsP$_3$R) [182]. As a result, BAX and BAK deficient cells have a dramatically reduced ER calcium level and decreased calcium uptake by mitochondria making them highly resistant to calcium-dependent death stimuli. Genetic correction of the ER calcium defect in double-knockout (DKO) cells by overexpressing sarcoplasmic–ER calcium adenosine triphosphatase (SERCA) restored apoptosis in response to calcium-mobilizing stimuli, including brefeldin A [179]. In addition, several studies

suggest that both BCL-2 and BCL-X$_L$ physically interact with the InsP$_3$R which sensitizes single InsP$_3$R channels in ER membranes, possibly through phosphorylation, resulting in a reduction of ER calcium content [182-184]. In contrast, the pro-apoptotic proteins BAX and tBID antagonize this effect by blocking the biochemical interaction of BCL-X$_L$ with the InsP$_3$R [184]. Therefore, decreased calcium release by reduced ER calcium content in ER-stressed cells may explain how overexpression of BCL-2 or BCL-X$_L$ protects cells from ER stress-induced apoptosis and why BAX and BAK double null MEFs are resistant to ER stress.

Recent studies provide evidence for a possible function of the BCL-2 protein family in the UPR. BAX and BAK modulate the amplitude of IRE1α signaling by controlling its autophosphorylation and oligomerization [185]. BAX and BAK double-knockout (DKO) mice showed a decreased expression of IRE1α-downstream signals, including JNK phosphorylation and spliced XBP-1 expression under experimental ER-stress conditions [185]. At the biochemical level, BAX and BAK form a protein complex with the cytosolic domain of IRE1α, in a manner that requires their conserved BH1 and BH3 domains [185]. These findings suggest a new role for proapoptotic family members as accessory factors to instigate certain UPR signaling events.

BAX inhibitor-1 (BI-1) is an antiapoptotic protein that contains several transmembrane domains, localizes to ER membranes [186], and is conserved in both animal and plant species [187]. BI-1 has no obvious homology with BCL-2-related proteins, yet it interacts with different members of the family such as BCL-XL and BCL-2 [186,187]. Recent reports show BI-1 protects from apoptosis induced by ER stress [188], possibly by modulating calcium signaling [188] and oxidative-stress response gene expression [189]. Cells isolated from *Bi-1* null mice exhibit selective hypersensitivity *in vitro* to apoptosis induced by ER stress [188]. Moreover, *Bi-1* null mice are more sensitive to renal tubule cell death induced by tunicamycin, and to stroke injury analyzed in a model of transient cerebral artery occlusion [190]. In addition BI-1 deficiency results in an ER stress phenotype, as manifested by induction of CHOP, XBP1-s, ATF6 cleavage, and phospho-JNK activation by IRE1α [190]. These data suggest that BI-1 has an inhibitory activity on the UPR, in contrast to the stimulatory effect that BAX and BAK have on the IRE1α pathway.

BIM (BCL-2-interacting mediator of cell death) translocates from the dynein-rich compartment to the ER membrane [134] and activates procaspase-12 in response to ER stress [169]. The antiapoptotic factor BCL-X$_L$ (BCL-2-like 1) binds to BIM and inhibits BIM translocation to the ER [169]. Consistent with this notion, BIM knockout cells and mice exhibit resistance to ER stress-induced death. ER stress activates BIM through two novel pathways, involving protein phosphatase 2A mediated dephosphorylation, which prevents its ubiquitination and proteasomal degradation, and through CHOP-C/EBPα-mediated direct transcriptional induction [170].

5. CONSEQUENCE OF UPR PATHWAY DEFICIENCY

In mammalian cells, the ER serves many specialized functions including calcium storage and gated release, biosynthesis of membrane and secretory proteins, and production of lipids and sterols. The UPR attempts to maintain ER homeostasis of these functions during ER stress. Therefore perturbation or deficiency of the UPR paralyzes ER functions and eventually induces death of affected cells. However, evidence from genetic manipulation of UPR genes supports the notion that components of the UPR are more essential to sustain the function of specialized secretory cells (such as insulin secreting-pancreatic beta cells, immunoglobulin producing-plasma cells, digestive enzyme secreting-acinar cells, and antimicrobial molecule secreting-intestinal epithelial cells) more than normal cells. In addition, studies suggest that some specialized secretory cells have adapted to chronic ER stress. In the past decade a significant amount of information regarding the UPR has been generated from genetic manipulation of the proximal UPR sensors and downstream genes in mouse models. Furthermore, studies using conditional knockout mouse models are now shedding light on the tissue-specific roles of individual UPR pathways in cell function. In the following section we will discuss the current understanding of how the proximal UPR sensors and downstream genes contribute to the UPR in several tissues.

BiP-null Mouse Model

A study using a transgenic mouse model bearing a *lacZ* reporter gene driven by 3 kb of the rat *Grp78* promoter, discovered that the *Grp78* promoter is activated in both the trophectoderm and inner cell mass (ICM) of embryos at embryonic day 3.5 via a mechanism requiring the ER stress elements (ERSE) [191,192]. The β-galactosidase activity of the reporter gene from the model is below the detection limit at the one-cell stage and is weakly detectable from the two-cell stage to the morula stage but is abundant at the blastocyst stage in the developing mouse embryo [193]. These results suggest a physiological need for the induction of GRP78 during the blastocyst stage. Furthermore, high levels of GRP78 were detected in the heart, somites, and neural tube of developing mouse embryos at day 9.5 and day 10.5 [194,195].

To understand GRP78 function *in vivo*, heterozygous and knockout mouse models were generated [191]. The targeted disruption of one allele of the *Grp78* gene caused a 50% reduction in the GRP78 protein level and specific upregulation of the ER proteins GRP94 and protein disulfide isomerase (PDI) at both the transcript and protein levels, while other UPR targets such as CHOP and XBP1 were not affected. However, *Grp78* knockout embryos displayed peri-implantation lethality [191]. These embryos did not hatch from the *zona pellucida in vitro,* failed to grow in culture, and exhibited proliferation defects with a massive apoptotic increase within the inner cell mass (ICM), which is the precursor of embryonic stem cells. These findings provide the first evidence that GRP78 is essential for embryonic cell growth and pluripotent cell survival. It was recently reported that genetic disruption of SIL1/BAP, which encodes an adenosine nucleotide exchange factor of GRP78, leads to protein accumulation, ER stress, and subsequent neurodegeneration [196]. While this result strongly implicates GRP78 in neuroprotection, SIL/BAP is not an obligatory cochaperone for GRP78 during early development.

Ire1α-null Mouse Model

Two different groups including our laboratory generated *Ire1α* knockout mouse models [41,132,197]. Both experiments revealed that IRE1α is required for embryonic development. In our study, most homozygous *Ire1α*-null embryos died between 12.5 and 13 days of gestation [197]. By embryonic 13 days, the *Ire1α*-null embryos could be recognized by their small size, growth retardation, and pale coloration. Histological inspection of the *Ire1α*-null mice identified fetal liver hypoplasia with prevalent apoptotic cell death and reduced expression of several acute-phase response genes [197]. Therefore, the failure of fetal liver development is likely to be one major cause of early embryonic death in *Ire1α*-null mice. However, why IRE1α is required for fetal liver development is unknown. MEF studies revealed that there is a complete lack of *Xbp1* mRNA splicing and JNK pathway activation in response to ER stress in *Ire1α*-null cells [41,132,198]. Another defective phenotype in *Ire1α*-null cells was shown by reconstitution of recombinase-activating gene2– deficient (*Rag2*-null) mice with *Ire1α*-null hematopoietic cells [197]. It was revealed that the IRE1α kinase and RNase catalytic activities are required for terminal differentiation of mature B cells into antibody-secreting plasma cells which came as no surprise because it had already been shown that *Xbp1*-null mice display the same defects in B cell differentiation [199,200]. Although, IRE1α-deficient hematopoietic stem cells can proliferate and give rise to pro-B cells that reside in bone marrow [197]. However, IRE1α, but not its kinase or RNase catalytic activities, is required for immunoglobulin (Ig) gene rearrangement (VDJ recombination) and production of B cell receptors (BCRs). The reduced expression of *Rag1*, *Rag2*, and *TdT* transcripts could account, at least partially, for the defective rearrangement of Ig genes in the IRE1α- deficient lymphocytes [197]. These results suggest that the IRE1α cytoplasmic domain provides an additional function different from *Xbp1* mRNA splicing in regulating B cell development. This study raised two fundamental questions. First, how is the UPR connected to early B cell differentiation? Second, how does IRE1α regulate induction of *Rag1*, *Rag2*, and *TdT* genes during VDJ recombination of Ig genes? These questions should be answered by further studies.

Ire1β-null Mouse Model

As described earlier, the expression of IRE1β is restricted to the epithelium of the gastrointestinal tract [201]. Expression of IRE1β was significantly weaker in the small intestine than in the stomach or colon. *Ire1β*-null mice develop normally, can reproduce and are indistinguishable from wild-type littermates [201]. However, BiP protein, a marker of ER stress, was elevated in the colonic mucosa of *Ire1β*-null mice. In addition, dextran sodium sulfate (DSS)-induced inflammatory bowel disease developed 3-5 days earlier in *Ire1β*-null mice compared to wild-type mice [201]. Despite these findings several questions remain. For instance, what does IRE1β do in the epithelium of the gastrointestinal tract that have all UPR pathways

intact, including IRE1α? and what are the direct downstream targets of IRE1β?

Recently Iqbal J. *et al.* [55] demonstrated that high-cholesterol or high-fat diets fed to *Ire1β*-null mice induced pronounced hyperlipidemia compared to wild-type mice due to an increased intestinal secretion of chylomicrons that transport large quantities of dietary fat and fat-soluble vitamins. *Ire1β*-null mice expressed more intestinal microsomal triglyceride transfer protein (MTP, an essential chaperone and a rate-limiting factor for chylomicron assembly) [55]. As a result, intestines from *Ire1β*-null mice secrete more lipids into the circulatory system. The study showed that MTP mRNA, protein, and activity are increased in the intestines of *Ire1β* null mice due to decreased *Mtp* and *28S rRNA* mRNA posttranscriptional degradation. In addition, high-fat diet treatment induced the UPR but reduced *Ire1β* mRNA levels, suggesting that enterocytes optimize fat absorption by activating the ER stress response but downregulating IRE1β. By upregulating the ER stress response, the ER is protected from the increased load of synthesizing and packaging of chylomicrons and by downregulating IRE1β, chylomicron assembly is maximized by enhancing MTP. These findings raise the possibility that upregulation of IRE1β may be beneficial to avoid diet-induced hyperlipidemia.

Xbp1-null Mouse Model

XBP1 is the most highly chaaracterized factor among the components of UPR pathway. As a direct substrate of activated IRE1α, *Xbp1*-null mice show very similar embryonic phenotypes to those of *Ire1α* knockout mice. *Xbp1* mRNA is highly expressed in the liver bud at E10.5 which is a time point before significant population of the liver by hematopoietic cells [202]. This supports a role for XBP1 in liver growth rather than in hematopoietic cell division and differentiation. Most *Xbp1*-null embryos die between 12.5 and 14.5 days of gestation [202] and it was reported that mice lacking XBP-1 displayed hypoplastic fetal livers with reduced hematopoiesis resulting in death from anemia. Specific target genes of XBP1 in the liver were identified as α-fetoprotein (αFP), which may be a regulator of hepatocyte growth, and three acute phase protein family members (α1- antitrypsin (α1*AT*), transthyretin, apolipoprotein A1 (*apoA-1*) [202]. Taken together these findings demonstrate XBP1 is a transcription factor essential for fetal hepatocyte growth. However, why the IRE1α-XBP1 pathway is required for fetal liver development is unknown and UPR activation in embryonic liver development has not been reported.

In order to assess the effects of XBP1 deficiency on the immune system, Reimold A. M. *et al.* used the recombination activating gene-2 (*Rag2*) blastocyst complementation system to bypass the embryonic lethality of *Xbp1*-null mice [200]. *Xbp1*-null ES cells were generated and injected into Rag2-null blastocysts, and then Xbp1/Rag22 null chimeric mice were generated upon implantation into pseudopregnant females. These chimeric animals developed B cells normally, expressed Ig genes and performed isotype switching, but exhibited defective Ig secretion and plasma cell differentiation [200]. Expression of spliced XBP1 was sufficient to restore the phenotypes, demonstrating an essential role for this factor in plasma cell biogenesis [199]. Signals involved in plasma cell differentiation, specifically interleukin-4, control the transcription of *Xbp1*, whereas IRE1α-mediated *Xbp1* splicing is dependent on synthesis of immunoglobulins during B cell differentiation [199]. XBP1 is also involved in controlling the production of interleukin-6, a cytokine that is essential for plasma cell survival. These studies provided the first link between the UPR and secretory cell function [199].

Another function of XBP1 in the immune system was described in dendritic cells (DC) [203]. Dendritic cells play a critical role in the initiation, maintenance, and resolution of an immune response. DC survival is tightly controlled by extracellular stimuli such as cytokines and Toll-like receptor (TLR) signaling [204]. Lymphoid chimeras lacking XBP1 possess decreased numbers of both conventional and plasmacytoid DCs with reduced baseline survival in response to TLR signaling [203]. Overexpression of XBP1 in hematopoietic progenitors rescued and enhanced DC development. Remarkably, the XBP1 pathway was constitutively activated in immature DCs providing an indirect clue as to why *Xbp1*-null DCs die and suggesting that some specialized secretory cells are adapted to ER stress. Therefore, identifying the factors that evoke constitutive UPR activation before maturing into DC that have a multi-layered ER and secrete large amounts of protein will be of great interest.

The embryonic lethality of *Xbp1*-null mice precluded analysis of its role in adult mice. To circumvent the lethal liver phenotype, Lee A-H *et* *al.* targeted an *Xbp1* transgene back into the liver using a hepatocyte-specific promoter [205]. Liver specific expression of the *Xbp1* transgene rescued embryonic lethality of *Xbp1*-null mice but these transgenic mice still displayed abnormalities exclusively in secretory organs such as the exocrine pancreas and salivary glands that led to early postnatal lethality due to impaired production of pancreatic digestive enzymes [205]. However, XBP1 deficiency didn't affect the development or secretory function of the endocrine pancreas during the early postnatal stage. Ultrastructural analysis of *Xbp1*-null acinar cells showed ER expansion was severely impaired resulting in a complete disorganization of the ER network [205]. This *in vivo* observation is consistent with evidence that spliced XBP1 is required for ER membrane expansion by increasing phosphatidylcholine biosynthesis due to enhanced activities of the choline cytidylyltransferase (CCT) and cholinephosphotransferase enzymes [45]. In addition, the number and size of mature zymogen granules in *Xbp1*-null acinar cells was drastically decreased concomitant with decreased amylase and trypsin production [45,205]. These events correlate with decreased expression of certain ER chaperones (*Sec61a, Edem, Pdi-p,* and *Pdi*) in the affected pancreas. However, *Erdj4* and *Pdi-p5* mRNA levels that are highly dependent on XBP1 in both MEFs and B lymphocytes were not compromised in the *Xbp1*-null pancreas. In addition, the expression of *Grp78, Grp94, Herp, Grp58,* and *Ero1α*, which are upregulated by enforced expression of spliced XBP1 in B lymphocytes, was either increased or unaltered in the *Xbp1*-null pancreas. These results indicate that IRE1α/XBP1 UPR signaling pathway may control different programs of gene expression in different cell types or ER stress induced by *Xbp1* deletion may lead to activation of the PERK and ATF6 UPR pathways.

The conditional knockout mouse model to investigate the role of XBP1 in postnatal hepatic function established a new link between XBP1 and lipid metabolism, showing XBP1 as a novel transcription factor governing hepatic lipogenesis [206]. Surprisingly, mice that lacked XBP1 in the liver postnatally did not show any noticeable gross abnormalities or liver damage although they demonstrated mild defects such as slightly decreased serum albumin and total protein levels, modestly down-regulated XBP1-dependent UPR target genes (*Edem, Erdj4,* and *Sec61a*) and increased IRE1α activation. In contrast, inducible, hepatocyte specific XBP1 deletion resulted in reduced hepatic fatty acid and cholesterol synthesis by ~85 to 90%, thus lowering concentrations of plasma cholesterol and triglycerides [206]. Surprisingly, ApoB (a major protein component of VLDL) secretion from the liver was unaffected by the loss of XBP1. Instead, the hypolipidemia was associated with decreased expression of select XBP1-dependent genes involved in lipogenesis namely, three genes involved in fatty acid and triglyceride synthesis; diacylglycerol O-acyltransferase 2 (*Dgat2*), stearoyl-Coenzyme A desaturase 1 (*Scd1*), and acetyl–coenzyme A carboxylase 2 (*Acc2*) [206]. In contrast, the expression of genes encoding the fatty acid and cholesterol biosynthetic enzymes ACC1, fatty acid synthase, HMG-CoA reductase and HMG-CoA synthase were not reduced. Nevertheless, the overall rates of hepatic fatty acid and sterol synthesis were markedly reduced. These observations raise the possibility that in addition to the transcriptional changes observed in the *Xbp1*-null livers, posttranscriptional regulatory mechanisms may contribute to the phenotype. These results have raised several questions for the future study. Why is XBP1 required for survival of embryonic liver but not adult liver? Is the embryonic requirement related to UPR signaling? In addition, why is there no obvious UPR-related defect conferred by XBP1 deficiency in postnatal hepatocytes?

Finally, a new function of XBP1 in secretory cells was recently described in intestinal epithelial cells [207]. To examine the role played by the transcription factor XBP1 in the survival of intestinal epithelial cells (IEC), Kaser A *et al.* generated conditional-null mice in which *Xbp1* was specifically deleted in IEC. In these mice, *Xbp1* deletion in IEC leads to ER stress (elevated basal *GrP78* and *Chop* levels) and spontaneous enteritis [207]. Similarly it had been previously shown that *Ire1β* knockout mice were susceptible to experimental colitis induced by DSS [201]. The *Xbp1*-null epithelium showed absent paneth cells (specialized epithelial cells that have the capacity to secrete antimicrobial peptides and the cytokine interleukin-1 (IL-1) in response to bacteria) and reduced goblet cells (the glandular epithelial cells that are responsible for mucus secretion) [201]. *Xbp1* deletion impairs mucosal defense to oral *Listeria monocytogenes* infection and leads to increased susceptibility to experimental colitis induced by DSS. This report showed human colon mucosa from both inflammatory bowel diseases (IBD) (Crohn's disease (CD) and ulcerative colitis (UC) exhibit increased *BiP* and spliced *Xbp1*

expression level as indications of ER stress. In addition, these observations led the authors to uncover human variants of the *Xbp1* gene that maybe associated with inflammatory bowel disease. These findings suggest that in the highly secretory IECs, the ER stress response may be constitutively triggered by microbes in the gut lumen. The activation of ER stress markers in conjunction with intestinal inflammation in the mice with *Xbp1*-null IECs suggests that inflammatory bowel disease should also be added to the list of disorders associated with the UPR.

Although heterozygous *Xbp1*-null mice have no metabolic defects, high fat diet challenge leads to increased ER stress and impaired insulin signaling in liver, resulting in impaired glucose homeostasis [208]. This study suggests the ER attempts to cope with stress by activating the XBP1 pathway but when this response fails to restore homeostasis, IRE1α activates JNK1 leading to serine phosphorylation of IRS1, and impaired insulin signaling. This suggests that ER stress may be a central feature of peripheral insulin resistance and type 2 diabetes at the molecular, cellular, and organismal levels.

Perk-null Mouse Model

Two independent *Perk* knockout mice have been produced and show a phenotype remarkably similar to human Wolcott-Rallison syndrome (WRS) caused by mutations in *EIF2AK3* which encodes the human eIF2α kinase equivalent to rodent PERK [209,210]. WRS is a rare autosomal recessive disorder characterized by neonatal or early-infancy insulin-dependent diabetes, epiphyseal dysplasia and developmental delay that becomes apparent at later ages [211-213]. In contrast to the *Ire1α*- and *Xbp1*-null animals, *Perk*-null mice have no obvious development problems yet approximately half of the *Perk*-null mice die prenatally regardless of genetic background difference [209,210]. The cause of death is not fully understood but may be caused by hypoglycemia associated with defective gluconeogenesis and glycogen storage as shown in mice with homozygous Ser51Ala *eIF2α* mutation at the PERK phosphorylation site [78]. The surviving newborn *Perk*-null mice suffer from a multitude of metabolic and growth abnormalities including hyperglycemia, growth retardation, skeletal defects, and atrophy of the exocrine pancreas. The importance of PERK-mediated translational control was further demonstrated by studies of knock-in mice with a homozygous

Ser51Ala mutation in *eIF2α* [78]. The homozygous Ser51Ala *eIF2α* mutant mice showed more severe phenotypes than that of *Perk*-null mice. Newborn pups of homozygous Ser51Ala *eIF2α*mutant mice were observed at the expected Mendelian ratio and phenotypically indistinguishable from their wild-type and heterozygous littermates at birth. However, the homozygous Ser51Ala *eIF2α* mutant neonates died within 24 hr after birth due to hypoglycemia associated with defective gluconeogenesis (low PEPCK activity) and reduced glycogen storage. In addition, homozygous mutant embryos and neonates displayed a deficiency in pancreatic beta cells [78].

As of now, there hasn't been a detailed analysis regarding how deficiency of eIF2α phosphorylation in *Perk*-null and Ser51Ala *eIF2α* homozygous mice causes liver dysfunction or whether the UPR is related with the defect. With regard to the loss of pancreatic beta cells, two different explanations have been suggested. The first explanation is that the reduction of beta cell mass is due to ER stress-mediated cell death [78,209]. The support for this hypothesis is based on the notion that ER stress is associated with increased insulin production in pancreatic beta cells in response to elevated blood glucose concentration. Proinsulin synthesis imposes a heavy biosynthetic burden upon the beta cell as approximately 1×10^6 proinsulin molecules are synthesized per minute upon glucose stimulation [214]. Accumulation of misfolded proteins within the lumen of the ER in beta cells may occur as a consequence of increased proinsulin translation [39]. Whereas wild-type pancreatic beta cells can effectively remove misfolded protein by activating the UPR, beta cells with defective eIF2α-mediated translational control are susceptible to accumulation of misfolded proteins in the ER due uncontrollable translation and insufficient expression of UPR genes [78,209]. It is postulated that the eIF2α phosphorylation deficiency results in heightened ER stress that then mediates beta cell death [78,209]. In support of this hypothesis, *Perk*-null and Ser51Ala *eIF2α*homozygous cells are sensitive to treatment with ER stress inducers. The importance of the PERK-eIF2α pathway is also exhibited by the fact that heterozygous *eIF2α Ser51Ala* mutant mice become obese and diabetic on a high-fat diet. Profound glucose intolerance due to reduced insulin secretion was accompanied by abnormal distension of the ER lumen, accumulation of misfolded proinsulin, defective

trafficking of proinsulin, and a reduced number of insulin granules in beta cells [215]. However, no clear evidence of UPR activation in pancreatic beta cells of *Perk*-null mice, homozygous Ser51Ala *eIF2α*, and diabetic heterozygous Ser51Ala *eIF2α* mice exists to date. It may be that eIF2α phosphorylation deficient cells are unable to induce a majority of ER stress response genes [78,81,145]. Interestingly, mice lacking ATF4, which is responsible for induction of 36% of the PERK target genes in MEFs [81,145], have no reported defects in glycemic control and have normal endocrine pancreata [216-218]. Therefore, decreased *Atf4* mRNA translation due to defective eIF2α phosphorylation in *Perk*-null and Ser51Ala *eIF2α* homozygous mutant mice doesn't seem to be the primary cause for the beta cell failure. In contrast, it was reported that *Atf4*-null mice exhibit postnatal exocrine pancreatic deficiency [219]. Taken together, these findings suggest that additional PERK-eIF2α dependent pathways/ mechanisms, other than ATF4, are responsible for the defects in beta cell function in *Perk*-null and Ser51Ala *eIF2α* homozygous mutant mice.

A second explanation for the pancreatic beta cell deficiency observed in *Perk*-null mice was suggested to result from impaired beta cell differentiation and proliferation, as opposed to ER stress-mediated cell death [210]. This reasoning is supported because beta cell mass increased only 2-fold in *Perk* null mice, compared to a 20.3-fold increase in wild-type mice during late fetal and neonatal development [220]. Microarray analysis of postnatal day 2 neonatal islets revealed that of the 42 genes that exhibit a 2-fold or greater decrease in expression in *Perk*-null mice, 22 genes encoded cell-cycle or proliferation factors, including genes with critical functions in G2 and M stages (including of cyclin A, CDK1, and TOP2A), whereas expression of the G1 cyclins D1, D2, and D3 as well as CDK4 was not significantly different. In addition, expression of the insulin genes and *Pdx1* and *MafA*, the key markers of beta cell differentiation and regulators of *Ins1* and *Ins2* transcription were significantly decreased in the fetal and postnatal stages, suggesting that differentiation of beta cells is impaired in *Perk*-null mice. Furthermore, PERK expression was not required in adult mice to maintain beta cell function and glucose homeostasis, as the beta cell-specific *Perk*-null mice (βPKO) did not become diabetic. However, the phenotypes of beta cell-specific *Perk*-null mice (βPKO) could be due to compensatory pathways that promote adaptation in response to PERK deficiency. The ability to adapt was suggested by the observation that abnormal proinsulin accumulated in neonatal mice with *Perk* deletion, but this was not observed in *Perk*-null mice at 30 days after birth [220]. This suggests that a compensatory pathway, possibly mediated by increased signaling through alternative eIF2α kinases, may restore function to *Perk*-deleted beta cells. Indeed, Western blot analysis revealed that phosphorylated eIF2α exists in the Perk-null pancreatic lysates and other studies suggest that GCN2 and PKR may phosphorylate eIF2α in response to ER stress [71,72,221]. However, these compensatory eIF2α kinase signaling pathways would not be functional in homozygous *Ser51Ala eIF2α* mutant cells. To address whether compensatory pathways utilizing alternative eIF2α kinases will require analysis of eIF2α phosphorylation-deficient beta cells.

The beta cells in *Perk*-null mice exhibit highly distended, electron-dense ER lumina caused by abnormal retention of misfolded secretory proteins such as proinsulin and glucose transporter 2 (Glut2). Surprisingly, increased ER stress-response gene expression was not detected [220]. The lack of UPR induction in islets lacking PERK can be partially reconciled by the fact that there is a fundamental defect in UPR gene expression in *Perk*-null MEFs as well [81,145]. Therefore, it is possible that *Perk*-null beta cells experience ER stress even though increased UPR gene expression is not detected. All together, these findings suggest that insulin secreting beta cells require PERK during the fetal and early neonatal period as a prerequisite for postnatal glucose homeostasis. This conclusion can be applied to the deficiency of embryonic beta cells in Ser51Ala *eIF2α* homozygous mice as well, albeit the phenotype is more severe. Important questions that arise as a result of these findings include why do *Perk*-null beta cells have reduced expression of cell-cycle and proliferation factors, key markers of beta cell differentiation, and regulators of *Ins1* and *Ins2* transcription? These genes have not been described as ER stress-inducible. The differences between *Perk*-null and Ser51Ala *eIF2α* homozygous phenotypes indicate that PERK has additional substrates, in addition to eIF2α, that may play important roles.

Deletion of PERK in humans and mice also causes postnatal exocrine pancreatic atrophy exhibited by a reduction in the synthesis of several major digestive enzymes and massive apoptosis [209,210]. Just as the beta cells in the endocrine

pancreas, acinar cells of the exocrine pancreas synthesize, store and secrete copious quantities of the major digestive enzymes, and are poised to respond to episodic feeding events. Pro-enzymes (zymogens) are folded and processed in the rough ER and Golgi complex and then packaged into zymogen granules. Therefore, acinar cells may be highly prone to ER stress just as pancreatic beta cells, and thereby *Perk*-null acinar cells might have heightened ER stress. The hypothesis is supported by postnatal exocrine pancreatic atrophy in *Atf4*-null [219] and *Xbp1*-null mice [205]. However, it is unknown whether translational control mediated by eIF2α phosphorylation is important to maintain function and/or viability of acinar cells. Iida K. *et al.* suggested there was no evidence for ER perturbation in *Perk*-null acinar cells that succumb to a non-apoptotic form of cell death, oncosis, that is associated with a pronounced inflammatory response and induction of the pancreatitis associated stress-response genes [219]. Therefore, further work is required to elucidate whether ER stress and UPR signaling provide important functions in pancreatic acinar cells.

Perk-null mice display severe osteopenia as neonates, that is caused by a defect in osteoblast differentiation leading to a reduced number of mature osteoblasts and reduced type I collagen secretion [210]. Impaired differentiation of osteoblasts in *Perk*-null mice was associated with decreased expression of *Runx2* and *Osterix*, key regulators of osteoblast development [222]. Gene expression analysis revealed that reduced cell proliferation and reduced expression of key cell cycle factors including cyclin D, cyclin E, cyclin A, Cdc2, and CDK2 occur in parallel with the differentiation defect in mutant osteoblasts. In addition, the trafficking and secretion of type I collagen was compromised by abnormal retention of procollagen I in the ER leading to reduced mature collagen production and mineralization. Taken together, these studies identify PERK as a novel regulator of skeletal development and osteoblast biology. *Atf4*, a PERK-eIF2α downstream gene, is also known as a critical regulator of osteoblast differentiation and function [223,224]. Similarly, *Atf4* null mice exhibit skeletal dysplasia like that of *Perk*-null mice. Although both *Atf4*- and *Perk*-null mice experience osteopenia, the decrease in bone mass may result from different mechanisms. In *Perk*-null mice, both *Runx2* and *Osterix* (key regulators of osteoblast development) are reduced. In addition a secretion defect of type I collagen may be responsible for the phenotype [210]. In contrast, *Atf4*-null mice have no change of *Runx2* and *Osterix* levels but experience reduced synthesis of Type I collagen due to a decrease in amino acid import, a function regulated by ATF4 in other cell types [223,224]. Thus, the osteoblast defects seen in *Perk*-null mice cannot be described as identical to the defects the *Atf4*-null mice.

ATF6 Deficient Mouse Model

Recently two groups, Wu J. *et al.* [146] and Yamamoto K. et al [121] described the generation of mice with the targeted deletion of the *Atf6α* gene. Surprisingly, ATF6α is neither essential for basal expression of ER protein chaperone genes nor for embryonic or postnatal development. Both groups unraveled the protective role of ATF6-mediated signaling during ER stress *in vitro* as ATF6α-deficient cells demonstrated reduced survival in response to ER stress. Furthermore, Wu *et al.* showed that ATF6α deficiency resulted in increased sensitivity to chronic stress in mice challenged with an inhibitor of N-linked glycosylation, tunicamycin. Because ATF6α is responsible for transcriptional induction of many ER chaperones and heterodimerizes with XBP1 for the induction of ER-associated degradation components, it was suggested that ATF6α is required to optimize protein folding, secretion, and degradation during ER stress and thus facilitate recovery from acute stress and confer tolerance to chronic stress. Like ATF6α, ATF6β is neither essential for expression of ER stress inducible genes nor for embryonic or postnatal development. However, *Atf6β*-null MEFs were slightly more sensitive to tunicamycin treatment than wild-type MEFs. Interestingly, the double knockout of *Atf6α* and *Atf6β* causes early embryonic lethality. The embryonic lethality of the double knockout suggests these isoforms play redundant roles in early embryogenesis. Further studies are required to identify the function(s) of these factors in embryogeneis and the role of the N-terminal fragment of ATF6β during ER stress.

6. FUTURE DIRECTIONS

Over the past few decades, considerable progress has been made towards understanding the signaling pathways and the physiological significance of the UPR. Collectively these studies revealed that the mammalian cell has evolved a complex and intertwined set of signaling pathways to respond to both physiological and pathological ER stresses. Nonetheless, much remains unknown about the UPR. It is not still clear how the proximal UPR sensors discriminate various ER stresses, both physiological and pathological. Similarly, understanding how the adaptive response and apoptotic pathways of the UPR integrate during and after ER stresses of different types, severity and duration will help to determine the expressional context that ultimately "decides" whether the cell lives or dies. In addition, there is increasing evidence that some specific cell types or tissues are under ER stress naturally but don't develop pathological conditions. This context raises the question of how these professional secretory cells activate the UPR productively throughout their cellular lifetime without mediating ER stress-induced cell death. In future studies, tissue-specific deletion of stress sensing molecules and their downstream effectors in the mouse, in combination with genetic or environmental challenge, will reveal the cell-type- and tissue-specific functions of each molecule in the UPR. The answers to these questions will give us clues as to how ER stress-related diseases can be manipulated in order to prevent the death of specific cell types thereby preserving and possibly improving organismal function.

7. ACKNOWLEDGEMENTS

This work was supported in part by the National Institutes of Health grants DK042394, HL052173, and HL057346 to principle investigator R.J. Kaufman. R.J. Kaufman is an investigator at the Howard Hughes Medical Institute. We thank J. L. Mitchell for her efforts in preparing the document and materials for submission.

8. ABBREVIATIONS

ACC2	=	Acetyl–coenzyme A (CoA) carboxylase 2
ADP	=	Adenosine diphosphate
ASK1	=	Apoptosis signal-regulating kinase 1
ATF	=	Activating transcription factor
ATP	=	Adenosine triphosphate
Bad	=	Bcl-xL/Bcl-2 associated death promoter
BAG-1	=	Bcl-2 associated athanogene protein 1
Bak	=	Bcl-2 homologous antagonist/killer
BAP	=	BiP-associated protein
Bax	=	Bcl-2 associated X protein

Bcl-2	=	B cell leukemia/lymphoma 2
Bcl-Xl	=	Bcl-x long
Bcl-xS	=	splice variant of Bcl-xL
BCR	=	B cell receptor
BI1	=	Bax inhibitor 1
Bim	=	Bcl-2 interacting mediator of cell death
BiP	=	Heavy chain binding protein
bZIP	=	Basic leucine zipper
C/EBP	=	CCAAT-enhancer binding protein
c-Abl	=	Cellular Abelson murine leukemia virus transforming protein
cAMP	=	Cyclic adenosine monophosphate
cat-1	=	Cationic amino acid transporter
CD	=	Crohn's disease
CHOP	=	C/EBP homologous protein
CRE	=	cAMP response element
CREB	=	CRE binding protein
CREB-RP	=	CREB related protein
CreP	=	Constitutive repressor of eIF2α phosphorylation
Dgat2	=	Diacylglycerol O-acyltransferase 2
DSS	=	Dextran sodium sulfate
ER	=	Endoplasmic reticulum
eIF2α	=	Eukaryotic initiation factor 2α
ERAD	=	ER associated degradation
ERSE	=	ER stress response element
ES	=	Embryonic stem
GADD153	=	Growth arrest and DNA damage-inducible gene 153
GCN2	=	General control of nitrogen metabolism kinase 2
HAC1	=	Homologous to ATF/CREB1
HRI	=	Heme-regulated inhibitor kinase
IBD	=	Inflammatory bowel diseases
IEC	=	Intestinal epithelial cells
IκB	=	Inhibitor of NF-κB
IKK	=	IκB kinase
IL-4	=	Interleukin 4
IRE1	=	Inositol requiring 1
IRES	=	Internal ribosomal entry site

JAB1	=	Jun activation domain binding protein-1
JNK	=	Jun N-terminal kinase
LZIP	=	Long bZIP
NF-κB	=	Nuclear factor κB
NF-Y	=	Nuclear factor Y
OASIS	=	Old astrocyte specifically induced substance
ORF	=	Open reading frame
P58^{IPK}	=	58 kDa inhibitor of PKR
PDI	=	Protein disulfide isomerase
PEPCK	=	Phosphoenolpyruvate carboxykinase
PERK	=	PKR like endoplasmic reticulum kinase
PKR	=	doUble stranded RNA activated Protein kinase
PP1	=	Protein phosphatase 1, PP1c
Puma	=	p53 Upregulated modulator of apoptosis
RAG-2	=	Recombination-activating gene 2
RNase	=	Ribonuclease
S1P	=	Site-1 protease
S2P	=	Site-2 protease
Scd1	=	Stearoyl-Coenzyme A desaturase 1
TRAF2	=	Tumor necrosis factor receptor associated factor 2
TRB3	=	Tribbles-related protein 3
tRNA	=	Transfer RNA
uORF	=	Upstream open reading frame
UC	=	Ulcerative colitis
UPR	=	Unfolded protein response
UPRE	=	UPR element
XBP1	=	X box binding protein 1

9. REFERENCES

1.   Voeltz GK, Rolls MM, Rapoport TA. Structural organization of the endoplasmic reticulum. EMBO Rep. 2002;3(10):944-50.
2.   Ellgaard L, Molinari M, Helenius A. Setting the standards: quality control in the secretory pathway. Science. 1999;286(5446):1882-8.

3.   McMaster CR. Lipid metabolism and vesicle trafficking: more than just greasing the transport machinery. Biochem Cell Biol. 2001;79(6):681-92.

4.   Meldolesi J, Pozzan T. The endoplasmic reticulum Ca2+ store: a view from the lumen. Trends Biochem Sci. 1998;23(1):10-4.

5.   Meusser B, Hirsch C, Jarosch E, Sommer T. ERAD: the long road to destruction. Nat Cell Biol. 2005;7(8):766-72.

6.   Romisch K. Endoplasmic reticulum-associated degradation. Annu Rev Cell Dev Biol. 2005;21:435-56.

7.   Lin JH, Walter P, Yen TS. Endoplasmic reticulum stress in disease pathogenesis. Annu Rev Pathol. 2008;3:399-425.

8.   Malhotra JD, Kaufman RJ. The endoplasmic reticulum and the unfolded protein response. Semin Cell Dev Biol. 2007;18(6):716-31.

9.   Otsu M, Sitia R. Diseases originating from altered protein quality control in the endoplasmic reticulum. Curr Med Chem. 2007;14(15):1639-52.

10.   Ron D, Walter P. Signal integration in the endoplasmic reticulum unfolded protein response. Nat Rev Mol Cell Biol. 2007;8(7):519-29.

11.   Yoshida H. ER stress and diseases. FEBS J. 2007;274(3):630-58.

12.   Boyce M, Yuan J. Cellular response to endoplasmic reticulum stress: a matter of life or death. Cell Death Differ. 2006;13(3):363-73.

13.   Rutkowski DT, Kaufman RJ. That which does not kill me makes me stronger: adapting to chronic ER stress. Trends Biochem Sci. 2007;32(10):469-76.

14.   Szegezdi E, Logue SE, Gorman AM, Samali A. Mediators of endoplasmic reticulum stress-induced apoptosis. EMBO Rep. 2006;7(9):880-5.

15.   Xu C, Bailly-Maitre B, Reed JC. Endoplasmic reticulum stress: cell life and death decisions. J Clin Invest. 2005;115(10):2656-64.

16.   Schroder M, Kaufman RJ. The mammalian unfolded protein response. Annu Rev Biochem. 2005;74:739-89.

17.   Cox JS, Shamu CE, Walter P. Transcriptional induction of genes encoding endoplasmic reticulum resident proteins requires a transmembrane protein kinase. Cell. 1993;73(6):1197-206.

18.   Mori K, Ma W, Gething MJ, Sambrook J. A transmembrane protein with a cdc2+/CDC28-related kinase activity is required for signaling from the ER to the nucleus. Cell. 1993;74(4):743-56.

19.   Mori K, Kawahara T, Yoshida H, Yanagi H, Yura T. Signalling from endoplasmic reticulum to nucleus: transcription factor with a basic-leucine zipper motif is required for the unfolded protein-response pathway. Genes Cells. 1996;1(9):803-17.

20.   Cox JS, Walter P. A novel mechanism for regulating activity of a transcription factor that controls the unfolded protein response. Cell. 1996;87(3):391-404.

21.   Sidrauski C, Cox JS, Walter P. tRNA ligase is required for regulated mRNA splicing in the unfolded protein response. Cell. 1996;87(3):405-13.

22.   Sidrauski C, Walter P. The transmembrane kinase Ire1p is a site-specific endonuclease that initiates mRNA splicing in the unfolded protein response. Cell. 1997;90(6):1031-9.

23.   Welihinda AA, Kaufman RJ. The unfolded protein response pathway in Saccharomyces cerevisiae. Oligomerization and trans-phosphorylation of Ire1p (Ern1p) are required for kinase activation. J Biol Chem. 1996;271(30):18181-7.

24.   Kimata Y, Kimata YI, Shimizu Y, Abe H, Farcasanu IC, Takeuchi M, Rose MD, Kohno K. Genetic evidence for a role of BiP/Kar2 that regulates Ire1 in

25.   response to accumulation of unfolded proteins. Mol Biol Cell. 2003;14(6):2559-69.

25.   Liu CY, Wong HN, Schauerte JA, Kaufman RJ. The protein kinase/endoribonuclease IRE1alpha that signals the unfolded protein response has a luminal N-terminal ligand-independent dimerization domain. J Biol Chem. 2002;277(21):18346-56.

26.   Liu CY, Xu Z, Kaufman RJ. Structure and intermolecular interactions of the luminal dimerization domain of human IRE1alpha. J Biol Chem. 2003;278(20):17680-7.

27.   Okamura K, Kimata Y, Higashio H, Tsuru A, Kohno K. Dissociation of Kar2p/BiP from an ER sensory molecule, Ire1p, triggers the unfolded protein response in yeast. Biochem Biophys Res Commun. 2000;279(2):445-50.

28.   Bertolotti A, Zhang Y, Hendershot LM, Harding HP, Ron D. Dynamic interaction of BiP and ER stress transducers in the unfolded-protein response. Nat Cell Biol. 2000;2(6):326-32.

29.   Shamu CE, Walter P. Oligomerization and phosphorylation of the Ire1p kinase during intracellular signaling from the endoplasmic reticulum to the nucleus. EMBO J. 1996;15(12):3028-39.

30.   Ruegsegger U, Leber JH, Walter P. Block of HAC1 mRNA translation by long-range base pairing is released by cytoplasmic splicing upon induction of the unfolded protein response. Cell. 2001;107(1):103-14.

31.   Chapman RE, Walter P. Translational attenuation mediated by an mRNA intron. Curr Biol. 1997;7(11):850-9.

32.   Casagrande R, Stern P, Diehn M, Shamu C, Osario M, Zuniga M, Brown PO, Ploegh H. Degradation of proteins from the ER of S. cerevisiae requires an intact unfolded protein response pathway. Mol Cell. 2000;5(4):729-35.

33.   Friedlander R, Jarosch E, Urban J, Volkwein C, Sommer T. A regulatory link between ER-associated protein degradation and the unfolded-protein response. Nat Cell Biol. 2000;2(7):379-84.

34.   Travers KJ, Patil CK, Wodicka L, Lockhart DJ, Weissman JS, Walter P. Functional and genomic analyses reveal an essential coordination between the unfolded protein response and ER-associated degradation. Cell. 2000;101(3):249-58.

35.   Patil C, Walter P. Intracellular signaling from the endoplasmic reticulum to the nucleus: the unfolded protein response in yeast and mammals. Curr Opin Cell Biol. 2001;13(3):349-55.

36.   Kaufman RJ. Regulation of mRNA translation by protein folding in the endoplasmic reticulum. Trends Biochem Sci. 2004;29(3):152-8.

37.   Ma Y, Hendershot LM. The unfolding tale of the unfolded protein response. Cell. 2001;107(7):827-30.

38.   Mori K. Tripartite management of unfolded proteins in the endoplasmic reticulum. Cell. 2000;101(5):451-4.

39.   Scheuner D, Kaufman RJ. The Unfolded Protein Response: A Pathway That Links Insulin Demand with {beta}-Cell Failure and Diabetes. Endocr Rev. 2008;29(3):317-33.

40.   Back SH, Lee K, Vink E, Kaufman RJ. Cytoplasmic IRE1alpha-mediated XBP1 mRNA splicing in the absence of nuclear processing and endoplasmic reticulum stress. J Biol Chem. 2006;281(27):18691-706.

41.   Lee K, Tirasophon W, Shen X, Michalak M, Prywes R, Okada T, Yoshida H, Mori K, Kaufman RJ. IRE1-mediated unconventional mRNA splicing and S2P-mediated ATF6 cleavage merge to regulate XBP1 in

signaling the unfolded protein response. Genes Dev. 2002;16(4):452-66.

42.   Yoshida H, Matsui T, Yamamoto A, Okada T, Mori K. XBP1 mRNA is induced by ATF6 and spliced by IRE1 in response to ER stress to produce a highly active transcription factor. Cell. 2001;107(7):881-91.

43.   Lee AH, Iwakoshi NN, Glimcher LH. XBP-1 regulates a subset of endoplasmic reticulum resident chaperone genes in the unfolded protein response. Mol Cell Biol. 2003;23(21):7448-59.

44.   Shaffer AL, Shapiro-Shelef M, Iwakoshi NN, Lee A-H, Qian SB, Zhao H, Yu X, Yang L, Tan BK, Rosenwald A, Hurt EM, Petroulakis E, Sonenberg N, Yewdell JW, Calame K, Glimcher LH, Staudt LM. XBP1, downstream of Blimp-1, expands the secretory apparatus and other organelles, and increases protein synthesis in plasma cell differentiation. Immunity. 2004;21(1):81-93.

45.   Sriburi R, Jackowski S, Mori K, Brewer JW. XBP1: a link between the unfolded protein response, lipid biosynthesis, and biogenesis of the endoplasmic reticulum. J Cell Biol. 2004;167(1):35-41.

46.   Oikawa D, Tokuda M, Iwawaki T. Site-specific cleavage of CD59 mRNA by endoplasmic reticulum-localized ribonuclease, IRE1. Biochem Biophys Res Commun. 2007;360(1):122-7.

47.   Tirasophon W, Lee K, Callaghan B, Welihinda A, Kaufman RJ. The endoribonuclease activity of mammalian IRE1 autoregulates its mRNA and is required for the unfolded protein response. Genes Dev. 2000;14(21):2725-36.

48.   Hollien J, Weissman JS. Decay of endoplasmic reticulum-localized mRNAs during the unfolded protein response. Science. 2006;313(5783):104-7.

49.   Tirasophon W, Welihinda AA, Kaufman RJ. A stress response pathway from the endoplasmic reticulum to the nucleus requires a novel bifunctional protein kinase/endoribonuclease (Ire1p) in mammalian cells. Genes Dev. 1998;12(12):1812-24.

50.   Wang XZ, Harding HP, Zhang Y, Jolicoeur EM, Kuroda M, Ron D. Cloning of mammalian Ire1 reveals diversity in the ER stress responses. EMBO J. 1998;17(19):5708-17.

51.   Iwawaki T, Hosoda A, Okuda T, Kamigori Y, Nomura-Furuwatari C, Kimata Y, Tsuru A, Kohno K. Translational control by the ER transmembrane kinase/ribonuclease IRE1 under ER stress. Nat Cell Biol. 2001;3(2):158-64.

52.   Urano F, Wang X, Bertolotti A, Zhang Y, Chung P, Harding HP, Ron D. Coupling of stress in the ER to activation of JNK protein kinases by transmembrane protein kinase IRE1. Science. 2000;287(5453):664-6.

53.   Calfon M, Zeng H, Urano F, Till JH, Hubbard SR, Harding HP, Clark SG, Ron D. IRE1 couples endoplasmic reticulum load to secretory capacity by processing the XBP-1 mRNA. Nature. 2002;415(6867):92-6.

54.   Imagawa Y, Hosoda A, Sasaka S, Tsuru A, Kohno K. RNase domains determine the functional difference between IRE1alpha and IRE1beta. FEBS Lett. 2008;582(5):656-60.

55.   Iqbal J, Dai K, Seimon T, Jungreis R, Oyadomari M, Kuriakose G, Ron D, Tabas I, Hussain MM. IRE1beta inhibits chylomicron production by selectively degrading MTP mRNA. Cell Metab. 2008;7(5):445-55.

56.   Harding HP, Calfon M, Urano F, Novoa I, Ron D. Transcriptional and translational control in the mammalian unfolded protein response. Annu Rev Cell Dev Biol. 2002;18:575-99.

57.   Credle JJ, Finer-Moore JS, Papa FR, Stroud RM, Walter P. On the mechanism of sensing unfolded protein in the endoplasmic reticulum. Proc Natl Acad Sci U S A. 2005;102(52):18773-84.

58.   Zhou J, Liu CY, Back SH, Clark RL, Peisach D, Xu Z, Kaufman RJ. The crystal structure of human IRE1 luminal domain reveals a conserved dimerization interface required for activation of the unfolded protein response. Proc Natl Acad Sci U S A. 2006;103(39):14343-8.

59.   Kimata Y, Ishiwata-Kimata Y, Ito T, Hirata A, Suzuki T, Oikawa D, Takeuchi M, Kohno K. Two regulatory steps of ER-stress sensor Ire1 involving its cluster formation and interaction with unfolded proteins. J Cell Biol. 2007;179(1):75-86.

60.   Lee KP, Dey M, Neculai D, Cao C, Dever TE, Sicheri F. Structure of the dual enzyme Ire1 reveals the basis for catalysis and regulation in nonconventional RNA splicing. Cell. 2008;132(1):89-100.

61.   Papa FR, Zhang C, Shokat K, Walter P. Bypassing a kinase activity with an ATP-competitive drug. Science. 2003;302(5650):1533-7.

62.   Acosta-Alvear D, Zhou Y, Blais A, Tsikitis M, Lents NH, Arias C, Lennon CJ, Kluger Y, Dynlacht BD. XBP1 controls diverse cell type- and condition-specific transcriptional regulatory networks. Mol Cell. 2007;27(1):53-66.

63.   Harding HP, Zhang Y, Ron D. Protein translation and folding are coupled by an endoplasmic-reticulum-resident kinase. Nature. 1999;397(6716):271-4.

64.   Liu CY, Schroder M, Kaufman RJ. Ligand-independent dimerization activates the stress response kinases IRE1 and PERK in the lumen of the endoplasmic reticulum. J Biol Chem. 2000;275(32):24881-5.

65.   Shi Y, Vattem KM, Sood R, An J, Liang J, Stramm L, Wek RC. Identification and characterization of pancreatic eukaryotic initiation factor 2 α-subunit kinase, PEK, involved in translational control. Mol Cell Biol. 1998;18(12):7499-509.

66.   Proud CG. eIF2 and the control of cell physiology. Semin Cell Dev Biol. 2005;16(1):3-12.

67.   Chen JJ. Regulation of protein synthesis by the heme-regulated eIF2alpha kinase: relevance to anemias. Blood. 2007;109(7):2693-9.

68.   Dong J, Qiu H, Garcia-Barrio M, Anderson J, Hinnebusch AG. Uncharged tRNA activates GCN2 by displacing the protein kinase moiety from a bipartite tRNA-binding domain. Mol Cell. 2000;6(2):269-79.

69.   Hinnebusch A. Mechanism and regulation of initiator methionyl-tRNA binding to ribosomes. In Translational Control of Gene Expression (Sonenberg, N et al, eds), Cold Spring Harbor Laboratory Press. 2000:pp. 185–244.

70.   Garcia MA, Gil J, Ventoso I, Guerra S, Domingo E, Rivas C, Esteban M. Impact of protein kinase PKR in cell biology: from antiviral to antiproliferative action. Microbiol Mol Biol Rev. 2006;70(4):1032-60.

71.   Jiang HY, Wek SA, McGrath BC, Lu D, Hai T, Harding HP, Wang X, Ron D, Cavener DR, Wek RC. Activating transcription factor 3 is integral to the eukaryotic initiation factor 2 kinase stress response. Mol Cell Biol. 2004;24(3):1365-77.

72.   Hamanaka RB, Bennett BS, Cullinan SB, Diehl JA. PERK and GCN2 contribute to eIF2alpha phosphorylation and cell cycle arrest after activation of the unfolded protein response pathway. Mol Biol Cell. 2005;16(12):5493-501.

73. Brewer JW, Diehl JA. PERK mediates cell-cycle exit during the mammalian unfolded protein response. Proc Natl Acad Sci U S A. 2000;97(23):12625-30.

74. Raven JF, Baltzis D, Wang S, Mounir Z, Papadakis AI, Gao HQ, Koromilas AE. PKR and PKR-like endoplasmic reticulum kinase induce the proteasome-dependent degradation of cyclin D1 via a mechanism requiring eukaryotic initiation factor 2alpha phosphorylation. J Biol Chem. 2008;283(6):3097-108.

75. Fernandez J, Yaman I, Sarnow P, Snider MD, Hatzoglou M. Regulation of internal ribosomal entry site-mediated translation by phosphorylation of the translation initiation factor eIF2alpha. J Biol Chem. 2002;277(21):19198-205.

76. Yaman I, Fernandez J, Liu H, Caprara M, Komar AA, Koromilas AE, Zhou L, Snider MD, Scheuner D, Kaufman RJ, Hatzoglou M. The zipper model of translational control: a small upstream ORF is the switch that controls structural remodeling of an mRNA leader. Cell. 2003;113(4):519-31.

77. Harding HP, Novoa I, Zhang Y, Zeng H, Wek R, Schapira M, Ron D. Regulated translation initiation controls stress-induced gene expression in mammalian cells. Mol Cell. 2000;6(5):1099-108.

78. Scheuner D, Song B, McEwen E, Liu C, Laybutt R, Gillespie P, Saunders T, Bonner-Weir S, Kaufman RJ. Translational control is required for the unfolded protein response and in vivo glucose homeostasis. Mol Cell. 2001;7(6):1165-76.

79. Vattem KM, Wek RC. Reinitiation involving upstream ORFs regulates ATF4 mRNA translation in mammalian cells. Proc Natl Acad Sci U S A. 2004;101(31):11269-74.

80. Lu PD, Harding HP, Ron D. Translation reinitiation at alternative open reading frames regulates gene expression in an integrated stress response. J Cell Biol. 2004;167(1):27-33.

81. Harding HP, Zhang Y, Zeng H, Novoa I, Lu PD, Calfon M, Sadri N, Yun C, Popko B, Paules R, Stojdl DF, Bell JC, Hettmann T, Leiden JM, Ron D. An integrated stress response regulates amino acid metabolism and resistance to oxidative stress. Mol Cell. 2003;11(3):619-33.

82. Luo S, Baumeister P, Yang S, Abcouwer SF, Lee AS. Induction of Grp78/BiP by translational block: activation of the Grp78 promoter by ATF4 through and upstream ATF/CRE site independent of the endoplasmic reticulum stress elements. J Biol Chem. 2003;278(39):37375-85.

83. Ma Y, Brewer JW, Diehl JA, Hendershot LM. Two distinct stress signaling pathways converge upon the CHOP promoter during the mammalian unfolded protein response. J Mol Biol. 2002;318(5):1351-65.

84. Ma Y, Hendershot LM. ER chaperone functions during normal and stress conditions. J Chem Neuroanat. 2004;28(1-2):51-65.

85. Gerlitz G, Jagus R, Elroy-Stein O. Phosphorylation of initiation factor-2 alpha is required for activation of internal translation initiation during cell differentiation. Eur J Biochem. 2002;269(11):2810-9.

86. Fernandez J, Lopez AB, Wang C, Mishra R, Zhou L, Yaman I, Snider MD, Hatzoglou M. Transcriptional control of the arginine/lysine transporter, cat-1, by physiological stress. J Biol Chem. 2003;278(50):50000-9.

87. Cullinan SB, Zhang D, Hannink M, Arvisais E, Kaufman RJ, Diehl JA. Nrf2 is a direct PERK substrate and effector of PERK-dependent cell survival. Mol Cell Biol. 2003;23(20):7198-209.

88. Cullinan SB, Diehl JA. Coordination of ER and oxidative stress signaling: the PERK/Nrf2 signaling pathway. Int J Biochem Cell Biol. 2006;38(3):317-32.

89. Nguyen T, Sherratt PJ, Pickett CB. Regulatory mechanisms controlling gene expression mediated by the antioxidant response element. Annu Rev Pharmacol Toxicol. 2003;43:233-60.

90. Itoh K, Wakabayashi N, Katoh Y, Ishii T, Igarashi K, Engel JD, Yamamoto M. Keap1 represses nuclear activation of antioxidant responsive elements by Nrf2 through binding to the amino-terminal Neh2 domain. Genes Dev. 1999;13(1):76-86.

91. Cullinan SB, Diehl JA. PERK-dependent activation of Nrf2 contributes to redox homeostasis and cell survival following endoplasmic reticulum stress. J Biol Chem. 2004;279(19):20108-17.

92. Marciniak SJ, Yun CY, Oyadomari S, Novoa I, Zhang Y, Jungreis R, Nagata K, Harding HP, Ron D. CHOP induces death by promoting protein synthesis and oxidation in the stressed endoplasmic reticulum. Genes Dev. 2004;18(24):3066-77.

93. Song B, Scheuner D, Ron D, Pennathur S, Kaufman RJ. Chop deletion reduces oxidative stress, improves beta cell function, and promotes cell survival in multiple mouse models of diabetes. J Clin Invest. 2008;118(10):3378-89.

94. Brush MH, Weiser DC, Shenolikar S. Growth arrest and DNA damage-inducible protein GADD34 targets protein phosphatase 1 alpha to the endoplasmic reticulum and promotes dephosphorylation of the alpha subunit of eukaryotic translation initiation factor 2. Mol Cell Biol. 2003;23(4):1292-303.

95. Jousse C, Oyadomari S, Novoa I, Lu P, Zhang Y, Harding HP, Ron D. Inhibition of a constitutive translation initiation factor 2α phosphatase, *CReP*, promotes survival of stressed cells. J Cell Biol. 2003;163(4):767-75.

96. Kojima E, Takeuchi A, Haneda M, Yagi A, Hasegawa T, Yamaki K, Takeda K, Akira S, Shimokata K, Isobe K. The function of GADD34 is a recovery from a shutoff of protein synthesis induced by ER stress: elucidation by GADD34-deficient mice. FASEB J. 2003;17(11):1573-5.

97. Ma Y, Hendershot LM. Delineation of a negative feedback regulatory loop that controls protein translation during endoplasmic reticulum stress. J Biol Chem. 2003;278(37):34864-73.

98. Haze K, Okada T, Yoshida H, Yanagi H, Yura T, Negishi M, Mori K. Identification of the G13 (cAMP-response-element-binding protein-related protein) gene product related to activating transcription factor 6 as a transcriptional activator of the mammalian unfolded protein response. Biochem J. 2001;355(1):19-28.

99. Haze K, Yoshida H, Yanagi H, Yura T, Mori K. Mammalian transcription factor ATF6 is synthesized as a transmembrane protein and activated by proteolysis in response to endoplasmic reticulum stress. Mol Biol Cell. 1999;10(11):3787-99.

100. Yoshida H, Okada T, Haze K, Yanagi H, Yura T, Negishi M, Mori K. ATF6 activated by proteolysis binds in the presence of NF-Y (CBF) directly to the *cis*-acting element responsible for the mammalian unfolded protein response. Mol Cell Biol. 2000;20(18):6755-67.

101. Chen X, Shen J, Prywes R. The luminal domain of ATF6 senses endoplasmic reticulum (ER) stress and causes translocation of ATF6 from the ER to the Golgi. J Biol Chem. 2002;277(15):13045-52.

102. Shen J, Chen X, Hendershot L, Prywes R. ER stress regulation of ATF6 localization by dissociation of

BiP/GRP78 binding and unmasking of Golgi localization signals. Dev Cell. 2002;3(1):99-111.

103.   Ye J, Rawson RB, Komuro R, Chen X, Dave UP, Prywes R, Brown MS, Goldstein JL. ER stress induces cleavage of membrane-bound ATF6 by the same proteases that process SREBPs. Mol Cell. 2000;6(6):1355-64.

104.   Shen J, Prywes R. Dependence of site-2 protease cleavage of ATF6 on prior site-1 protease digestion is determined by the size of the luminal domain of ATF6. J Biol Chem. 2004;279(41):43046-51.

105.   Okada T, Yoshida H, Akazawa R, Negishi M, Mori K. Distinct roles of activating transcription factor 6 (ATF6) and double-stranded RNA-activated protein kinase-like endoplasmic reticulum kinase (PERK) in transcription during the mammalian unfolded protein response. Biochem J. 2002;366(2):585-94.

106.   Yoshida H, Okada T, Haze K, Yanagi H, Yura T, Negishi M, Mori K. Endoplasmic reticulum stress-induced formation of transcription factor complex ERSF including NF-Y (CBF) and activating transcription factors 6alpha and 6beta that activates the mammalian unfolded protein response. Mol Cell Biol. 2001;21(4):1239-48.

107.   Shen JS, Snapp EL, Lippincott-Schwartz J, Prywes R. Stable binding of ATF6 to BiP in the endoplasmic reticulum stress response. Mol Cell Biol. 2005;25(3):921-32.

108.   Nadanaka S, Okada T, Yoshida H, Mori K. Role of disulfide bridges formed in the luminal domain of ATF6 in sensing endoplasmic reticulum stress. Mol Cell Biol. 2007;27(3):1027-43.

109.   Luebke-Wheeler J, Zhang K, Battle M, Si-Tayeb K, Garrison W, Chhinder S, Li J, Kaufman RJ, Duncan SA. Hepatocyte nuclear factor 4alpha is implicated in endoplasmic reticulum stress-induced acute phase response by regulating expression of cyclic adenosine monophosphate responsive element binding protein H. Hepatology. 2008;48(4):1242-50.

110.   Zhang K, Shen X, Wu J, Sakaki K, Saunders T, Rutkowski DT, Back SH, Kaufman RJ. Endoplasmic reticulum stress activates cleavage of CREBH to induce a systemic inflammatory response. Cell. 2006;124(3):587-99.

111.   Kondo S, Murakami T, Tatsumi K, Ogata M, Kanemoto S, Otori K, Iseki K, Wanaka A, Imaizumi K. OASIS, a CREB/ATF-family member, modulates UPR signalling in astrocytes. Nat Cell Biol. 2005;7(2):186-94.

112.   Kondo S, Saito A, Hino S, Murakami T, Ogata M, Kanemoto S, Nara S, Yamashita A, Yoshinaga K, Hara H, Imaizumi K. BBF2H7, a novel transmembrane bZIP transcription factor, is a new type of endoplasmic reticulum stress transducer. Mol Cell Biol. 2007;27(5):1716-29.

113.   Nagamori I, Yabuta N, Fujii T, Tanaka H, Yomogida K, Nishimune Y, Nojima H. Tisp40, a spermatid specific bZip transcription factor, functions by binding to the unfolded protein response element via the Rip pathway. Genes Cells. 2005;10(6):575-94.

114.   Liang G, Audas TE, Li Y, Cockram GP, Dean JD, Martyn AC, Kokame K, Lu R. Luman/CREB3 induces transcription of the endoplasmic reticulum (ER) stress response protein Herp through an ER stress response element. Mol Cell Biol. 2006;26(21):7999-8010.

115.   Raggo C, Rapin N, Stirling J, Gobeil P, Smith-Windsor E, O'Hare P, Misra V. Luman, the cellular counterpart of herpes simplex virus VP16, is processed by regulated intramembrane proteolysis. Mol Cell Biol. 2002;22(16):5639-49.

116.   Stirling J, O'Hare P. CREB4, a transmembrane bZip transcription factor and potential new substrate for regulation and cleavage by S1P. Mol Biol Cell. 2006;17(1):413-26.

117.   Roy B, Lee AS. The mammalian endoplasmic reticulum stress response element consists of an evolutionarily conserved tripartite structure and interacts with a novel stress-inducible complex. Nucleic Acids Res. 1999;27(6):1437-43.

118.   Yoshida H, Haze K, Yanagi H, Yura T, Mori K. Identification of the *cis*-acting endoplasmic reticulum stress response element responsible for transcriptional induction of mammalian glucose-regulated proteins. Involvement of basic leucine zipper transcription factors. J Biol Chem. 1998;273(50):33741-9.

119.   Yamamoto K, Yoshida H, Kokame K, Kaufman RJ, Mori K. Differential contributions of ATF6 and XBP1 to the activation of endoplasmic reticulum stress-responsive *cis*-acting elements ERSE, UPRE and ERSE-II. J Biochem (Tokyo). 2004;136(3):343-50.

120.   Wang Y, Shen J, Arenzana N, Tirasophon W, Kaufman RJ, Prywes R. Activation of ATF6 and an ATF6 DNA binding site by the endoplasmic reticulum stress response. J Biol Chem. 2000;275(35):27013-20.

121.   Yamamoto K, Sato T, Matsui T, Sato M, Okada T, Yoshida H, Harada A, Mori K. Transcriptional Induction of Mammalian ER Quality Control Proteins Is Mediated by Single or Combined Action of ATF6alpha and XBP1. Dev Cell. 2007;13(3):365-76.

122.   Kokame K, Agarwala KL, Kato H, Miyata T. Herp, a new ubiquitin-like membrane protein induced by endoplasmic reticulum stress. J Biol Chem. 2000;275(42):32846-53.

123.   Kokame K, Kato H, Miyata T. Identification of ERSE-II, a new *cis*-acting element responsible for the ATF6-dependent mammalian unfolded protein response. J Biol Chem. 2001;276(12):9199-205.

124.   Fawcett TW, Martindale JL, Guyton KZ, Hai T, Holbrook NJ. Complexes containing activating transcription factor (ATF)/cAMP-responsive-element-binding protein (CREB) interact with the CCAAT/enhancer-binding protein (C/EBP)-ATF composite site to regulate *Gadd153* expression during the stress response. Biochem J. 1999;339(1):135-41.

125.   Ubeda M, Habener JF. CHOP gene expression in response to endoplasmic-reticular stress requires NFY interaction with different domains of a conserved DNA-binding element. Nucleic Acids Res. 2000;28(24):4987-97.

126.   Harding HP, Zhang Y, Bertolotti A, Zeng H, Ron D. *Perk* is essential for translational regulation and cell survival during the unfolded protein response. Mol Cell. 2000;5(5):897-904.

127.   van Laar T, Schouten T, Hoogervorst E, van Eck M, van der Eb AJ, Terleth C. The novel MMS-inducible gene Mif1/KIAA0025 is a target of the unfolded protein response pathway. FEBS Lett. 2000;469(1):123-31.

128.   Ma Y, Hendershot LM. Herp is dually regulated by both the endoplasmic reticulum stress-specific branch of the unfolded protein response and a branch that is shared with other cellular stress pathways. J Biol Chem. 2004;279(14):13792-9.

129.   Adachi Y, Yamamoto K, Okada T, Yoshida H, Harada A, Mori K. ATF6 is a transcription factor specializing in the regulation of quality control proteins in the endoplasmic reticulum. Cell Struct Funct. 2008;33(1):75-89.

130.   Kang SW, Rane NS, Kim SJ, Garrison JL, Taunton J, Hegde RS. Substrate-specific translocational

attenuation during ER stress defines a pre-emptive quality control pathway. Cell. 2006;127(5):999-1013.

131. Rutkowski DT, Arnold SM, Miller CN, Wu J, Li J, Gunnison KM, Mori K, Sadighi Akha AA, Raden D, Kaufman RJ. Adaptation to ER stress is mediated by differential stabilities of pro-survival and pro-apoptotic mRNAs and proteins. PLoS Biol. 2006;4(11):e374.

132. Urano F, Bertolotti A, Ron D. IRE1 and efferent signaling from the endoplasmic reticulum. J Cell Sci. 2000;113 Pt 21:3697-702.

133. Nishitoh H, Matsuzawa A, Tobiume K, Saegusa K, Takeda K, Inoue K, Hori S, Kakizuka A, Ichijo H. ASK1 is essential for endoplasmic reticulum stress-induced neuronal cell death triggered by expanded polyglutamine repeats. Genes Dev. 2002;16(11):1345-55.

134. Lei K, Davis RJ. JNK phosphorylation of Bim-related members of the Bcl2 family induces Bax-dependent apoptosis. Proc Natl Acad Sci U S A. 2003;100(5):2432-7.

135. Putcha GV, Le S, Frank S, Besirli CG, Clark K, Chu B, Alix S, Youle RJ, LaMarche A, Maroney AC, Johnson EM, Jr. JNK-mediated BIM phosphorylation potentiates BAX-dependent apoptosis. Neuron. 2003;38(6):899-914.

136. Yamamoto K, Ichijo H, Korsmeyer SJ. BCL-2 is phosphorylated and inactivated by an ASK1/Jun N-terminal protein kinase pathway normally activated at G(2)/M. Mol Cell Biol. 1999;19(12):8469-78.

137. Kaneko M, Niinuma Y, Nomura Y. Activation signal of nuclear factor-kappa B in response to endoplasmic reticulum stress is transduced via IRE1 and tumor necrosis factor receptor-associated factor 2. Biol Pharm Bull. 2003;26(7):931-5.

138. Leonardi A, Vito P, Mauro C, Pacifico F, Ulianich L, Consiglio E, Formisano S, Di Jeso B. Endoplasmic reticulum stress causes thyroglobulin retention in this organelle and triggers activation of nuclear factor-kappa B via tumor necrosis factor receptor-associated factor 2. Endocrinology. 2002;143(6):2169-77.

139. Mauro C, Crescenzi E, De Mattia R, Pacifico F, Mellone S, Salzano S, de Luca C, D'Adamio L, Palumbo G, Formisano S, Vito P, Leonardi A. Central role of the scaffold protein tumor necrosis factor receptor-associated factor 2 in regulating endoplasmic reticulum stress-induced apoptosis. J Biol Chem. 2006;281(5):2631-8.

140. Hu P, Han Z, Couvillon AD, Kaufman RJ, Exton JH. Autocrine tumor necrosis factor alpha links endoplasmic reticulum stress to the membrane death receptor pathway through IRE1alpha-mediated NF-kappaB activation and down-regulation of TRAF2 expression. Mol Cell Biol. 2006;26(8):3071-84.

141. Luo D, He Y, Zhang H, Yu L, Chen H, Xu Z, Tang S, Urano F, Min W. AIP1 is critical in transducing IRE1-mediated endoplasmic reticulum stress response. J Biol Chem. 2008;283(18):11905-12.

142. Oono K, Yoneda T, Manabe T, Yamagishi S, Matsuda S, Hitomi J, Miyata S, Mizuno T, Imaizumi K, Katayama T, Tohyama M. JAB1 participates in unfolded protein responses by association and dissociation with IRE1. Neurochem Int. 2004;45(5):765-72.

143. Yoneda T, Imaizumi K, Oono K, Yui D, Gomi F, Katayama T, Tohyama M. Activation of caspase-12, an endoplastic reticulum (ER) resident caspase, through tumor necrosis factor receptor-associated factor 2-dependent mechanism in response to the ER stress. J Biol Chem. 2001;276(17):13935-40.

144. Oyadomari S, Mori M. Roles of CHOP/GADD153 in endoplasmic reticulum stress. Cell Death Differ. 2004;11(4):381-9.

145. Lu PD, Jousse C, Marciniak SJ, Zhang Y, Novoa I, Scheuner D, Kaufman RJ, Ron D, Harding HP. Cytoprotection by pre-emptive conditional phosphorylation of translation initiation factor 2. EMBO J. 2004;23(1):169-79.

146. Wu J, Rutkowski DT, Dubois M, Swathirajan J, Saunders T, Wang J, Song B, Yau GD, Kaufman RJ. ATF6alpha Optimizes Long-Term Endoplasmic Reticulum Function to Protect Cells from Chronic Stress. Dev Cell. 2007;13(3):351-64.

147. Matsumoto M, Minami M, Takeda K, Sakao Y, Akira S. Ectopic expression of CHOP (GADD153) induces apoptosis in M1 myeloblastic leukemia cells. FEBS Lett. 1996;395(2-3):143-7.

148. McCullough KD, Martindale JL, Klotz LO, Aw TY, Holbrook NJ. Gadd153 sensitizes cells to endoplasmic reticulum stress by down-regulating Bcl2 and perturbing the cellular redox state. Mol Cell Biol. 2001;21(4):1249-59.

149. Zinszner H, Kuroda M, Wang X, Batchvarova N, Lightfoot RT, Remotti H, Stevens JL, Ron D. CHOP is implicated in programmed cell death in response to impaired function of the endoplasmic reticulum. Genes Dev. 1998;12(7):982-95.

150. Tajiri S, Oyadomari S, Yano S, Morioka M, Gotoh T, Hamada JI, Ushio Y, Mori M. Ischemia-induced neuronal cell death is mediated by the endoplasmic reticulum stress pathway involving CHOP. Cell Death Differ. 2004;11(4):403-15.

151. Yamaguchi H, Wang HG. CHOP is involved in endoplasmic reticulum stress-induced apoptosis by enhancing DR5 expression in human carcinoma cells. J Biol Chem. 2004;279(44):45495-502.

152. Ohoka N, Yoshii S, Hattori T, Onozaki K, Hayashi H. *TRB3*, a novel ER stress-inducible gene, is induced via ATF4- CHOP pathway and is involved in cell death. EMBO J. 2005;24(6):1243-55.

153. Sok J, Wang XZ, Batchvarova N, Kuroda M, Harding H, Ron D. CHOP-Dependent stress-inducible expression of a novel form of carbonic anhydrase VI. Mol Cell Biol. 1999;19(1):495-504.

154. Adler HT, Chinery R, Wu DY, Kussick SJ, Payne JM, Fornace AJ, Jr., Tkachuk DC. Leukemic HRX fusion proteins inhibit GADD34-induced apoptosis and associate with the GADD34 and hSNF5/INI1 proteins. Mol Cell Biol. 1999;19(10):7050-60.

155. Dias-Gunasekara S, Benham AM. Defining the protein-protein interactions of the mammalian endoplasmic reticulum oxidoreductases (EROs). Biochem Soc Trans. 2005;33(Pt 6):1382-4.

156. Cheung HH, Lynn Kelly N, Liston P, Korneluk RG. Involvement of caspase-2 and caspase-9 in endoplasmic reticulum stress-induced apoptosis: a role for the IAPs. Exp Cell Res. 2006;312(12):2347-57.

157. Dahmer MK. Caspases-2, -3, and -7 are involved in thapsigargin-induced apoptosis of SH-SY5Y neuroblastoma cells. J Neurosci Res. 2005;80(4):576-83.

158. Di Sano F, Ferraro E, Tufi R, Achsel T, Piacentini M, Cecconi F. Endoplasmic reticulum stress induces apoptosis by an apoptosome-dependent but caspase 12-independent mechanism. J Biol Chem. 2006;281(5):2693-700.

159. Hitomi J, Katayama T, Eguchi Y, Kudo T, Taniguchi M, Koyama Y, Manabe T, Yamagishi S, Bando Y, Imaizumi K, Tsujimoto Y, Tohyama M. Involvement of caspase-4 in endoplasmic reticulum stress-induced

apoptosis and Aβ-induced cell death. J Cell Biol. 2004;165(3):347-56.

160.   Nakagawa T, Zhu H, Morishima N, Li E, Xu J, Yankner BA, Yuan J. Caspase-12 mediates endoplasmic-reticulum-specific apoptosis and cytotoxicity by amyloid-β. Nature. 2000;403(6765):98-103.

161.   Nakagawa T, Yuan J. Cross-talk between two cysteine protease families. Activation of caspase-12 by calpain in apoptosis. J Cell Biol. 2000;150(4):887-94.

162.   Rao RV, Hermel E, Castro-Obregon S, del Rio G, Ellerby LM, Ellerby HM, Bredesen DE. Coupling endoplasmic reticulum stress to the cell death program. Mechanism of caspase activation. J Biol Chem. 2001;276(36):33869-74.

163.   Fischer H, Koenig U, Eckhart L, Tschachler E. Human caspase 12 has acquired deleterious mutations. Biochem Biophys Res Commun. 2002;293(2):722-6.

164.   Masud A, Mohapatra A, Lakhani SA, Ferrandino A, Hakem R, Flavell RA. Endoplasmic reticulum stress-induced death of mouse embryonic fibroblasts requires the intrinsic pathway of apoptosis. J Biol Chem. 2007;282(19):14132-9.

165.   Obeng EA, Boise LH. Caspase-12 and caspase-4 are not required for caspase-dependent endoplasmic reticulum stress-induced apoptosis. J Biol Chem. 2005;280(33):29578-87.

166.   Cory S, Adams JM. The Bcl2 family: regulators of the cellular life-or-death switch. Nat Rev Cancer. 2002;2(9):647-56.

167.   Thomenius MJ, Wang NS, Reineks EZ, Wang Z, Distelhorst CW. Bcl-2 on the endoplasmic reticulum regulates Bax activity by binding to BH3-only proteins. J Biol Chem. 2003;278(8):6243-50.

168.   Wang NS, Unkila MT, Reineks EZ, Distelhorst CW. Transient expression of wild-type or mitochondrially targeted Bcl-2 induces apoptosis, whereas transient expression of endoplasmic reticulum-targeted Bcl-2 is protective against Bax-induced cell death. J Biol Chem. 2001;276(47):44117-28.

169.   Morishima N, Nakanishi K, Tsuchiya K, Shibata T, Seiwa E. Translocation of Bim to the endoplasmic reticulum (ER) mediates ER stress signaling for activation of caspase-12 during ER stress-induced apoptosis. J Biol Chem. 2004;279(48):50375-81.

170.   Puthalakath H, O'Reilly LA, Gunn P, Lee L, Kelly PN, Huntington ND, Hughes PD, Michalak EM, McKimm-Breschkin J, Motoyama N, Gotoh T, Akira S, Bouillet P, Strasser A. ER stress triggers apoptosis by activating BH3-only protein Bim. Cell. 2007;129(7):1337-49.

171.   Germain M, Mathai JP, McBride HM, Shore GC. Endoplasmic reticulum BIK initiates DRP1-regulated remodelling of mitochondrial cristae during apoptosis. EMBO J. 2005;24(8):1546-56.

172.   Germain M, Mathai JP, Shore GC. BH-3-only BIK functions at the endoplasmic reticulum to stimulate cytochrome c release from mitochondria. J Biol Chem. 2002;277(20):18053-60.

173.   Luo X, He Q, Huang Y, Sheikh MS. Transcriptional upregulation of PUMA modulates endoplasmic reticulum calcium pool depletion-induced apoptosis via Bax activation. Cell Death Differ. 2005;12(10):1310-8.

174.   Reimertz C, Kogel D, Rami A, Chittenden T, Prehn JH. Gene expression during ER stress-induced apoptosis in neurons: induction of the BH3-only protein Bbc3/PUMA and activation of the mitochondrial apoptosis pathway. J Cell Biol. 2003;162(4):587-97.

175.   Wei MC, Zong WX, Cheng EH, Lindsten T, Panoutsakopoulou V, Ross AJ, Roth KA, MacGregor GR, Thompson CB, Korsmeyer SJ. Proapoptotic BAX

176.   Zong WX, Lindsten T, Ross AJ, MacGregor GR, Thompson CB. BH3-only proteins that bind pro-survival Bcl-2 family members fail to induce apoptosis in the absence of Bax and Bak. Genes Dev. 2001;15(12):1481-6.

177.   Upton JP, Austgen K, Nishino M, Coakley KM, Hagen A, Han D, Papa FR, Oakes SA. Caspase-2 cleavage of BID is a critical apoptotic signal downstream of endoplasmic reticulum stress. Mol Cell Biol. 2008;28(12):3943-51.

178.   Korsmeyer SJ, Wei MC, Saito M, Weiler S, Oh KJ, Schlesinger PH. Pro-apoptotic cascade activates BID, which oligomerizes BAK or BAX into pores that result in the release of cytochrome c. Cell Death Differ. 2000;7(12):1166-73.

179.   Scorrano L, Oakes SA, Opferman JT, Cheng EH, Sorcinelli MD, Pozzan T, Korsmeyer SJ. BAX and BAK regulation of endoplasmic reticulum Ca^{2+}: a control point for apoptosis. Science. 2003;300(5616):135-9.

180.   Zong WX, Li C, Hatzivassiliou G, Lindsten T, Yu Q-C, Yuan J, Thompson CB. Bax and Bak can localize to the endoplasmic reticulum to initiate apoptosis. J Cell Biol. 2003;162(1):59-69.

181.   Nutt LK, Pataer A, Pahler J, Fang B, Roth J, McConkey DJ, Swisher SG. Bax and Bak promote apoptosis by modulating endoplasmic reticular and mitochondrial Ca2+ stores. J Biol Chem. 2002;277(11):9219-25.

182.   Oakes SA, Scorrano L, Opferman JT, Bassik MC, Nishino M, Pozzan T, Korsmeyer SJ. Proapoptotic BAX and BAK regulate the type 1 inositol trisphosphate receptor and calcium leak from the endoplasmic reticulum. Proc Natl Acad Sci U S A. 2005;102(1):105-10.

183.   Chen R, Valencia I, Zhong F, McColl KS, Roderick HL, Bootman MD, Berridge MJ, Conway SJ, Holmes AB, Mignery GA, Velez P, Distelhorst CW. Bcl-2 functionally interacts with inositol 1,4,5-trisphosphate receptors to regulate calcium release from the ER in response to inositol 1,4,5-trisphosphate. J Cell Biol. 2004;166(2):193-203.

184.   White C, Li C, Yang J, Petrenko NB, Madesh M, Thompson CB, Foskett JK. The endoplasmic reticulum gateway to apoptosis by Bcl-X(L) modulation of the InsP3R. Nat Cell Biol. 2005;7(10):1021-8.

185.   Hetz C, Bernasconi P, Fisher J, Lee AH, Bassik MC, Antonsson B, Brandt GS, Iwakoshi NN, Schinzel A, Glimcher LH, Korsmeyer SJ. Proapoptotic BAX and BAK modulate the unfolded protein response by a direct interaction with IRE1alpha. Science. 2006;312(5773):572-6.

186.   Xu Q, Reed JC. Bax inhibitor-1, a mammalian apoptosis suppressor identified by functional screening in yeast. Mol Cell. 1998;1(3):337-46.

187.   Chae HJ, Ke N, Kim HR, Chen S, Godzik A, Dickman M, Reed JC. Evolutionarily conserved cytoprotection provided by Bax Inhibitor-1 homologs from animals, plants, and yeast. Gene. 2003;323:101-13.

188.   Chae HJ, Kim HR, Xu C, Bailly-Maitre B, Krajewska M, Krajewski S, Banares S, Cui J, Digicaylioglu M, Ke N, Kitada S, Monosov E, Thomas M, Kress CL, Babendure JR, Tsien RY, Lipton SA, Reed JC. BI-1 regulates an apoptosis pathway linked to endoplasmic reticulum stress. Mol Cell. 2004;15(3):355-66.

189.   Lee GH, Kim HK, Chae SW, Kim DS, Ha KC, Cuddy M, Kress C, Reed JC, Kim HR, Chae HJ. Bax

inhibitor-1 regulates endoplasmic reticulum stress-associated reactive oxygen species and heme oxygenase-1 expression. J Biol Chem. 2007;282(30):21618-28.

190. Bailly-Maitre B, Fondevila C, Kaldas F, Droin N, Luciano F, Ricci JE, Croxton R, Krajewska M, Zapata JM, Kupiec-Weglinski JW, Farmer D, Reed JC. Cytoprotective gene bi-1 is required for intrinsic protection from endoplasmic reticulum stress and ischemia-reperfusion injury. Proc Natl Acad Sci U S A. 2006;103(8):2809-14.

191. Luo S, Mao C, Lee B, Lee AS. GRP78/BiP is required for cell proliferation and protecting the inner cell mass from apoptosis during early mouse embryonic development. Mol Cell Biol. 2006;26(15):5688-97.

192. Mao C, Dong D, Little E, Luo S, Lee AS. Transgenic mouse model for monitoring endoplasmic reticulum stress in vivo. Nat Med. 2004;10(10):1013-4; author reply 4.

193. Kim SK, Kim YK, Lee AS. Expression of the glucose-regulated proteins (GRP94 and GRP78) in differentiated and undifferentiated mouse embryonic cells and the use of the GRP78 promoter as an expression system in embryonic cells. Differentiation. 1990;42(3):153-9.

194. Barnes JA, Smoak IW. Glucose-regulated protein 78 (GRP78) is elevated in embryonic mouse heart and induced following hypoglycemic stress. Anat Embryol (Berl). 2000;202(1):67-74.

195. Mao C, Tai WC, Bai Y, Poizat C, Lee AS. In vivo regulation of Grp78/BiP transcription in the embryonic heart: role of the endoplasmic reticulum stress response element and GATA-4. J Biol Chem. 2006;281(13):8877-87.

196. Zhao L, Longo-Guess C, Harris BS, Lee JW, Ackerman SL. Protein accumulation and neurodegeneration in the woozy mutant mouse is caused by disruption of SIL1, a cochaperone of BiP. Nat Genet. 2005;37(9):974-9.

197. Zhang K, Wong HN, Song B, Miller CN, Scheuner D, Kaufman RJ. The unfolded protein response sensor IRE1alpha is required at 2 distinct steps in B cell lymphopoiesis. J Clin Invest. 2005;115(2):268-81.

198. Lin JH, Li H, Yasumura D, Cohen HR, Zhang C, Panning B, Shokat KM, Lavail MM, Walter P. IRE1 signaling affects cell fate during the unfolded protein response. Science. 2007;318(5852):944-9.

199. Iwakoshi NN, Lee A-H, Vallabhajosyula P, Otipoby KL, Rajewsky K, Glimcher LH. Plasma cell differentiation and the unfolded protein response intersect at the transcription factor XBP-1. Nat Immunol. 2003;4(4):321-9.

200. Reimold AM, Iwakoshi NN, Manis J, Vallabhajosyula P, Szomolanyi-Tsuda E, Gravallese EM, Friend D, Grusby MJ, Alt F, Glimcher LH. Plasma cell differentiation requires the transcription factor XBP-1. Nature. 2001;412(6844):300-7.

201. Bertolotti A, Wang X, Novoa I, Jungreis R, Schlessinger K, Cho JH, West AB, Ron D. Increased sensitivity to dextran sodium sulfate colitis in IRE1β-deficient mice. J Clin Invest. 2001;107(5):585-93.

202. Reimold AM, Etkin A, Clauss I, Perkins A, Friend DS, Zhang J, Horton HF, Scott A, Orkin SH, Byrne MC, Grusby MJ, Glimcher LH. An essential role in liver development for transcription factor XBP-1. Genes Dev. 2000;14(2):152-7.

203. Iwakoshi NN, Pypaert M, Glimcher LH. The transcription factor XBP-1 is essential for the development and survival of dendritic cells. J Exp Med. 2007;204(10):2267-75.

204. Zenke M, Hieronymus T. Towards an understanding of the transcription factor network of dendritic cell development. Trends Immunol. 2006;27(3):140-5.

205. Lee AH, Chu GC, Iwakoshi NN, Glimcher LH. XBP-1 is required for biogenesis of cellular secretory machinery of exocrine glands. EMBO J. 2005;24(24):4368-80.

206. Lee AH, Scapa EF, Cohen DE, Glimcher LH. Regulation of hepatic lipogenesis by the transcription factor XBP1. Science. 2008;320(5882):1492-6.

207. Kaser A, Lee AH, Franke A, Glickman JN, Zeissig S, Tilg H, Nieuwenhuis EE, Higgins DE, Schreiber S, Glimcher LH, Blumberg RS. XBP1 links ER stress to intestinal inflammation and confers genetic risk for human inflammatory bowel disease. Cell. 2008;134(5):743-56.

208. Ozcan U, Cao Q, Yilmaz E, Lee AH, Iwakoshi NN, Ozdelen E, Tuncman G, Gorgun C, Glimcher LH, Hotamisligil GS. Endoplasmic reticulum stress links obesity, insulin action, and type 2 diabetes. Science. 2004;306(5695):457-61.

209. Harding HP, Zeng H, Zhang Y, Jungries R, Chung P, Plesken H, Sabatini DD, Ron D. Diabetes mellitus and exocrine pancreatic dysfunction in *Perk-/-* mice reveals a role for translational control in secretory cell survival. Mol Cell. 2001;7(6):1153-63.

210. Zhang P, McGrath B, Li S, Frank A, Zambito F, Reinert J, Gannon M, Ma K, McNaughton K, Cavener DR. The PERK eukaryotic initiation factor 2 alpha kinase is required for the development of the skeletal system, postnatal growth, and the function and viability of the pancreas. Mol Cell Biol. 2002;22(11):3864-74.

211. Biason-Lauber A, Lang-Muritano M, Vaccaro T, Schoenle EJ. Loss of kinase activity in a patient with Wolcott-Rallison syndrome caused by a novel mutation in the EIF2AK3 gene. Diabetes. 2002;51(7):2301-5.

212. Delepine M, Nicolino M, Barrett T, Golamaully M, Lathrop GM, Julier C. EIF2AK3, encoding translation initiation factor 2-alpha kinase 3, is mutated in patients with Wolcott-Rallison syndrome. Nat Genet. 2000;25(4):406-9.

213. Senee V, Vattem KM, Delepine M, Rainbow LA, Haton C, Lecoq A, Shaw NJ, Robert JJ, Rooman R, Diatloff-Zito C, Michaud JL, Bin-Abbas B, Taha D, Zabel B, Franceschini P, Topaloglu AK, Lathrop GM, Barrett TG, Nicolino M, Wek RC, Julier C. Wolcott-Rallison Syndrome: clinical, genetic, and functional study of EIF2AK3 mutations and suggestion of genetic heterogeneity. Diabetes. 2004;53(7):1876-83.

214. Schuit FC, In't Veld PA, Pipeleers DG. Glucose stimulates proinsulin biosynthesis by a dose-dependent recruitment of pancreatic beta cells. Proc Natl Acad Sci U S A. 1988;85(11):3865-9.

215. Scheuner D, Mierde DV, Song B, Flamez D, Creemers JW, Tsukamoto K, Ribick M, Schuit FC, Kaufman RJ. Control of mRNA translation preserves endoplasmic reticulum function in beta cells and maintains glucose homeostasis. Nat Med. 2005;11(7):757-64.

216. Hettmann T, Barton K, Leiden JM. Microphthalmia due to p53-mediated apoptosis of anterior lens epithelial cells in mice lacking the CREB-2 transcription factor. Dev Biol. 2000;222(1):110-23.

217. Masuoka HC, Townes TM. Targeted disruption of the activating transcription factor 4 gene results in severe fetal anemia in mice. Blood. 2002;99(3):736-45.

218. Tanaka T, Tsujimura T, Takeda K, Sugihara A, Maekawa A, Terada N, Yoshida N, Akira S. Targeted disruption of ATF4 discloses its essential role in the formation of eye lens fibres. Genes Cells. 1998;3(12):801-10.

219. Iida K, Li Y, McGrath BC, Frank A, Cavener DR. PERK eIF2 alpha kinase is required to regulate the viability of the exocrine pancreas in mice. BMC Cell Biol. 2007;8:38.

220. Zhang W, Feng D, Li Y, Iida K, McGrath B, Cavener DR. PERK EIF2AK3 control of pancreatic beta cell differentiation and proliferation is required for postnatal glucose homeostasis. Cell Metab. 2006;4(6):491-7.

221. Srivastava SP, Davies MV, Kaufman RJ. Calcium depletion from the endoplasmic reticulum activates the double-stranded RNA-dependent protein kinase (PKR) to inhibit protein synthesis. J Biol Chem. 1995;270(28):16619-24.

222. Wei J, Sheng X, Feng D, McGrath B, Cavener DR. PERK is essential for neonatal skeletal development to regulate osteoblast proliferation and differentiation. J Cell Physiol. 2008;217(3):693-707.

223. Elefteriou F, Benson MD, Sowa H, Starbuck M, Liu X, Ron D, Parada LF, Karsenty G. ATF4 mediation of NF1 functions in osteoblast reveals a nutritional basis for congenital skeletal dysplasiae. Cell Metab. 2006;4(6):441-51.

224. Yang X, Matsuda K, Bialek P, Jacquot S, Masuoka HC, Schinke T, Li L, Brancorsini S, Sassone-Corsi P, Townes TM, Hanauer A, Karsenty G. ATF4 is a substrate of RSK2 and an essential regulator of osteoblast biology; implication for Coffin-Lowry Syndrome. Cell. 2004;117(3):387-98.

CHAPTER 3

The ER Chaperone GRP78 and Cancer

Risheng Ye, Yi Zhang and Amy S. Lee

Department of Biochemistry and Molecular Biology, USC/Norris Comprehensive Cancer Center, University of Southern California Keck School of Medicine, 1441 Eastlake Avenue, Los Angeles, California 90089, USA

Address correspondence to: Dr. Amy S. Lee, USC/Norris Comprehensive Cancer Center, University of Southern California Keck School of Medicine, 1441 Eastlake Avenue, Los Angeles, California 90089, USA; Tel.: 323-865-0507; Fax: 323-865-0094; E-mail: amylee@ccnt.usc.edu.

Abstract: The unfolded protein response (UPR) is emerging as a major contributor to cancer cell adaptation to the pathophysiological stress of tumorigenesis. As a major endoplasmic reticulum (ER) chaperone, GRP78/BiP is induced by the UPR, and functions as a master regulator of the UPR signaling pathways. In this review, recent global analysis of *Grp78* mRNA level in specific human tissues and its role in ER stress signaling and cell survival are discussed. Very recently the dynamic molecular events during the transcriptional induction of *Grp78* were elucidated, providing kinetics of factor occupancy along the *Grp78* promoter in cells subjected to ER stress. In addition to its established function of an apoptotic protein, a regulatory role of GRP78 in stress-induced autophagy in mammalian cells is also recently defined. In multiple cancer models, both *in vitro* and *in vivo*, GRP78 confers growth advantage and drug resistance to solid tumors. Finally, the newly discovered cell surface GRP78 provides potential cancer specific therapy.

1. INTRODUCTION

Tumorigenesis progresses through initial activation of oncogene, proliferation of tumor cells resulting in tumor growth and potentially metastasis. Throughout this process, the transformed tumor cells are subjected to immune attack as part of the host's defense mechanism. At the same time, the rapid growth of the tumor in the absence of adequate tumor vasculature supply creates metabolic stress which could lead to apoptosis, as well as autophagy. For survival, tumor cells utilize multiple mechanisms to overcome these adverse pathophysiological conditions. For example, apoptotic pathways are often inactivated in tumor cells through mutations, and concomitantly, prosurvival pathways are activated. One of the rapidly emerging research areas is the adaptation of cancer cells to the physiological stress of tumorigenesis through induction of the unfolded protein response (UPR), an evolutionarily conserved mechanism protecting cells against stress targeting the endoplasmic reticulum (ER). Within the ER resides a major chaperone protein GRP78 which also functions as a key rheostat for ER homeostasis. The role of ER stress and GRP78 in cancer has been the topic of several recent reviews [1-4]. This review focuses on exciting new developments that expand and advance our understanding on the mechanisms whereby GRP78 contributes to tumor cell proliferation, inhibition of apoptosis and resistance to anti-cancer therapy.

2. GRP78 IS A MASTER REGULATOR OF ER HOMEOSTASIS

The ER is a specialized perinuclear organelle where secretory and membrane proteins, as well as lipids, are synthesized. It is also a major intracellular storage compartment for Ca^{2+}, which involves multiple pathways of signal transduction in multiple cell types. ER stress is defined as an imbalance between protein load and folding capacity of ER, which triggers the evolutionarily conserved mechanism referred to as the UPR [5]. Within the lumen of the ER, protein chaperones such as GRP78, GRP94, calnexin and calreticulin assist in folding of newly synthesized polypeptides and prevent aggregation of unfolded or misfolded protein [6]. GRP78 has also been implicated in transporting misfolded proteins in the ER lumen to the cytosol for proteasome-mediated degradation [6, 7]. Cells that are specialized for a high secretory capacity, such as plasma cells, liver cells and pancreatic beta cells, are known to expand their ER capacities to adapt to the increased demand in protein folding.

Recently, it is also recognized that obesity induces ER stress in peripheral tissues [8, 9]. Further, differentiated adipocytes act as potent endocrine cells, secreting large amounts of peptides and lipid mediators such as leptin and adiponectin [10]. Biosynthesis of these adipocytokines requires molecular chaperones and folding enzymes in the

ER. Thus, ER stress experienced by various cell types may play a significant role in human diseases and understanding the contribution of the UPR will be important towards the development of effective preventive and therapeutic strategies.

The glucose regulated protein, GRP78, is commonly referred to as BiP, the immunoglobulin heavy chain binding protein [7], or HSPA5, denoting that it is a member of the 70 kilodalton heat shock protein family. As a major molecular chaperone located primarily in the ER, GRP78 facilitates proper protein folding, maintains proteins in a folded state and prevents protein folding intermediates from aggregating [7, 11]. Among the peripheral tissues, GRP78 expression is readily detected in adult adipose tissues and liver, but is very low in muscle. Global analysis of Grp78 mRNA levels in specific human tissues revealed relatively high expression of Grp78 in hormone- or enzyme-producing tissues, including islets of Langerhans, thyroid, pituitary and exocrine pancreas, consistent with the requirement of GRP78 to assist the specified cellular function in protein folding and secretion (http://amazonia.montp. inserm.fr). Interestingly, low level of GRP78 is expressed in adult skeletal muscle, brain, skin, appendix and oocyte. Among tissue culture cell lines, GRP78 expression is high in embryonic stem (ES) cells, myelogenous leukemic cell lines HL60 and K562, and low in the lymphoblastic leukemic cell line MOLT4. Although how the expression of GRP78 is regulated in various organs, tissues and cell types remains to be determined, this could be due to differential demands of various tissues on protein folding, secretion and energy source utilization. The latter is demonstrated by high level of GRP78 expression in the day 11 embryonic heart where glucose is a major source of energy and subsides in later development [12, 13].

A large amount of work has established that induction of GRP78 is indicative of ER stress. In addition to the chemical inducers, ER stress can occur under various physiological settings that have significant implications in health and disease [3, 4, 6, 14]. For example, similar to the early embryonic heart, GRP78 expression is commonly elevated in solid tumors [3]. This could result from both the high glucose consumption rate and the poor perfusion of glucose and oxygen in the microenvironment [4].

Why is GRP78 such an integral part of ER stress and the UPR? The answer may lie in the multiple functional roles of GRP78. In addition to being an essential and major chaperone protein, GRP78 binds Ca^{2+} and serves as an ER stress signaling regulator [7, 11]. It is well accepted that GRP78 is a key rheostat in controlling ER homeostasis. In mammalian cells, several ER-resident transmembrane proteins have been identified that act as transducers of ER stress signaling: the serine/ threonine kinase and endoribonuclease IRE1, the PERK serine/threonine kinase (also referred to as PEK) and the basic leucine-zipper transcription factor ATF6 [14, 15]. In non-stressed cells, GRP78 binds to all three transducers which are maintained in an inactive state. Upon ER stress, all three sensors are released from GRP78. Therefore, GRP78 is a key regulator of ER stress transducers since their activation upon ER stress is dependent on their release from GRP78.

A fraction of GRP78 can exist as a transmembrane ER protein [16, 17]. This implies that GRP78 can potentially interact directly with the cytosolic components. For example, GRP78 has been reported to form complexes with pro-apoptotic BH3 domain protein, BIK, and caspases such as caspase-7 and mouse caspase-12 that associate with the outer ER membrane. Through these interactions, either directly or indirectly, GRP78 regulates the balance between cell survival and apoptosis in ER-stressed cells. The parallel role of GRP78 as a regulator of the UPR and ER-initiated apoptosis is summarized in Fig. (**1**).

While GRP78 is a key master regulator of ER function, how its depletion affects the UPR pathways and cell survival appears to be cell specific and may be related to the basal expression of GRP78 level. For example, HeLa cells that express high level of GRP78 are highly sensitive to GRP78 depletion [18]. Previously we observed that in mouse embryos, *Grp78* heterozygosity is associated with upregulation of ER chaperone GRP94 and the ER folding enzyme protein disulphide isomerase (PDI), without the concomitant induction of other branches of the UPR such as CHOP and XBP-1 splicing [19]. This observation has recently been extended to the tumor associated endothelial cells [20].

Collectively, these new findings reveal that specific cells can induce GRP78 without full activation of the UPR and some cells under stress can elicit compensatory protective responses such as upregulation of ER chaperones as a result of the genetic alteration of *Grp78*. Most recently, it has been reported that a small molecule BIX, that preferentially induces GRP78, and slight induction

Role of GRP78 as a Regulator of UPR

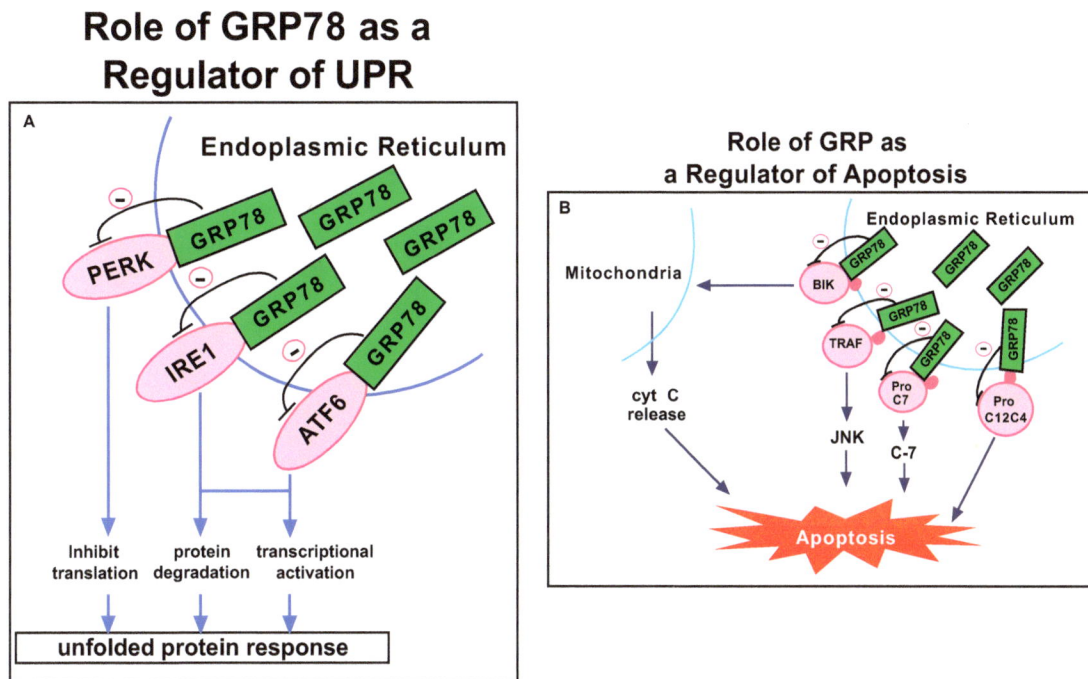

Fig. (1). GRP78 regulates ER stress signaling pathways of the UPR and survival. (A) In non-stressed cells, the ER-transmembrane signaling molecules (ATF6, IRE1, PERK) are maintained in an inactive state through binding to GRP78. Following ER stress such as protein misfolding, GRP78 is titrated away and the UPR is triggered. (B) In non-stressed cells, GRP78 either directly or indirectly interacts with ER-associated BIK and caspases (murine caspase-12/human caspase 4) and blocks their activation. However, when the stress is too severe, GRP78 is titrated away and apoptotic responses are triggered which eventually lead to cell death.

of GRP94 and calreticulin can protect neurons from ER stress [21]. This therapeutic benefit may also be applied to other organs that require increase in protein folding capacity for maintenance of ER homeostasis in survival against stress.

3. DYNAMIC LOADING OF FACTORS AND CHROMATIN IN *Grp78* TRANSCRIPTIONAL INDUCTION

ER stress induction of *Grp78* transcription is primarily mediated through the ER stress response element (ERSE). Upstream of the TATA box on the Grp78 promoter, there are three successive copies of ERSE, with the consensus sequence of CCAAT(N_9)CCACG. Under non-stress status, the transcription factors NF-Y and Sp1 bind ERSE. Upon ER stress, a series of activators, including TFII-I, cleaved ATF6 nuclear form, YY1, p300 and

PRMT1, are recruited on ERSE and cooperate with NF-Y and Sp1 to activate *Grp78* transcription [3, 22-28].

Further, the chromatin organization of the *Grp78* promoter, as well as the dynamic loading of transcription factors onto ERSE during its activation process, was captured by single molecule footprinting [29]. Taking advantage that the TATA containing rat *Grp78* promoter has a highly defined transcription start site, the locations of the three ERSE elements are well defined, the CpG islands of the promoter are unmethylated, and methyltransferase treatment followed by bisulfite sequencing for CpG island methylation allows detection of precise DNA regions protected by nucleosomes or transcription factor binding. It was demonstrated that under basal, non-stressed conditions, the ERSEs of the rat Grp78 promoter are devoid of nucleosomes, and the TATA box is frequently occupied, probably by TBP. After ER stress, the three copies of ERSE are sequentially loaded with transcription factors, from downstream to upstream. Afterwards, the general transcription machinery is recruited to the transcription initiation site, which in turn releases the transcription factors on ERSEs [29].

Grp78 promoter can also be induced by an ERSE-independent pathway. Associating with CREB1, ATF4 activates Grp78 transcription through binding to a conserved site (TGACGTGA) upstream of the ERSEs [30-32]. During ER stress, ATF4 is positively regulated by phosphorylation of PERK and eIF2α. While in tissue culture cells, the IRE1-activated transcription factor, XBP-1, appears to activate Grp78 transcription [33-35], in XBP-1 knockout MEFs, ER stress induction of Grp78 is minimally affected [36]. In contrast, MEFs knockout of ATF6 reduced Grp78 induction [37].

4. NEW OBLIGATORY ROLE OF GRP78 IN STRESS-INDUCED AUTO-PHAGY

Autophagy is a catabolic process for the degradation and recycling of cytosolic, long-lived or aggregated proteins, and excess of defective organelles. During nutrition starvation, autophagy is activated and it functions in cell survival by enabling the use of intracellular resources under starvation conditions; nonetheless, autophagy could also lead to death in the context dependent manner. Thus, autophagy plays a important role in high eukaryotes as a cellular adaptive response to pathological conditions [38].

In mammalian cells, ER stress has recently been shown to induce autophagy and the induction requires UPR signaling pathways [39, 40]. Interestingly, whereas ER stress-induced autophagy was suppressed by PI3KC3 inhibitor 3-methyladenine (3-MA), wortmannin and knockdown of Beclin1 using siRNA, only 3-MA suppressed UPR activation [41]. This same study further revealed that GRP78 is required for stress-induced autophagy. In cells where GRP78 expression was knockdown by siRNA, despite spontaneous activation of UPR pathways and LC3 conversion, autophagosome formation induced by ER stress as well as by nutrition starvation was inhibited. Electron microscopic analysis showed that the ER, a putative membrane source for generating autophagosomal double membrane, was

massively expanded and disorganized in cells where GRP78 was knockdown. ER expansion is known to be dependent on the UPR transcription factor XBP-1. Simultaneous knockdown of GRP78 and XBP-1 recovered normal levels of stress-induced autophagosome formation.

Collectively, these new studies uncover 3-MA as an inhibitor of UPR activation and establish GRP78 as a novel obligatory component of autophagy in mammalian cells. The integrated role of GRP78 in UPR and autophagy is summarized in Fig. (**2**).

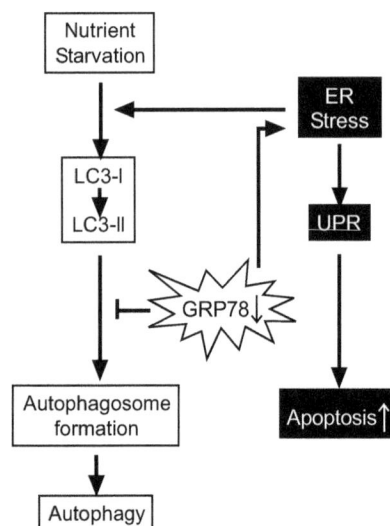

Fig. (2). GRP78 controls UPR and autophagosome formation. Nutrient starvation as well as ER stress leads to LC3 conversion and autophagosome formation. Knockdown of GRP78 results in ER stress, activation of the UPR pathways and massive ER expansion and disorganization. In GRP78-depleted cells, autophagosome formation induced by both nutrient starvation and ER stress is inhibited.

5. GRP78 PROMOTES BREAST CANCER PROGRESSION AND RESISTANCE TO ANTIHORMONAL THERAPY

High level of GRP78 is commonly associated with malignancy, metastasis as well as drug resistance in multiple types of cancer, including breast cancer [42, 43], lung cancer [44], gastric cancer [45], liver cancer [46], prostate cancer [47, 48], and glioma [49]. However, the mechanisms on how GRP78 promotes endogenous cancer in the context of a whole organism are just emerging.

Recently, heterozygous mice of Grp78 with about 50% expression of wild-type level of GRP78 have been created that are fertile and viable, in contrast to homogenous deletion of Grp78 which results in early embryonic lethality [19]. Utilizing such mice and the wild-type siblings as control, the physiological role of GRP78 in *in situ* generated tumor and the consequence of its suppression on normal organs were examined in a genetic model of breast cancer [50]. The fact that GRP78 expression was reduced by about half in *Grp78* heterozygous mice mimics anti-GRP78 agents that achieve partial suppression of GRP78 expression. These studies showed that *Grp78* heterozygosity has no effect on organ development or antibody production, but prolongs the latency period and significantly impedes tumor growth through three major mechanisms: enhancement of tumor cell proliferation, protection against apoptosis and promotion of tumor angiogenesis [50]. Importantly, while partial reduction of GRP78 in the *Grp78* heterozygous mice substantially reduces the tumor microvessel density, it has no effect on vasculature of normal organs. These findings establish that GRP78 is preferably required for pathophysiological conditions such as tumor proliferation, survival and angiogenesis, and its potential value as a novel therapeutic target for dual anti-tumor and anti-angiogenesis activity.

The recent development of hormonal therapy that blocks estrogen synthesis represents a major advance in the treatment of estrogen receptor positive breast cancer. Despite early responses, cancer cells often acquire adaptations resulting in resistance. BIK, an apoptotic BH-3-only protein located primarily at the ER, has been implicated in estrogen-starvation induced apoptosis of breast cancer cells, and was found to selectively form complex with GRP78 [51]. GRP78 overexpression decreases apoptosis induced by ER-targeted BIK and inhibits estrogen-starvation induced BAX activation and apoptosis. Conversely, knockdown of endogenous GRP78 by siRNA sensitizes MCF-7/BUS cells to estrogen-starvation induced apoptosis in a BIK dependent manner [51]. Thus, not only does GRP78 confer resistance to a wide variety of chemotherapy regimens [3], GRP78 also suppresses estrogen-starvation induced apoptosis in breast cancer. These results further suggest that GRP78 expression level in the tumor biopsies may serve as a novel prognostic marker for responsiveness to hormonal therapy based on estrogen starvation and that combination therapy targeting GRP78 may enhance efficacy and reduce resistance.

6. DUAL ROLE OF GRP78 IN CHEMORESISTANCE OF GLIOMA AND TUMOR VASCULATURE

Glioma is one of the deadliest forms of human cancer. Poor chemosensitivity and the development of chemoresistance remain major obstacles to successful chemotherapy of malignant gliomas. A recent study showed that GRP78 is expressed at low levels in normal adult brain, but is significantly elevated in malignant glioma specimens and human malignant glioma cell lines, correlating with their rate of proliferation [52]. Downregulation of GRP78 by siRNA leads to a slow down in glioma cell growth, induces CHOP and sensitizes gliomas to temozolomide (TMZ), the chemotherapeutic agent of choice for treatment of malignant gliomas, whereas overexpression of GRP78 confers higher resistance. Knockdown of GRP78 also sensitizes glioma cells to 5-FU and CPT-11. Treatment of glioma cells with (-)-epigallocatechin gallate (EGCG), which targets the ATP-binding domain of GRP78 and blocks its protective function, sensitizes glioma cells to TMZ. These results imply that suppressing GRP78 with conventional agents such as TMZ might represent a novel approach to eliminate residual tumor cells after surgery and increase the effectiveness of malignant glioma chemotherapy.

The tumor vasculature is essential for tumor growth and survival, and is a key target for anticancer therapy. Primary cultures of human brain endothelial cells, derived from blood vessels of malignant glioma tissues (TuBEC), are physiologically and functionally different from endothelial cells derived from non-malignant brain tissues (BEC) and are substantially more resistant to apoptosis. Recently, it was discovered that in addition to high GRP78 expression in brain tumor cells, it was also highly elevated in the vasculature derived from human glioma specimens, both *in situ* in tissue and *in vitro* in primary cell cultures, as compared to minimal GRP78 expression in normal brain tissues and blood vessels [20]. Interestingly, TuBEC constitutively overexpresses GRP78 without concomitant induction of other major UPR targets. Resistance of TuBEC to chemotherapeutic agents such as CPT-11, etoposide and TMZ can be overcome by knockdown of GRP78 using siRNA or chemical inhibition of its catalytic site by EGCG. These studies provide the proof-of-principle that targeting GRP78 will sensitize the tumor vasculature as well tumor cells to chemotherapeutic drugs. Further studies involving animal studies will confirm these important findings.

7. DISCOVERY OF SURFACE GRP78 AND CANCER SPECIFIC THERAPY

While GRP78 is traditionally regarded as an ER lumenal protein due to retrieval capacity through KDEL retention motif, evidence is emerging that in specific cell lines and tissues, and particularly under pathological conditions, a small fraction of GRP78 cellular pool can translocate to the cell surface membrane. Global profiling of cell surface proteome of tumor cells disclosed a relative abundance of chaperone heat shock and glucose-regulated proteins, including GRP78 [53]. The conformation and orientation of GRP78 in the cell membrane is not well characterized. Interestingly, antibody directed against both the NH2 and COOH termini of GRP78 altered the binding of virus to the cell surface [54], suggesting that both the NH2 and COOH termini of GRP78 are accessible at the cell surface.

The discovery that GRP78 can form complex with other proteins on the cell surface hints at a new functional role of GRP78 outside the ER compartment in mediating cell surface receptor initiated signaling transduction. Several GRP78 binding partners have been identified recently. For example, cell surface GRP78 may be involved in the promotion of survival and metastasis of prostate cancer by activation of α2-macroglobulin as receptor. Furthermore, it is reported that Galphaq11 forms tertiary signaling complex with GRP78 and MTJ-1 on plasma membrane of α2-macroglobulin stimulated cells, indicating the signaling cascade is mediated via G protein and tyrosine phosphorylated receptor [55]. Other cell surface proteins, like Cripto, a multifunctional cell surface protein which is key to vertebrate embryogenesis and human tumor progression, was bound to cell surface GRP78 [56]. The complex of Cripto and GRP78 can enhance tumor growth via inhibition of TGF-β signaling. Surface GRP78 is also reported to associate with GPI-anchored T-cadherin contributing to survival of human endothelial cells [57].

Overexpression of GRP78 on the surface of human cancer cells or in cells under stress provides a potential for cell surface GRP78 acting as a specific therapeutic target of cancer. The antiangiogenic and proapoptotic activity of Kringle 5, a human plasminogen, depends on a high-affinity binding interaction with GRP78 exposed on the surface of stimulated endothelial cells and on hypoxic and cytotoxic stressed tumor cells [58]. In both breast and prostate cancer, surface GRP78 can be recognized by peptide ligand linked to cytoxic agents [47]. In another study, peptide Pep42 was identified to bind to the cell surface GRP78 and can be internalized into the tumor cells [59]. This highly specific GRP78-pep42 interaction can be utilized for drug delivery for cancer therapy. Moreover, human antibody Ab39, discovered through phage display, directs against COOH terminus of cell surface GRP78 in cancer cells but not normal cells/tissues [60]. Further, an 82kDa tumor specific variant of GRP78 offers a new target for antibody-based therapy [61]. The epitope is an O-linked carbohydrate moiety and is specific for malignant cells, which prevents GRP78 from immune surveillance and immune response. The generality of this observation in other types of cancer remains to be determined.

8. CONCLUSIONS

GRP78, originally discovered as an ER luminal chaperone protein primarily involved in protein folding, is now established as a multifunctional protein with surface localization. ER stress induction results in highly ordered, sequential loading of transcription factors onto the ER stress response elements of the *Grp78* promoter followed by recruitment of the transcriptional machinery. GRP78 is pivotal in controlling ER stress pathways and the balance between cell survival and apoptosis. Its requirement for maintaining ER integrity extends its role in regulating stress-induced autophagy. In multiple types of cancer, induction of GRP78 contributes to the tumor progression and drug resistance by promoting tumor cell proliferation and angiogenesis, and protecting against apoptosis induced by chemotherapy and anti-hormonal therapy. In addition, GRP78 is required for drug resistance of tumor associated endothelial cells. The discovery of cell surface GRP78 in tumor but not normal cells opens up new possibilities for cancer specific drug delivery and targeted immune therapy. GRP78 may represent a major adaptive mechanism for cancer to escape host defense and anti-caner treatment, leading to the prediction that its suppression in cancer will greatly sensitize cancer cells and the tumor vasculature to anti-cancer therapy.

9. ABBREVIATIONS

EGCG   = (-)-Epigallocatechin gallate

ER   = Endoplasmic reticulum

ERSE   = ER stress response element

3-MA   = 3-Methyladenine

TMZ   = Temozolomide

TuBEC   = Tumor-associated endothelial cells derived from gliomas

UPR   = Unfolded protein response

10. ACKNOWLEDGEMENTS

The authors gratefully acknowledge grant support from the National Institutes of Health (CA27607, CA11700), the US Army Medical Research and Material Command (BC060145) and the L.K. Whittier Foundation. We thank Miao Wang for helpful discussions and Ms. Sarah Olivo for assistance in the preparation of this manuscript.

11. REFERENCES

1. Ma Y, Hendershot LM. The role of the unfolded protein response in tumour development: friend or foe? Nat Rev Cancer 2004;4(12):966-977.
2. Fu Y, Lee AS. Glucose regulated proteins in cancer progression, drug resistance and immunotherapy. Cancer Biol Ther 2006;5(7):741-744.
3. Li J, Lee AS. Stress induction of GRP78/BiP and its role in cancer. Curr Mol Med 2006;6(1):45-54.
4. Lee AS. GRP78 induction in cancer: therapeutic and prognostic implications. Cancer Res 2007;67(8):3496-3499.
5. Kaufman RJ, Scheuner D, Schroder M, Shen X, Lee K, Liu CY, Arnold SM. The unfolded protein response in nutrient sensing and differentiation. Nat Rev Mol Cell Biol 2002;3(6):411-421.
6. Ni M, Lee AS. ER chaperones in mammalian development and human diseases. FEBS Lett 2007;581(19):3641-3651.
7. Hendershot LM. The ER function BiP is a master regulator of ER function. Mt Sinai J Med 2004;71(5):289-297.
8. Ozcan U, Yilmaz E, Ozcan L, Furuhashi M, Vaillancourt E, Smith RO, Gorgun CZ, Hotamisligil GS. Chemical chaperones reduce ER stress and restore glucose homeostasis in a mouse model of type 2 diabetes. Science 2006;313(5790):1137-1140.
9. Gregor MF, Hotamisligil GS. Thematic review series: Adipocyte Biology. Adipocyte stress: the endoplasmic reticulum and metabolic disease. J Lipid Res 2007;48(9):1905-1914.
10. Rosen ED, Spiegelman BM. Adipocytes as regulators of energy balance and glucose homeostasis. Nature 2006;444(7121):847-853.
11. Lee AS. The glucose-regulated proteins: stress induction and clinical applications. Trends Biochem Sci 2001;26(8):504-510.
12. Barnes JA, Smoak IW. Glucose-regulated protein 78 (GRP78) is elevated in embryonic mouse heart and induced following hypoglycemic stress. Anat Embryol (Berl) 2000;202(1):67-74.
13. Mao C, Dong D, Little E, Luo S, Lee AS. Transgenic mouse models for monitoring endoplasmic reticulum stress in vivo. Nat Med 2004;10(10):1013-1014.
14. Rutkowski DT, Kaufman RJ. A trip to the ER: coping with stress. Trends Cell Biol 2004;14(1):20-28.
15. Sommer T, Jarosch E. BiP binding keeps ATF6 at bay. Dev Cell 2002;3(1):1-2.
16. Rao RV, Castro-Obregon S, Frankowski H, Schuler M, Stoka V, del Rio G, Bredesen DE, Ellerby HM. Coupling endoplasmic reticulum stress to the cell death program. An Apaf-1-independent intrinsic pathway. J Biol Chem 2002;277(24):21836-21842.
17. Reddy RK, Mao C, Baumeister P, Austin RC, Kaufman RJ, Lee AS. Endoplasmic reticulum chaperone protein GRP78 protects cells from apoptosis induced by topoisomerase inhibitors: role of ATP binding site in suppression of caspase-7 activation. J Biol Chem 2003;278(23):20915-20924.
18. Suzuki T, Lu J, Zahed M, Kita K, Suzuki N. Reduction of GRP78 expression with siRNA activates unfolded protein response leading to apoptosis in HeLa cells. Arch Biochem Biophys 2007;468(1):1-14.
19. Luo S, Mao C, Lee B, Lee AS. GRP78/BiP is required for cell proliferation and protecting the inner cell mass from apoptosis during early mouse embryonic development. Mol Cell Biol 2006;26(15):5688-5697.
20. Virrey JJ, Dong D, Stiles C, Patterson JB, Pen L, Ni M, Schönthal AH, Chen TC, Hofman FM, Lee AS. Stress chaperone GRP78/BiP confers chemoresistance to tumor-associated endothelial cells. Mol Cancer Res 2008;6(8):1268-1275.
21. Kudo T, Kanemoto S, Hara H, Morimoto N, Morihara T, Kimura R, Tabira T, Imaizumi K, Takeda M. A molecular chaperone inducer protects neurons from ER stress. Cell Death Differ 2008;15(2):364-375.
22. Li WW, Hsiung Y, Zhou Y, Roy B, Lee AS. Induction of the mammalian GRP78/BiP gene by Ca2+ depletion and formation of aberrant proteins: activation of the conserved stress-inducible grp core promoter element by the human nuclear factor YY1. Mol Cell Biol 1997;17(1):54-60.
23. Li M, Baumeister P, Roy B, Phan T, Foti D, Luo S, Lee AS. ATF6 as a transcription activator of the endoplasmic reticulum stress element: thapsigargin stress-induced changes and synergistic interactions with NF-Y and YY1. Mol Cell Biol 2000;20(14):5096-5106.
24. Yoshida H, Okada T, Haze K, Yanagi H, Yura T, Negishi M, Mori K. ATF6 activated by proteolysis binds in the presence of NF-Y (CBF) directly to the cis-acting element responsible for the mammalian unfolded protein response. Mol Cell Biol 2000;20(18):6755-6767.
25. Parker R, Phan T, Baumeister P, Roy B, Cheriyath V, Roy AL, Lee AS. Identification of TFII-I as the endoplasmic reticulum stress response element binding factor ERSF: its autoregulation by stress and interaction with ATF6. Mol Cell Biol 2001;21(9):3220-3233.
26. Abdelrahim M, Liu S, Safe S. Induction of endoplasmic reticulum-induced stress genes in Panc-1 pancreatic cancer cells is dependent on Sp proteins. J Biol Chem 2005;280(16):16508-16513.
27. Baumeister P, Luo S, Skarnes WC, Sui G, Seto E, Shi Y, Lee AS. Endoplasmic reticulum stress induction of the Grp78/BiP promoter: activating mechanisms mediated by YY1 and its interactive chromatin modifiers. Mol

Cell Biol 2005;25(11):4529-4540.

28. Hong M, Lin MY, Huang JM, Baumeister P, Hakre S, Roy AL, Lee AS. Transcriptional regulation of the Grp78 promoter by endoplasmic reticulum stress: role of TFII-I and its tyrosine phosphorylation. J Biol Chem 2005;280(17):16821-16828.

29. Gal-Yam EN, Jeong S, Tanay A, Egger G, Lee AS, Jones PA. Constitutive nucleosome depletion and ordered factor assembly at the GRP78 promoter revealed by single molecule footprinting. PLoS Genet 2006;2(9):e160.

30. Yoshida H, Haze K, Yanagi H, Yura T, Mori K. Identification of the *cis*-acting endoplasmic reticulum stress response element responsible for transcriptional induction of mammalian glucose-regulated proteins. Involvement of basic leucine zipper transcription factors. J Biol Chem 1998;273(50):33741-33749.

31. Roy B, Lee AS. The mammalian endoplasmic reticulum stress response element consists of an evolutionarily conserved tripartite structure and interacts with a novel stress-inducible complex. Nucleic Acids Res 1999;27(6):1437-1443.

32. Luo S, Baumeister P, Yang S, Abcouwer SF, Lee AS. Induction of Grp78/BiP by translational block: activation of the Grp78 promoter by ATF4 through an upstream ATF/CRE site independent of the endoplasmic reticulum stress elements. J. Biol. Chem. 2003;278(39):37375-37385.

33. Harding HP, Novoa I, Zhang Y, Zeng H, Wek R, Schapira M, Ron D. Regulated translation initiation controls stress-induced gene expression in mammalian cells. Mol Cell 2000;6(5):1099-1108.

34. Yoshida H, Okada T, Haze K, Yanagi H, Yura T, Negishi M, Mori K. Endoplasmic reticulum stress-induced formation of transcription factor complex ERSF including NF-Y (CBF) and activating transcription factors 6α and 6β that activates the mammalian unfolded protein response. Mol Cell Biol 2001;21(4):1239-1248.

35. Lee AH, Iwakoshi NN, Glimcher LH. XBP-1 regulates a subset of endoplasmic reticulum resident chaperone genes in the unfolded protein response. Mol Cell Biol 2003;23(21):7448-7459.

36. Lee AH, Iwakoshi NN, Glimcher LH. XBP-1 regulates a subset of endoplasmic reticulum resident chaperone genes in the unfolded protein response. Mol Cell Biol 2003;23(21):7448-7459.

37. Wu J, Rutkowski DT, Dubois M, Swathirajan J, Saunders T, Wang J, Song B, Yau GD, Kaufman RJ. ATF6alpha optimizes long-term endoplasmic reticulum function to protect cells from chronic stress. Dev Cell 2007;13(3):351-364.

38. Kundu M, Thompson CB. Autophagy: basic principles and relevance to disease. Annu Rev Pathol 2008;3:427-455.

39. Ogata M, Hino S, Saito A, Morikawa K, Kondo S, Kanemoto S, Murakami T, Taniguchi M, Tanii I, Yoshinaga K, Shiosaka S, Hammarback JA, Urano F, Imaizumi K. Autophagy is activated for cell survival after endoplasmic reticulum stress. Mol Cell Biol 2006;26(24):9220-9231.

40. Kouroku Y, Fujita E, Tanida I, Ueno T, Isoai A, Kumagai H, Ogawa S, Kaufman RJ, Kominami E, Momoi T. ER stress (PERK/eIF2alpha phosphorylation) mediates the polyglutamine-induced LC3 conversion, an essential step for autophagy formation. Cell Death Differ 2007;14(2):230-239.

41. Li J, Ni M, Lee B, Barron E, Hinton DR, Lee AS. The unfolded protein response regulator GRP78/BiP is required for endoplasmic reticulum integrity and stress-

induced autophagy in mammalian cells. Cell Death Differ 2008;15(9):1460-1471.

42. Fernandez PM, Tabbara SO, Jacobs LK, Manning FC, Tsangaris TN, Schwartz AM, Kennedy KA, Patierno SR. Overexpression of the glucose-regulated stress gene GRP78 in malignant but not benign human breast lesions. Breast Cancer Res Treat 2000;59(1):15-26.

43. Lee E, Nichols P, Spicer D, Groshen S, Yu MC, Lee AS. GRP78 as a novel predictor of responsiveness to chemotherapy in breast cancer. Cancer Res 2006;66(16):7849-7853.

44. Koomagi R, Mattern J, Volm M. Glucose-related protein (GRP78) and its relationship to the drug-resistance proteins P170, GST-pi, LRP56 and angiogenesis in non-small cell lung carcinomas. Anticancer Res 1999;19(5B):4333-4336.

45. Song MS, Park YK, Lee JH, Park K. Induction of glucose-regulated protein 78 by chronic hypoxia in human gastric tumor cells through a protein kinase C-epsilon/ERK/AP-1 signaling cascade. Cancer Res 2001;61(22):8322-8330.

46. Shuda M, Kondoh N, Imazeki N, Tanaka K, Okada T, Mori K, Hada A, Arai M, Wakatsuki T, Matsubara O, Yamamoto N, Yamamoto M. Activation of the ATF6, XBP1 and grp78 genes in human hepatocellular carcinoma: a possible involvement of the ER stress pathway in hepatocarcinogenesis. J Hepatol 2003;38(5):605-614.

47. Arap MA, Lahdenranta J, Mintz PJ, Hajitou A, Sarkis AS, Arap W, Pasqualini R. Cell surface expression of the stress response chaperone GRP78 enables tumor targeting by circulating ligands. Cancer Cell 2004;6(3):275-284.

48. Misra UK, Deedwania R, Pizzo SV. Binding of activated alpha2-macroglobulin to its cell surface receptor GRP78 in 1-LN prostate cancer cells regulates PAK-2-dependent activation of LIMK. J Biol Chem 2005;280(28):26278-26286.

49. Lee HK, Xiang C, Cazacu S, Finniss S, Kazimirsky G, Lemke N, Lehman NL, Rempel SA, Mikkelsen T, Brodie C. GRP78 is overexpressed in glioblastomas and regulates glioma cell growth and apoptosis. Neuro Oncol 2008;10(3):236-243.

50. Dong D, Ni M, Li J, Xiong S, Ye W, Virrey JJ, Mao C, Ye R, Wang M, Pen L, Dubeau L, Groshen S, Hofman FM, Lee AS. Critical role of the stress chaperone GRP78/BiP in tumor proliferation, survival and tumor angiogenesis in transgene-induced mammary tumor development. Cancer Res 2008;68(2):498-505.

51. Fu Y, Li J, Lee AS. GRP78/BiP inhibits endoplasmic reticulum BIK and protects human breast cancer cells against estrogen-starvation induced apoptosis. Cancer Res 2007;67(8):3734-3740.

52. Pyrko P, Schonthal AH, Hofman FM, Chen TC, Lee AS. The unfolded protein response regulator GRP78/BiP as a novel target for increasing chemosensitivity in malignant gliomas. Cancer Res 2007;67(20):9809-9816.

53. Shin BK, Wang H, Yim AM, Le Naour F, Brichory F, Jang JH, Zhao R, Puravs E, Tra J, Michael CW, Misek DE, Hanash SM. Global profiling of the cell surface proteome of cancer cells uncovers an abundance of proteins with chaperone function. J Biol Chem 2003;278(9):7607-7616.

54. Jindadamrongwech S, Thepparit C, Smith DR. Identification of GRP 78 (BiP) as a liver cell expressed receptor element for dengue virus serotype 2. Arch Virol 2004;149(5):915-927.

55. Misra UK, Pizzo SV. Heterotrimeric Galphaq11 co-immunoprecipitates with surface-anchored GRP78

from plasma membranes of alpha2M*-stimulated macrophages. J Cell Biochem 2008;104(1):96-104.

56.   Shani G, Fischer WH, Justice NJ, Kelber JA, Vale W, Gray PC. GRP78 and Cripto form a complex at the cell surface and collaborate to inhibit transforming growth factor beta signaling and enhance cell growth. Mol Cell Biol 2008;28(2):666-677.

57.   Philippova M, Ivanov D, Joshi MB, Kyriakakis E, Rupp K, Afonyushkin T, Bochkov V, Erne P, Resink TJ. Identification of proteins associating with glycosylphosphatidylinositol- anchored T-cadherin on the surface of vascular endothelial cells: role for Grp78/BiP in T-cadherin-dependent cell survival. Mol Cell Biol 2008;28(12):4004-4017.

58.   Davidson DJ, Haskell C, Majest S, Kherzai A, Egan DA, Walter KA, Schneider A, Gubbins EF, Solomon L, Chen Z, Lesniewski R, Henkin J. Kringle 5 of human plasminogen induces apoptosis of endothelial and tumor cells through surface-expressed glucose-regulated protein 78. Cancer Res 2005;65(11):4663-4672.

59.   Liu Y, Steiniger SC, Kim Y, Kaufmann GF, Felding-Habermann B, Janda KD. Mechanistic studies of a peptidic GRP78 ligand for cancer cell-specific drug delivery. Mol Pharm 2007;4(3):435-447.

60.   Jakobsen CG, Rasmussen N, Laenkholm AV, Ditzel HJ. Phage display derived human monoclonal antibodies isolated by binding to the surface of live primary breast cancer cells recognize GRP78. Cancer Res 2007;67(19):9507-9517.

61.   Rauschert N, Brandlein S, Holzinger E, Hensel F, Muller-Hermelink HK, Vollmers HP. A new tumor-specific variant of GRP78 as target for antibody-based therapy. Lab Invest 2008;88(4):375-386.

CHAPTER 4

Endoplasmic Reticulum Stress and Protein Misfolding in Amyotrophic Lateral Sclerosis

A.K. Walker, B.J. Turner and J.D. Atkin*

Howard Florey Institute, University of Melbourne, Parkville, Victoria 3010, Australia

Abstract: The accumulation of ubiquitinated protein inclusions is a hallmark of amyotrophic laterals sclerosis (ALS), a rapidly progressing fatal neurodegenerative disease primarily affecting motor neurons. However, the exact cause of motor neuron death in ALS remains unclear. The unfolded protein response (UPR) is a homeostatic mechanism, which is activated in response to endoplasmic reticulum (ER) stress caused by unfolded or misfolded proteins within the ER lumen. The UPR activates three signalling pathways that lead to an up-regulation of protein chaperones and a block in general protein synthesis. However, chronic UPR activation promotes cell death via apoptosis. Here we review evidence from human patients and experimental models implicating ER-stress induced cell death in ALS. Recently, activation of all three UPR transduction pathways was shown in spinal cords of patients affected by ALS, including up-regulation of protein disulfide isomerase (PDI), an important ER chaperone, and activation of the ER stress-specific apoptotic factor caspase-4. Similarly, expression of mutant superoxide dismutase 1 (SOD1) proteins, which cause 20% of familial ALS cases, leads to activation of the UPR in neuronal cell culture and transgenic mutant SOD1 mice, which are the most widely accepted animal model of disease. Microsomal localisation and SNARE complex-regulated secretion of SOD1 implies entry into the ER-Golgi secretory pathway, and we discuss the disruptive effects of mutant SOD1 on the Golgi apparatus and general protein export. Importantly, the links between ER stress and other pathways implicated in ALS, including autophagy, oxidative stress and the ubiquitin-proteasome system, are becoming increasingly recognised, suggesting that ER stress is a central mechanism in disease. These observations suggest novel potential therapeutic targets for ALS.

INTRODUCTION

Many neurodegenerative disorders, including Huntington's, Parkinson's, Creutzfeldt-Jacob and Alzheimer's diseases, are characterised by the accumulation of abnormal protein inclusions in affected central nervous system tissues. In amyotrophic lateral sclerosis (ALS), the presence of cytoplasmic inclusions correlates with motor neuron degeneration, although their involvement in the aetiology of disease remains debated. These inclusions take the morphology of skein-like or Lewy body-like ubiquitinated inclusions containing aggregated TAR DNA-binding protein 43 (TDP-43) [1, 2], small eosinophilic Bunina bodies containing cystatin-C or hyaline conglomerates containing neurofilament proteins [3]. Although the cause of neurodegeneration in the majority of sporadic ALS (SALS) cases remains unknown, familial ALS (FALS) can be caused by mutations to a number of genes, including those encoding Cu/Zn-superoxide dismutase (SOD1) [4], alsin (ALS2) [5], vesicle-associated membrane protein/synaptobrevin-associated membrane protein B (VAPB) [6], and TDP-43 [7].

Approximately 20% of FALS results from SOD1 mutations [4], and this form of ALS remains the most widely studied and best characterised. SOD1 is a highly expressed, ubiquitous antioxidant enzyme that exists as a 32 kDa homodimer comprising two 153 amino acid residue subunits [8-11]. Over 100 different mutations have been found that cause SOD1-linked ALS [10]. Originally, it was speculated that the mutations caused a disturbance in the protein's ability to catalyse the normal superoxide reaction, either by a loss-of-function, increase in activity or a dominant negative effect [4]. However the wide dispersion of mutations over the entire primary amino acid sequence and tertiary structure of the protein, and the fact that transgenic SOD1 knockout animals do not suffer motor neuron disease, indicates that loss of SOD1 function is not the cause of mutant SOD1-linked FALS [8]. Transgenic mice expressing mutant SOD1 develop disease reminiscent of human ALS [12], and many rodent models have now been developed [13].

Mutant SOD1 shows an increased propensity for misfolding, and high molecular weight oligomeric SOD1 species are found in the spinal cords of mutant SOD1 transgenic mice prior to symptom onset [14]. Recently, evidence was found suggesting that the unfolded protein response (UPR) is activated in mutant SOD1 rodent disease models [15]. Importantly, these findings led to the identification of UPR and endoplasmic reticulum (ER) stress in human SALS patient tissue [16, 17], suggesting that dysfunction of the ER and alterations in protein folding could be central to pathophysiology in ALS.

THE ENDOPLASMIC RETICULUM

The endoplasmic reticulum (ER) is an organelle with intimate links to the nucleus and Golgi apparatus (GA), which is important for the synthesis, post-translational modification and transport of secreted and transmembrane proteins [18]. Most of these proteins enter the secretory pathway by translocation into the ER as unfolded polypeptide chains [19]. Protein folding within the ER lumen is facilitated by the local environment and ER-resident chaperones which prevent aggregation of nascent proteins by channelling them into productive folding pathways [20]. Due to the intrinsic high rate of misfolding of proteins within the ER, endoplasmic reticulum-associated degradation (ERAD) pathways routinely transport defective proteins from the ER to the cytoplasm for degradation by the proteasome [21].

The ER lumen is an oxidising environment, relative to the cytosol, which facilitates the formation of disulfide bonds in maturing proteins to further stabilise structure [22]. The ER therefore constitutes a protein folding unit that imposes fine quality control on its products, ensuring that only properly assembled and functional proteins are delivered to their destinations. The protein folding capacity of the ER is dynamic and cells adjust their folding capacity according to requirements in order to maintain homeostasis [23].

ER STRESS AND THE UNFOLDED PROTEIN RESPONSE

When the ER is damaged or the burden of unfolded proteins is high, ER stress results, triggering specific signalling pathways collectively termed the unfolded protein response (UPR) [21, 22]. A number of cellular insults lead to increased protein misfolding in the ER, including changes in intracellular calcium concentration, alterations in the redox state of the ER, nutrient deprivation, failure of post-translational modification and increases in secretory protein synthesis [24]. However, the UPR is also activated physiologically in cells that secrete large quantities of proteins, such as antibody-producing plasma cells [25] and collagen-producing osteoblasts [26] The result of UPR activation is a decrease in the

level of unfolded proteins within the ER and an increase in the organelle's capacity to cope with misfolded proteins. This is achieved by inhibition of general protein translation and translocation into the ER, by an expansion in the volume of ER membrane, and by transcriptional activation of UPR target genes, including ER protein chaperones, as reviewed recently [18, 27]. The UPR also enhances ER-associated degradation (ERAD), a process whereby unfolded and unsalvageable proteins or polypeptides present in the ER lumen are returned to the cytosol for degradation by the ubiquitin-proteasome system [28]. Although these mechanisms are often sufficient to overcome short-term insult, when ER stress is protracted and the biosynthetic machinery is overwhelmed, cell death is triggered via apoptosis [29], as shown in Fig. (**1**).

ACTIVATION OF THE UPR

The UPR involves three distinct pathways, mediated by the proximal UPR sensors: activating transcription factor 6 (ATF6), PRKR-like endoplasmic reticulum kinase (PERK), and inositol-requiring kinase 1 (IRE1) [30-34]. In unstressed cells, the ER luminal chaperone immunoglobulin binding protein (BiP, also known as glucose regulated protein 78, Grp78) interacts with each upstream UPR sensor protein. When the load of unfolded proteins in the ER rises however leading to ER stress, BiP dissociates from each UPR sensor and binds preferentially to hydrophobic regions at the surface of misfolded proteins presumably in an attempt to facilitate their correct folding. This results in activation of ATF6, PERK and IRE1 [27]. The ER luminal domain of IRE1 is also able to directly interact with misfolded proteins, leading to activation independent of BiP [35].

Activation of all three UPR sensors occurs simultaneously, with one downstream response occurring through the PERK/eIF2α (eukaryotic translation initiation factor 2α) pathway [23]. Upon release from BiP, PERK dimerises and phosphorylates eIF2α to attenuate general translation initiation. This prevents further protein synthesis when the ER lumen is already overloaded and compromised in its folding capacity [36]. PERK activation also leads to the translation of selected mRNAs specific to the UPR, including that of activating transcription factor 4 (ATF4) [37, 38].

The second pathway of the UPR is mediated through IRE1. Upon activation, IRE1 dimerises and becomes auto-phosphorylated, which activates its endoribonuclease (RNase) activity [39]. As a

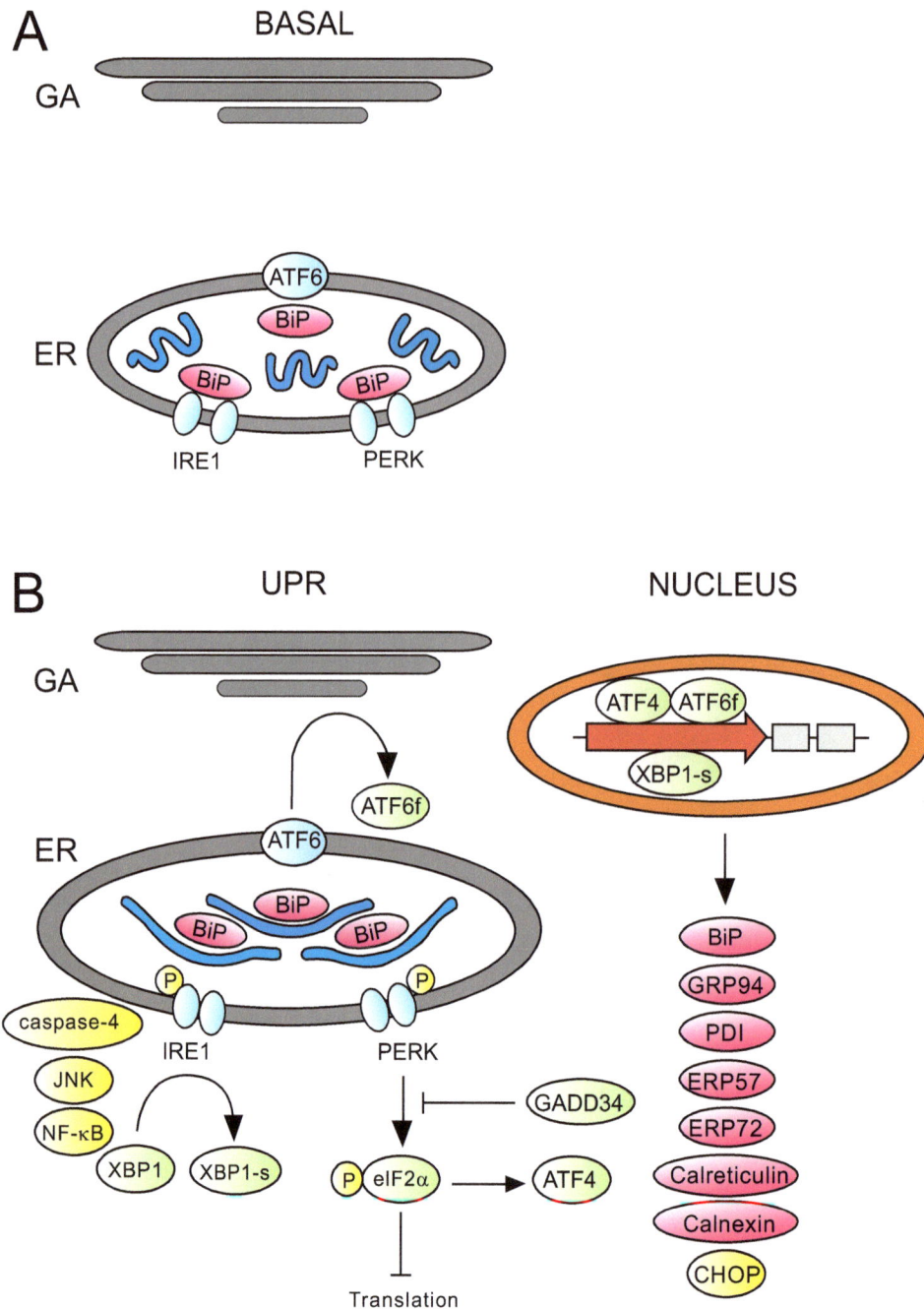

Fig. (1). Overview of major signalling pathways underlying ER stress and UPR-induced apoptosis in mammalian cells. (A) The ER chaperone BiP maintains interaction with stress transducers under normal conditions. (B) Upon ER damage or accumulation of unfolded/misfolded proteins, BiP detaches, thereby activating PERK, IRE1 and ATF6 UPR pathways. Prolonged ER stress results in transition to apoptosis mediated by CHOP, JNK and caspase-4.

result of the RNase activity, splicing of a 26-base intron from the mRNA of X box-binding protein 1 (XBP1) occurs. This splicing modification introduces a translational frame shift into XBP1 mRNA that alters the C-terminus of the protein to create a strong transcription factor [40, 41]. IRE1 also causes activation of the JNK pathway, leading to an expansion of ER volume by increasing phospholipid synthesis and ER membrane biogenesis [27].

Finally, ATF6 is initially present as an ER-resident transmembrane protein, but on activation it transits to the cis-Golgi compartment. The cytosolic N-terminal bZIP domain is then proteolytically cleaved by the proteases S1P and S2P and migrates to the nucleus [42]. Here ATF6 acts as a transcription factor increasing transcription from promoters containing the ER stress response elements (ERSE) [20].

The combined actions of ATF4, spliced XBP1 and ATF6 increase the expression of proteins that augment the ER folding capacity. These proteins include ER chaperones such as BiP, glucose regulated protein 94 (GRP94), calreticulin, calnexin and the protein disulfide isomerase (PDI) family members PDI and endoplasmic reticulum protein 57 (ERp57). As well as the three major sensor proteins other factors have been reported to play a role in transducing UPR signals, including OASIS in astrocytes [43], CREB-H in hepatocytes [44], Tisp40/AIbZIP in prostate and testis [45] and BBF2H7 in neuroblastoma cell lines [46].

ER STRESS-INDUCED APOPTOSIS

Apoptotic cell death is controlled by various signalling pathways involving a number of organelles, including mitochondria, the ER and lysosomes [47]. Prolonged ER stress triggers both mitochondria-dependent and independent forms of cell death [29, 48, 49]. Apoptosis is activated by a combination of signals from each of the three UPR branches as well as Ca^{2+} release from the ER [48]. The PERK and ATF6 UPR pathways both contribute to upregulation of C/EBP-homologous protein (CHOP, also known as growth arrest- and DNA damage-inducible protein 153, GADD153), which is under the transcriptional control of both ATF4 [37] and the cytoplasmic domain of ATF6 [50]. CHOP is a pro-apoptotic transcription factor that may act partly by inhibiting and down-regulating the expression of anti-apoptotic Bcl-2 [51-53]. CHOP is thought to play an important function in regulating the transition of the cell from pro-survival to pro-apoptosis [24, 54]. This is consistent with the recent finding that the activation of PERK continues later into the apoptotic phase of UPR activation due to prolonged ER stress compared to IRE1, since CHOP is a downstream target of PERK [55]. ER stress also initiates other pro-apoptotic events, such as IRE1 binding to TNF receptor-associated factor 2 (TRAF2), which is thought to subsequently induce the JNK cascade [30], p53 activation and disruption of cellular calcium homeostasis [23]. Recently, it was also demonstrated that IRE1 can bind directly to pro-apoptotic BAX and BAK, and that this interaction modulated cell survival [49].

Apoptosis also results in proteolytic activation of ER-localised caspases. In rodents, caspase-12 has been well studied, but since large deletions are present in the human caspase-12 gene homologue [56, 57], ER-localised caspase-4 may substitute in humans [58]. Caspase-9 and -3 are sequentially activated by caspase-12 independent of mitochondrial cytochrome-c. However, the role of

caspases-12 and -4 as initiators of ER-stress induced cell death is currently under debate [59]. It was recently demonstrated that the pro-apoptotic BH3-only family member BCL2 interacting mediator of cell death (BIM) translocates to the ER membrane and is essential for ER-stress induced apoptosis in several cell types, including macrophages, thymocytes and epithelial cells [60]. Evidence from other cell types suggests that other BH-3 proteins may also play a similar role, including Noxa and p53-upregulated modulator of apoptosis (PUMA) in neuroblastoma cells [61].

APOPTOTIC PATHWAYS IN ALS

Apoptosis is involved in motor neuron degeneration in ALS, and there is evidence for activation of both the extrinsic and intrinsic apoptotic programs exists in mutant SOD1 mice [62]. Fas receptor induced caspase-8 activation was reported in embryonic motor neuron cultures from multiple transgenic SOD1 mouse models [63]. Induction of TNF receptor 1 and p75 neurotrophin receptor levels was also noted in transgenic SOD1[G93A] mouse spinal cords, although the signalling consequences were not investigated [64, 65]. Molecular evidence for intrinsic apoptotic pathways mediated by pro-apoptotic factors released by mitochondria is compelling in FALS models [62]. Decreased Bcl-2 to Bax ratio, elevated cytosolic cytochrome-c levels, upstream caspase-1, -8 and -9 cleavage, as well as effector caspase-3, -7 and Bid activation was reported in transgenic mutant SOD1 mouse spinal cords [66-69]. Gould and co-workers recently provided evidence of a cell death independent role for Bax in facilitating mutant SOD1 provoked muscle denervation [70]. Genetic Bax deficiency extended lifespan and delayed the onset of motor dysfunction in transgenic SOD1[G93A] mice, consistent with a mechanism of Bax distinct from cell death activation. In accordance, Bax elimination delayed the onset of neuromuscular synaptic degeneration, long before the activation of cell death proteins in spinal cords [70].

In addition, a role for BIM in mutant SOD1-linked motor neuron death in ALS was recently described [71]. BIM was upregulated in SOD1[G93A] mice during the symptomatic stage of disease and *in vitro* analysis demonstrated that expression of BIM was highly neurotoxic to a motor neuron cell line and was required to trigger cell death induced by SOD1 mutations. Moreover, BIM deletion significantly delayed disease onset and extended lifespan in SOD1[G93A] mice, with diminished cellular apoptosis in the ventral horns of these mice [71]. Similarly, over-expression of X-linked inhibitor of apoptosis (XIAP) decreased caspase-12 activation and extended survival in SOD1^{G93A} mice [72, 73]. Also, deletion of ER-stress related ASK1 and PUMA significantly slowed UPR induction and disease progression in SOD1^{G93A} transgenic mice, as assessed by motor neuron loss, although there was no improvement in life span in these animals [74].

ER STRESS AND UPR IN MUTANT SOD1-LINKED ALS MODELS

Upregulation of BiP was initially reported in spinal motor neurons of presymptomatic transgenic SOD1^{H46R} and SOD1^{L84V} mice, as well as in COS7 cells transfected with mutant SOD1 constructs [75]. Despite finding activation of caspase-12 in SOD1^{G93A} mice, a subsequent study was unable to find any change in levels of BiP or CHOP [72], although an immunohistochemical study of the same model revealed CHOP induction in spinal motor neurons at disease onset, which co-incided with ATF3 and phospho c-Jun expression [76]. More recent studies have shown that BiP is an important player in ER stress in ALS. BiP was found to co-localise with SOD1-immunoreactive Lewy body-like inclusions, eosinophilic deposits and neuritic inclusions in spinal motor neurons from transgenic SOD1^{G93A} mice suggesting a possible association with mutant SOD1 [77]. This was confirmed by Kikuchi and colleagues [78], who demonstrated co-immunoprecipitation of BiP and insoluble high molecular weight forms of mutant SOD1, but not wild-type SOD1, from spinal microsomal fractions of mice. Moreover, the presence of cleaved ATF6, ATF4 and spliced XBP1 in transgenic SOD1^{G93A} and SOD1^{G85R} mice at symptom onset through to disease end stage in spinal cords, but not cerebellum, was also reported [78].

An analysis of the full spectrum of UPR proteins showed that UPR sensors IRE1, PERK and ATF6, chaperones BiP, PDI and ERp57, and apoptotic effectors caspase-12 and CHOP were all upregulated in SOD1^{G93A} mouse spinal cord tissues at disease onset, implying that ER stress plays a role in SOD1-mediated neurodegeneration [15]. This was consistent with the activation of downstream caspase-9 and the executioner caspase-3 by disease end-stage, correlating with previous reports [72]. This was confirmed in a subsequent study whereby IRE1, PDI and CHOP were upregulated in SOD1^{G93A} mouse spinal cord at 60 days of age, four weeks prior to the onset of symptoms [16]. Recent micro-array studies using laser-capture microdissected motor neurons from transgenic mutant SOD1 mice identified an up-regulation of CHOP in presymptomatic SOD1^{G37R}

mice as well as up-regulation of ATF4 and ATF3 at disease-onset stage [79]. Similarly ATF4 was upregulated in presymptomatic SOD1^{G93A} mice, while CHOP (Ddit3) was significantly upregulated at disease end-stage in these animals [80].

Two more recent studies examined the effect of modulation of ER stress on mutant SOD1 aggregation and toxicity *in vitro*. Treatment of neuroblastoma cells expressing mutant SOD1 with the ER stress inducers tunicamycin or thapsigargin increased the formation of ubiquitinated SOD1 hyaline inclusions, which partially co-localised with ER markers [81]. Expression of mutant SOD1 also activated the UPR in Neuro2a cells, and treatment with salubrinal, a specific ER stress inhibitor that prevents eIF2α dephosphorylation, decreased the formation of visible mutant SOD1 inclusions and improved cellular viability [82]. These studies imply that ER stress participates in mutant SOD1 aggregation and inclusion formation.

ER STRESS IN SPORADIC ALS

ER stress was recently described in human patients with SALS, thus implicating ER stress in general ALS pathophysiology [16, 17]. Upregulation of PDI and phosphorylation of PERK-target eIF2α was found in spinal cords of ALS patients [17]. This observation was confirmed with a comprehensive analysis of the UPR, which showed upregulation of UPR sensors, chaperones and apoptotic effectors caspase-4, CHOP, JNK and p38 in human lumbar spinal cord tissue from sporadic ALS patients [16]. PDI was also significantly increased in the cerebrospinal fluid of SALS cases, and immunohistochemical studies revealed that PDI was intimately associated with intracellular inclusions with abnormal distribution and aggregation in surviving motor neurons of SALS patients [16]. These studies confirm the link between inclusion formation and ER stress in human ALS.

ER-GOLGI ABNORMALITIES IN OTHER MOTOR NEURON DISEASES

Dysregulation of ER-related and trafficking processes have also been described in other condtions related to ALS. Missense mutations of vesicle-associated membrane protein-associated protein B (VAPB), a physiological regulator of the ER stress response, are linked with atypical ALS [6]. Mutant VAPB perturbs the UPR [83], and tubular VAPB aggregates are observed related to the ER [84]. More recently, VAPB was found to interact with and modulate the function of ATF6

[85], indicating that possible perturbation of its normal function could result in disease. Similarly, decreased levels of VAPB were found in SALS patient and SOD1^{G93A} mouse spinal cord [84], indicating that VAPB disturbance could be involved in other forms of ALS.

Mutations of charged multivesicular body protein 2B (CHMP2B) have also been associated with ALS [86], and loss-of-function mutations of ALS2/alsin, involved in endosome and vesicle trafficking that also modulates toxicity of mutant SOD1 *in vitro*, result in a form of upper motor neuron disease [5, 87, 88]. Mutant SOD1 expression also causes changes in levels of vesicle-associated and Golgi proteins such as KIF3B and c-Fes in cell culture [89]. Thus, involvement of these ER, Golgi and vesicular proteins in ALS indicates a generalised role of the secretory pathway in ALS pathophysiology.

Insights have also been made from studies of spontaneous mouse mutants showing neurodegeneration. The progressive motor neuronopathy (*pmn*) mouse shows accumulation of the mutant tubulin-specific chaperone TBCE in the cis-Golgi compartment [90], and the causative mutant protein in the ataxia neurodegenerative *woozy* mouse has been identified as Sil1, a co-chaperone of BiP [91]. In addition, the *wobbler* mouse develops a neurodegenerative motor neuron disease due to mutations in the vacuolar-vesicular protein sorting factor Vps54, which is involved in Golgi-associated vesicular trafficking [92].

Similarly, mutations to the gene encoding seipin, an ER transmembrane protein, cause distal hereditary motor neuronopathy [93], which has been suggested as a disease triggered by ER stress [94]. Expression of mutant seipin in neuroblastoma cell culture induces the UPR, including upregulation of CHOP, BiP and GRP94, and mutant protein also shows increased ubiquitination and ERAD degradation [93]. This study suggests that mutant SOD1 and mutant seipin could induce cell death via similar mechanisms involving ER stress, and that protecting cells from ER stress could be neuroprotective in ALS and other motor neuron degenerative diseases [93].

ER-ASSOCIATED DEGRADATION

ER-associated degradation (ERAD) is a distinct process which complements the UPR by removing misfolded proteins from the ER lumen [95]. ERAD involves the retrotranslocation of unfolded proteins from the ER to the cytosol, where they are targeted for degradation by the ubiquitin-proteosome system [21, 96]. Studies have revealed a functional link between ER stress induction and dysfunction of the ubiquitin-proteasome system. Pharmacological induction of ER stress leads to an accumulation of ERAD substrates and compromised function of the proteasome [97].

One important cytosolic ERAD protein involved in escorting ubiquitinated proteins to the proteasome is the AAA+ ATPase valosin containing protein (VCP; also known as p97) [98]. Mutations in VCP cause inclusion body myopathy associated with Paget disease of bone and frontotemporal dementia (IBMPFD) [99], and are associated with protein aggregation [100]. Interestingly, protein inclusions in affected brain regions of IBMPFD patients with VCP mutations have been shown to include TDP-43 [101], which was recently discovered as the hyperphosphorylated, ubiquitinated and fragmented protein present in inclusions of ALS and frontotemporal lobar degeneration (FTLD) [1, 2]. ALS and FTLD have been suggested to represent a spectrum of disorders, with clinical and pathological overlap [102, 103], suggesting that an association between altered VCP function and ALS could exist. Indeed, VCP binds to the cytosolic ER membrane via interactions with the ER transmembrane protein Derlin-1 [104], which interacts specifically with mutant SOD1, causing activation of the UPR in mutant SOD1 models of ALS [105]. Further investigation of the proteins and pathways involved in ERAD in ALS and related diseases will be required to identify if dysregulation of this system is important for causation of disease.

ER STRESS AND AUTOPHAGY

Autophagy (referring to macroautophagy as opposed to the distinct processes of microautophagy and chaperone-mediated autophagy) is a regulated degradation mechanism for clearance of long-lived proteins and damaged or unnecessary organelles (reviewed in [106, 107]). The direct interaction between autophagy, ER stress and neurodegeneration has been an area of recent intense research [107]. Autophagy is activated by ER stress, since pharmacologically induced ER stress leads to an increase in autophagosome formation in neuroblastoma cells, and this effect is inhibited by IRE1 deficiency [108]. ER stress also leads to an increase in activity of the autophagy protein Atg1 [109]. UPR activation and disruption of calcium homeostasis has also been linked with increased autophagy via alterations in mTor [110]. Similarly, transgenic mice with knockout of Atg7, which is essential for functional autophagy, show up-regulation of PDI and BiP in liver [111], while knockdown of BiP in cell culture leads to a decrease in ER stress-induced autophagosome formation [112]. Cross-talk between autophagy and apoptosis highlights the importance of this system in triggering cell death [73]. However the cellular context of ER stress-induced autophagy is important in determining cell survival since the process may either be cytoprotective or destructive depending on the environment [113, 114]

In order to investigate whether autophagy is directly involved in mutant SOD1-linked ALS, one study used pharmacological inhibitors of autophagy or the proteasome and analysed the effect on SOD1 clearance from neuronal and non-neuronal cells [73]. Both wild-type and mutant SOD1 were degraded equally by the proteasome and autophagy. Furthermore, autophagy inhibition led to cell toxicity in the presence of mutant but not wild-type SOD1 [73].

ER STRESS, OXIDATIVE STRESS AND EXCITOTOXICITY

Neuronal cell death due to excitotoxicity caused by over-stimulation of glutamate receptors has been proposed as causative in ALS [114]. Chronic excitotoxicity led to protein retention and aggregation in the ER of motor neurons suggesting a link to ER stress [115]. This was confirmed by a more recent study [116]. Neuronal degeneration and excitotoxic brain injury induced by kainic acid (KA) involved activation of PERK, ATF6, and IRE1, leading to cleavage of caspase-12, increased CHOP expression and downstream phospho c-Jun in hippocampal neurons [116]. KA also induced fragmentation of the ER membrane in neurons, which was attributable to increased calcium influx and activation of glutamate receptors. These findings correlate with previous studies showing that JNK3 is crucial for excitotoxic damage in the brain [117] and that expression of BiP protects neurons against glutamate-induced excitotoxicity [118].

ER stress leading to UPR activation can also increase reactive oxygen species (ROS) generation through an increased requirement for catalysis and oxidative folding of misfolded proteins [119]. Excessive ROS can lead to protein and organelle damage and stimulate cell death [120]. Importantly, a link between oxidative stress and ER stress has now been established in sporadic cases of human ALS [17]. UPR induction and increased protein oxidative damage were present in spinal cord samples of human ALS patients. This study also demonstrated that pharmacologically induced excitotoxicity in organotypic spinal cord cultures stimulates both protein oxidative damage and ER stress, further linking these processes in a common pathway towards cell death.

PROTEIN DISULFIDE ISOMERASE IN ALS

PDI is the prototypical member of an extended mammalian PDI family that is responsible for regulating the disulfide status of proteins, by forming, reducing and isomerasing disulfide bonds, to produce the correctly bonded structures (reviewed in [121, 122]). PDI consists of five main structural domains, nominally denoted as a, a', b, b' and c [123]. The a and a' domains are homologous and each contains an independent thioredoxin-like active site consisting of the sequence CGHC, responsible for the disulfide isomerase activity of the protein [123].

Recently we demonstrated that both PDI and another PDI family member, ERp57, are greatly upregulated in the spinal cords of transgenic SOD1^{G93A} ALS rodent models [15]. PDI is also induced in motor neuron-like NSC-34 cells upon mutant SOD1 transfection and co-localises with mutant SOD1 inclusions [15]. The association between PDI and mSOD1 suggests chaperone-like activity to prevent SOD1 misfolding and PDI upregulation may be a cellular defence against inclusion formation. Indeed, PDI is protective against SOD1 aggregation *in vitro* since pharmacologic inhibition of PDI increased inclusion burden in both wild-type and mutant SOD1 expressing NSC-34 cells [15], and conversely over-expression of PDI decreases inclusion formation (Walker et al., unpublished observations). Importantly, the upregulation of PDI in SOD1 rodents occurs prior to symptom onset, implying an active role in disease [16, 124].

PDI was recently shown to co-localise with inclusions of mutant VAPB in motor neurons of a Drosophila model of VAPB-linked ALS [125]. This correlates with our observations of altered PDI localisation in motor neurons of SALS patients [16], suggesting that PDI disturbance could be a feature of all forms of ALS. Indeed, increasing evidence suggests that ER stress leads to a redistribution of ER associated proteins, including BiP, which redistributes from the ER lumen to the cytosol [126]. The recent finding of pathological modification of PDI by S-nitrosylation on the active site cysteine residues in the brains of Parkinson's and Alzheimer's disease patients, which caused a loss of PDI's normally protective function, has also linked PDI with neurodegeneration [127]. The upregulation of PDI in both SALS and FALS, and its known role in neurodegeneration, suggests that PDI is an important defence against protein aggregation in neurons in general. PDI may be useful therefore as both a marker of neurodegeneration, and could offer a potential target for development of therapeutics for ALS and other nervous system disorders.

SOD1 DISULFIDE BONDING IN PROTEIN MISFOLDING

Aggregation of mutant SOD1 protein is a recognised feature of ALS, which is linked with disease development and cell death [126, 128]. The normal SOD1 homodimer is stabilised by the presence of intrasubunit disulfide bonds between cysteine residues Cys57 and Cys146 (reviewed in [10]). Cys57 is contained within the loop that also contributes to the formation of the dimer interface, and mutant SOD1 proteins show an increased susceptibility to disulfide bond reduction, and protein monomerisation and aggregation, suggesting that reduction of the SOD1 disulfide bond is important in mutant SOD1-linked ALS pathogenesis [129-134].

Recent studies have revealed that SOD1 aggregates contain abnormally disulfide crosslinked multimers in the spinal cord of affected transgenic mutant SOD1 mice [129, 130, 135]. Molecular approaches involving site directed mutagenesis of all four cysteine residues has shown that ablation of specific cysteine residues does lead to a decreased propensity for aggregation [131-133], although these findings have been disputed [134]. While the Cys57-Cys146 bond is involved in normal SOD1 dimerisation, the disulfide reduction caused by FALS mutation may allow the other SOD1 cysteine residues to become involved in aberrant disulfide bonding, creating multimeric disulfide-linked species, which could form the basis of protein aggregates [129].

However the mutant SOD1 aggregates arise, whether by abnormal disulfide bonding or some other mechanism, the formation of a destabilised form of the enzyme appears to be central to the start of this process. Therefore, stabilisation of the native SOD1 structure could provide a new therapeutic avenue in FALS. Recently, aggregation of the common and highly toxic SOD1^{A4V} mutant was shown to be decreased when an artificial disulfide bond that prevented dimer dissociation was introduced into the protein [136]. Similarly, *in silico* screening of over 1.5 million compounds for those that bind to the dimer interface of SOD1^{A4V}, which shows an increased hydrophobic cavity as compared to the wild-type protein, discovered a small set of molecules that were then shown to prevent unfolding and aggregation of the mutant SOD1 *in vitro* [137]. Further development of these lead molecules offers an exciting opportunity for FALS therapy.

GOLGI APPARATUS PATHOLOGY IN ALS

At the cellular level, abnormalities in the secretory GA feature prominently in ALS which is the second focus of this chapter. The Golgi complex consists of membranous cisternal stacks that house transport machinery and enzymes involved in sorting, phosphorylation and glycosylation of ER-derived secretory and membrane proteins to lysosomes, vacuoles and the cell surface [138]. This ER-GA dependent protein secretion is termed the classical or conventional pathway. In neurons, the GA is also crucial for axoplasmic anterograde, retrograde and trans-synaptic movement of organelles, proteins and other macromolecules using kinesin- and dynein-mediated microtubule based transport. Moreover, Golgi structure and stability relies on close association with the centrosome, a juxtanuclear organelle that serves as the mictotubule organising centre of cells [138]. Thus, GA disassembly or fragmentation occurs in dividing cells, but not post-mitotic cells in normal physiology [139].

Raising novel antibodies to probe GA structure in the human brain, Gonatas and co-workers discovered GA fragmentation in spinal motor neurons of SALS, but not non-neurological controls [140]. Occurring in about 30% of motor neurons, GA dispersion was independent of chromatolysis, alpha-tubulin, tau or phospho-neurofilament distribution, suggesting this was not secondary to gross cytoskeletal pathology in ALS [141]. GA fragmentation was next confirmed in spinal motor neurons of Guamanian SALS cases correlating with ubiquitin-positive skein and globular inclusions [142]. Disrupted Golgi complexes were also associated with neuronal basophilic inclusions in juvenile-onset SALS [143] and Bunina bodies in SALS [144], supporting a role of protein aggregates in GA abnormalities. Similar GA morphology was also described in anterior horn cells of FALS cases with SOD1 mutations and posterior column involvement [145]. Recently, GA fragmentation was tightly linked with TDP-43 positive inclusions and cytoplasmic redistribution in spinal motor neurons of SALS [146], implicating the Golgi complex as a common pathological substrate for rare genetic and common idiopathic forms of ALS. Importantly, GA pathology is not limited to lower motor neurons in ALS since affected corticospinal neurons were also reported in sporadic and familial patients [147]. It is now recognised that fragmentation of the GA occurs beyond ALS in neurons of prevalent neurological diseases [138, 139], suggesting this phenomenon is a wider hallmark pathologic feature of late-onset neurodegeneration.

GOLGI APPARATUS PATHOLOGY IN ALS MODELS

The question whether GA pathology represents a terminal event in dead neurons or actively contributes to degeneration was addressed in cellular and animal models of ALS. Expression of ALS-linked mutant SOD1 promoted GA pathology in transfected CHO cells [148] and motor neuronal NSC-34 cells [147, 149]. Furthermore, fragmented GA was not caused by apoptosis and caspase-dependent cleavage of the Golgi proteins GRASP55, p115 and GM130 in NSC-34 cells [147]. In primary motor neuron cultures, expression of SOD1 mutants induced cytoplasmic mislocalisation of dynein and Golgi dispersion, suggesting that disruption of the dynein-dynactin complex may be sufficient to cause GA abnormalities [150]. Golgi pathology was also found in COS7 cells expressing full-length or nonsense mutations of the peripheral endosomal membrane protein alsin associated with ALS2 [151]. Finally, abnormal Golgi complexes were a feature of hippocampal neurons expressing ALS8-linked mutant VAPB or depleted for endogenous VAPA [84], implicating GA disruption in many genetic models of ALS.

Investigations in ALS rodent models have established a potential role for GA lesions in disease progression. Intrathecal injection of cerebrospinal fluid (CSF) from SALS patients induced abnormal Golgi in spinal motor neurons of neonatal rats [152]. GA fragmentation was observed in spinal motor neurons of presymptomatic and symptomatic transgenic SOD1^{G93A} mice, but not age-matched transgenic SOD1^{WT} controls [153]. Importantly, GA abnormalities were first evident at 30 days of age in mouse mutants, suggesting this organelle is targeted early by mutant SOD1-induced toxicity, preceding known time points of distal (47 days) and proximal (100 days) motor neuron degeneration in this model. Neuronal Golgi dispersion was also confirmed in a low transgene copy number strain of SOD1^{G93A} mice with slowly progressive disease [154]. By contrast, GA fragmentation was not reported in motor neurons of transgenic mice overexpressing neurofilament heavy chain that develop ALS-like symptoms, reinforcing earlier suggestions that perikaryal neurofilament accumulation does not underlie Golgi pathology [154]. However, mutant SOD1 and ubiquitinated protein aggregates in the neuropil and soma of motor neurons did correlate

with fragmented GA in transgenic SOD1^{G93A} mice, again suggesting a potential causal relationship between protein inclusions and Golgi pathology [155]. Interestingly, dendritic and periaxonal aggregation of mutant SOD1 appeared sufficient for fragmented neuronal GA in the absence of perikaryal inclusions in young ALS mice [156]. It is noteworthy that GA fragmentation coincided with expression of late UPR markers including CHOP and JNK in spinal motor neurons of presymptomatic SOD1^{G93A} mice [76], suggesting that ER stress induction may promote GA pathology. Moreover, ER stress inhibition prevents induction of Golgi fragmentation *in vitro*, illustrating functional cross-talk between these cellular events in neurodegeneration [157].

Although the molecular mechanism by which mutant SOD1 promotes GA dispersion is unknown, increasing evidence points towards disruption of the neuronal dynein-dynactin complex. An aberrant interaction of mutant SOD1 with the dynein motor was reported in spinal cords transgenic ALS mice and rats, increasing with disease progression [158]. Next, intact dynein complexes were essential for microtubule dependent transport of mutant SOD1 to aggresome-like inclusions in culture since overexpression of the dynamitin p50 impeded aggregation in culture [159]. Importantly, aggresome formation and increasing size correlates with onset and severity of Golgi pathology, providing compelling evidence linking protein aggregation to GA fragmentation [160]. Thus, mutant SOD1 interaction with dynein may affect correct Golgi localisation, stabilisation and cargo trafficking through disruption of the microtubule organising centre. Indeed, inhibition of dynein through neuronal overexpression of truncated bicaudal D2, an adaptor protein of dynamitin, recently induced GA fragmentation in spinal motor neurons of transgenic mice [161]. Alternatively, mutant SOD1 may disrupt the microtubule network independently of dynein. Proteomic analysis of transgenic SOD1^{G93A} mouse spinal cord revealed dysregulation of one isoform of stathmin, a microtubule destabilising protein [162]. Cytoplasmic accumulation of stathmin correlated with dispersed Golgi in affected motor neurons of ALS mice and furthermore, stathmin overexpression induced disruption of microtubules and GA integrity in transfected HeLa cells [162]. Thus, mutant SOD1 damage to the dynein-mediated microtubule transport system may lead to GA alterations in ALS.

SECRETORY PATHWAY DYSFUNC-TION IN ALS

ER and GA pathology in affected neurons of ALS intuitively suggests that dysfunction of the secretory pathway may play a role in disease. Damage to the secretory machinery beyond the GA is also documented in ALS. Classic secretion of proteins from the GA is mediated by microvesicles (minivesicles), synaptic vesicles and secretory granules, also known as large core-dense vesicles (LDCVs). Vesicle fusion and exocytosis at the plasma membrane requires proteins of the soluble N-ethylmaleimide-sensitive factor attachment protein receptor (SNARE) family comprising vesicle membrane (v-SNARE) and target membrane (t-SNARE) proteins [163]. The SNARE core complex in neurons consists of synaptosome-associated protein of 25 kDa (SNAP25) and syntaxin on the presynaptic membrane and vesicle-associated membrane protein (VAMP), or synaptobrevin, on synaptic vesicles [163]. Tight interaction of coiled-coil domains between v-SNAREs and t-SNAREs leads to synaptic vesicle docking, membrane fusion and release of contents, followed by retrieval of vesicles by endocytosis. The ternary SNARE complex is not the minimal membrane fusion machinery though and requires calcium-sensitive synaptotagmin for vesicle docking and SNARE-associated proteins such as Munc18 and complexin 1 for cargo release [164]. Furthermore, synapsin and synaptophysin are components of small synaptic vesicles that regulate their trafficking to the presynapse. Finally, chromagranin A (CgA), chromagranin B (CgB) and secretogranins are constituents of LDCVs [165].

In SALS, synapsin levels were reduced in spinal ventral horns, while SNAP25 and syntaxin were preserved [166, 167]. Synaptophysin immunoreactivity was consistently found diminished in spinal motor neurons of patients [165-169], suggesting that synaptic vesicle formation or transport is slowed in disease. Decreased CgA expression was first reported in ALS spinal cord consistent with GA fragmentation [165]. In a recent study, CgA, CgB and secretogranin II were all downregulated in ALS, often co-localising with SOD1-positive aggregates in motor neurons [170]. These observations are consistent with loss of LDCVs and synaptic vesicles in disease progression, however the impact of secretory vesicle trafficking on ALS pathology is difficult to discern from these autopsy studies.

Nonetheless, secretion of angiotensin, growth hormone, vascular endothelial growth factor and endocrinal Vgf peptides are few examples of proteins reduced in serum or CSF of ALS patients [171-174], supporting some disturbance in the secretory pathway. Most recently, extracellular levels of SOD1 were investigated in CSF of ALS patients based on new evidence of secretion of this enzyme. Genotype-specific decrease of secreted SOD1 was reported amongst FALS patients from one study, while extracellular levels were unaltered in the SALS patients examined [175, 176].

SOD1 SECRETION IN CULTURE

SOD1 is one of three dismutases in mammalian cells. Mn-superoxide dismutase (SOD2) is a homotetramer of 23 kDa subunits located in the mitochondrial matrix. Extracellular Cu,Zn-superoxide dismutase (SOD3) is a homotetramer of 32 kDa and is secreted into plasma, lymph and CSF [177]. Although SOD1 is primarily considered the cytosolic isoform, localisation to other organelles such as nuclei, peroxisomes and mitochondria has been reported in cell culture [178, 179]. Recently, SOD1 distribution to secretory organelles, including microsome preparations and the GA, was described [15, 78, 180], implying potential entry into the conventional secretory pathway.

Mondola and colleagues first proposed that SOD1 is secreted from human cell lines. Radiolabelled SOD1 was detectable in conditioned medium from hepatocarcinoma HepG2 cells and fibroblasts at 8 hours and it accumulated thereafter independent of cellular SOD1 expression or leakage [181]. Next, extracellular SOD1 was detected in neuroblastoma SK-N-BE cells without concomitant release of cytoplasmic enolase [182]. Mild oxidative stress elevated cellular SOD1, but not extracellular levels, suggesting that secreted SOD1 may exert non-canonical autocrine or paracrine roles [182]. Treatment of SK-N-BE cells with brefeldin-A (BFA) which disrupts Golgi anterograde transport blocked SOD1 release. However, the endocytosis inhibitor methylamine did not, consistent with an ER-GA dependent secretory pathway for SOD1 which was ATP driven [183].

However, there are caveats to this proposal. Firstly, how is SOD1 export facilitated without an overt signal peptide? The presence of a cryptic secretion sequence within the SOD1 gene cannot be ruled out. Alternatively, involvement of non-classic pathways of secretion, as decribed for leaderless fibroblast growth factor 2 and interleukin-1β proteins, may be considered [184]. In fact, acute methylamine treatment appeared to promote SOD1 release in the above study [183], suggesting that endosomes may partially regulate SOD1 secretion. This was recently confirmed *in vitro* by association of SOD1 with exosomes which are secreted nanovesicles derived from multivesicular bodies in the endosome system [185]. Thus, SOD1 secretion may be partly mediated by Golgi and/or endosomal-dependent mechanisms.

Secondly, how does SOD1 enter the ER lumen to become secreted? Data are presently conflicting for an ER presence of SOD1. Using cell-free assays, recombinant monomeric apo-SOD1 appeared to translocate into liver microsomes in the presence of ATP [186]. However, microsomal-associated mutant SOD1 derived from transgenic ALS mouse spinal cord was displaced by alkaline buffer extraction, suggesting peripheral association with microsomes [105]. Indeed, mutant SOD1 interaction with Derlin-1 at the ER cytoplasmic membrane surface was sufficient for UPR signalling and ERAD inhibition [105]. Hence, the nature of ER-resident SOD1, whether intraluminal or surface membrane-associated, remains debated.

Despite this, recent evidence that SOD1 secretion is depolarisation-inducible and regulated through the SNARE complex suggests a vesicular store of this enzyme. Ca^{2+}-dependent SOD1 export into culture medium was achieved within 15 minutes in rat pituitary GH3 cells and brain synaptosomes, suggesting an inducible pathway for secretion [187]. Importantly, this effect was abolished by botulinum toxin A treatment, indicative of Ca^{2+}-sensitive SNAP25-mediated exocytosis of SOD1. To define the vesicles mediating SNARE-dependent SOD1 secretion, GH3 cells were co-fractionated for vesicular markers. SOD1 segregated with synaptotagmin, syntaxin and CgB, but not synaptophysin, meaning inducible SOD1 secretion is mediated by LDCVs rather than synaptic vesicles [187]. These findings are reinforced by immunolocalisation studies in mouse spinal motor neurons which revealed partial overlap of SOD1 and CgB [180]. Therefore, it appears that a vesicular pool of intracellular SOD1 is mobilised

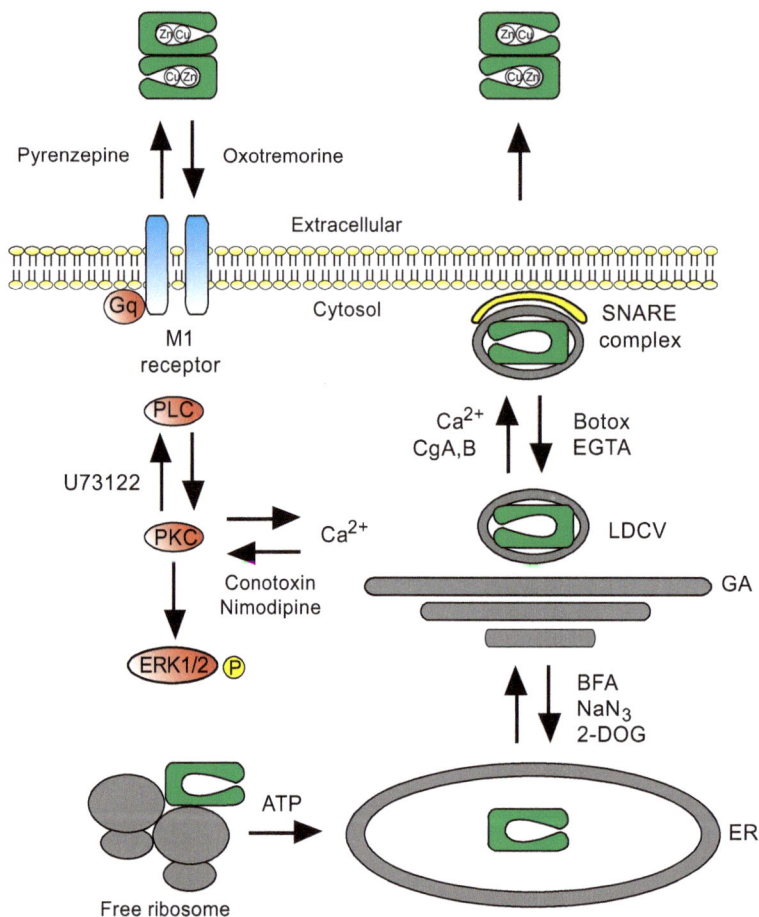

Fig. (2). Model for normal SOD1 secretion and extracellular activity in neurons. Intracellular SOD1 is synthesised at free ribosomes, however a proportion of monomeric apoprotein is believed to enter the ER-GA secretory pathway for loading into large-dense core vesicles (LDCVs) which subsequently dock at the SNARE complex for exocytosis which is activity-dependent and regulated by cytosolic Ca^{2+} levels. Extracellular SOD1 is proposed to interact and agonise muscarinic acetylcholine (M1) receptors leading to phospholipase C (PLC)-induced activation of protein kinase C (PKC) signalling, causing intracellular Ca^{2+} influx and repression of extracellular signal-regulated kinase (Erk1/2) activity.

for secretion in neurons via (1) minivesicles or nanovesicles under basal conditions and (2) LDCVs through activity-dependent SNARE driven exocytosis, as shown in Fig. (**2**). It is noteworthy that SOD1 secretion continues to be reported in various tissues, including human thymic cell lines, mouse primary astrocytes and mixed spinal neuronal-glial cultures [180, 188, 189], implying a generalised mechanism for most cells.

SOD1 SECRETION *IN VIVO*

In accordance with cellular models, SOD1 was detected in human plasma mainly in association with low and high density lipoproteins [190]. As previously stated, SOD1 was also present in human CSF contributing to 75% dismutase activity compared to SOD3 activity which contributes 25% and SOD2 less than 5% [175]. Furthermore, N-terminally truncated species of SOD1 corresponding to loss of the first 20 residues were found in these subjects, suggesting extracellular SOD1 may cleaved. We confirmed extracellular SOD1 presence in rodent CSF which increased with age [126], in accordance with central and peripheral circulating SOD1 *in vivo*.

EXTRACELLULAR ACTIVITY OF SOD1

SOD1 secretion appears both universal and regulated, suggesting that extracellular SOD1 may perform a physiological function. However, it is unclear whether SOD1 binds the cell surface or undergoes internalisation to exert activity. In earlier studies, uptake of exogenously applied SOD1 was essential to protect rat hepatocytes against oxidative injury [191]. Pretreatment of cultures with the endocytic inhibitors, methylamine, monensin and cytochalasin B, suppressed SOD1-mediated cytoprotection, consistent with receptor-mediated endocytosis of extracellular SOD1. Indeed, gold-labelled SOD1 was incorporated by hepatocytes via clathrin and vesicle dependent mechanisms in treated cell culture and rodents [192-194]. Recently, rapid endocytosis of fluorescent SOD1 by monocyte and endothelial cell cultures was observed within 5 minutes [195, 196]. The experiment was repeated with unconjugated SOD1, demonstrating equal propensity for cellular uptake by hepatocytes [193]. Although the receptor that mediates SOD1 internalisation remains unknown, this evidence collectively suggests that SOD1 may undergo active exo-endocytosis between cells.

Mondola and colleagues proposed the alternative hypothesis that secreted SOD1 may activate signal transduction pathways *in vitro*. Biotinylated SOD1

associated dose-dependently with the surface of SK-B-NE cells and was displaced by unlabelled SOD1, but not thyroglobulin or thryoperoxidase, suggesting a specific interaction with plasma membranes [197]. Furthermore, low dose exogenous SOD1 stimulated rapid phospholipase C (PLC)-dependent protein kinase C (PKC) activity, leading to increased cytosolic Ca^{2+} levels [197]. One consequence of SOD1-induced Ca^{2+} influx may be downregulation of extracellular signal-regulated kinase 1/2 (ERK1/2) phosphorylation and cell proliferation [198]. Treatment of rat GH3 cells with the muscarinic acetylcholine receptor antagonist, pyrenzepine, opposed SOD1-induced Ca^{2+} uptake and ERK1/2 dephosphorylation, suggesting that extracellular SOD1 action on cells may be mediated by modulation of muscarinic receptors [198]. In this scenario, secreted SOD1 may regulate neuronal excitability through PKC-dependent signalling as one function of extracellular SOD1, Fig. (**2**). Intriguingly, secretion and action of the classically intracellular zinc-binding protein metallothionein on low density lipoprotein and megalin receptors was recently found in neurons [199-201]. Extracellular metallothionein stimulated MAPK and PI3K pathways, potentially underlying its neuroprotective effects in brain injury.

SECRETORY PATHWAY DYSFUNCTION IN MUTANT SOD1-MEDIATED ALS

ER stress, GA fragmentation and secretory vesicle loss in ALS collectively suggests that defective protein secretion may contribute to disease, at least at the terminal phase. Investigations in experimental ALS have affirmed an early and critical role for the secretory pathway in pathogenesis. Transfection of CHO cells with mutant SOD1 slowed cell surface trafficking of CD4 [148], suggesting a decline in secretory function. Based on the evidence for extracellular SOD1 in cell lines, we hypothesised that SOD1 secretion may modulate toxicity in ALS. We first established that normal active SOD1 was exported by a BFA-dependent pathway in the motor neuron cell line NSC-34 [126]. More importantly, secretion of ALS-linked SOD1 mutants, ranging from dismutase active, inactive and truncated variants, relative to the normal enzyme, was impaired in culture. Further blockade of secretion by BFA treatment compounded toxicity, while upregulating extracellular mutant SOD1 rescued cell survival, strongly implicating disruption of mutant SOD1 secretion in the disease phenotype in culture. New studies in NSC-34 cells confirm these findings, since exosomal-associated mutant SOD1 levels were also reduced in conditioned medium [147]. Mutant SOD1 damage to the Golgi and endosomal secretory pathways may therefore deprive motor neurons of extracellular SOD1 and its putative signalling activities, leading to potential non cell-autonomous effects in ALS. Conversely, retention of secretory SOD1 in the ER-GA and endosome systems may induce protein aggregation and UPR causing cell-autonomous damage. We also detected extracellular mutant protein in transgenic SOD1^{G93A} rat CSF [126], although impaired secretion could not be assessed without corresponding transgenic SOD1^{WT} rat controls.

Secreted SOD1 mutants also have implications for non-cell autonomous toxicity in ALS. From a yeast-two hybrid assay, it was determined that CgB interacts with mutant SOD1, but not wild-type, via Hsp70-like domains that recognise misfolded protein conformation [180]. CgA and CgB overexpression upregulated mutant SOD1 secretion in cultured N2A cells. Exposure of microglial BV2 cells to this conditioned medium induced proinflammatory gene transcription of COX2, iNOS and TNFα [180]. Furthermore, extracellular recombinant mutant SOD1 was

directly toxic to spinal motor neuron cultures. It should be noted that intrathecal injection of mutant SOD1 induced inflammation without neurodegeneration in mice in later studies [202], supporting the proinflammatory nature of secreted SOD1 mutants. However, genetic ablation of iNOS and TNFα exerts no significant impact on disease progression in transgenic ALS mice, suggesting that extracellular mutant SOD1 may be toxic through other means [203, 204]. Nonetheless, these experiments suggest that secreted SOD1 mutants derived from LDCVs activate microglia which may influence motor neuron fate in ALS. This proposal was further evaluated using passive and active immunisation strategies targeting extracellular mutant SOD1 in transgenic SOD1^{G37R} and SOD1^{G93A} mice, respectively [205]. This yielded therapeutic benefits especially in the long-lived former model, assuming specificity of the polyclonal antibodies for mutant SOD1. Lastly, recent efforts from this group suggest that oxidative damage to wild-type SOD1 confers CgB binding and consequent toxic secretion similar to effects of ALS mutation [206].

How does one account for these apparently opposing data concerning impaired or permissive

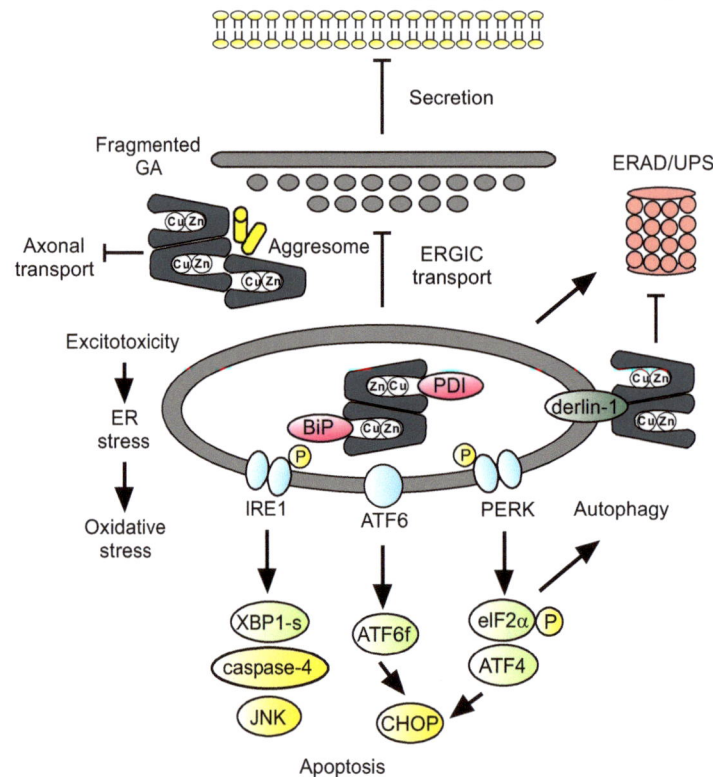

Fig. (3). A pathogenic model integrating ER stress, GA fragmentation and secretory pathway failure in mutant SOD1-mediated toxicity in ALS. Mutant SOD1 may trigger UPR signalling by directly binding ER luminal chaperones or interacting with derlin-1 on the ER cytoplasmic membrane, launching ER stress and apoptotic pathways in motor neurons. In addition, fragmentation of the Golgi complex may disrupt secretory protein transport, promoting ER intracellular protein retention, aggregation and inhibition of the proteasome, impairing ERAD and compounding ER stress.

SOD1 secretion in neurotoxicity? In the case of chromagranin-mediated export of SOD1 mutants, one consideration is that CgA and CgB are depleted in spinal motor neurons in ALS, perhaps subsequent to GA disruption [165, 170]. Thus, this toxic pathway relies on preserved and functional protein secretion which is undermined in ALS. However, a pathogenic model whereby impaired SOD1 mutant exocytosis and toxic secretion act in concert causing cell-autonomous and non-cell autonomous damage is not inconceivable. Genetic modifiers of chromagranin and SNARE proteins in transgenic ALS rodents would provide ample opportunity to test these possibilities.

SECRETORY PATHWAY DYSFUNC-TION IN MUTANT VAPB-MEDIA-TED ALS

Failure of protein secretion mechanisms is also implicated in disease caused by the ALS-linked VAPB mutation. The VAP family members (VAPA and VAPB) consist of an N-terminal major sperm protein (MSP) domain and localise to the ER membrane. New evidence suggests that VAPB is cleaved and secreted in humans and flies, releasing the MSP domain which binds Eph receptors responsible for Ephrin signalling of neuronal survival and death [125]. Importantly, mutant VAP secretion was impaired in a Drosophila model of ALS, leading to ER accumulation of ubiquitinated inclusions and UPR activation. Most recently, VAP overexpression inhibited ER to Golgi transport and lateral diffusion of membrane proteins in culture, suggesting that vesicular traffic from the ER is targeted in disease [207]. Thus, mutant VAPB with proposed extracellular signalling activity induces defective protein secretion analogous to SOD1 mutations.

CONCLUSION

The primary mechanisms mediating motor neuron degeneration in ALS remain unidentified, however it is clear that protein misfolding and aggregation is intimately linked with disease development. Increasing evidence suggests that the UPR, ER stress and secretory pathways are involved in pathophysiology, as summarised in Fig. (**3**). In the case of mutant SOD1, the changes seen in ER stress, Golgi apparatus and secretion occur early in disease, suggesting a critical involvement in disease development and progression. Importantly, similar activation of ER stress has now been found in human SALS. Future studies using genetic ablation of specific ER and secretory machinery

proteins in mice could confirm the importance of UPR and secretion in ALS pathogenesis. Ultimately, development of therapeutics aimed at preventing ER and secretory disturbances could be beneficial in treating ALS in the future.

ABBREVIATIONS

AIbZIP	=	Androgen-induced basic leucine zipper
ALS	=	Amyotrophic lateral sclerosis
ASK1	=	Apoptosis signal-regulating kinase 1
ATF4	=	Activating transcription factor 4
ATF6	=	Activating transcription factor 6
BAK	=	Bcl-2 homologous antagonist/killer
BAX	=	Bcl-2 associated X protein
Bcl-2	=	B cell lymphoma 2
BID	=	BH3 interacting domain death agonist
BIM	=	Bcl-2 interacting mediator of cell death
BiP	=	Immunoglobulin binding protein
bZIP	=	Basic leucine zipper
Cg	=	Chromagranin
CHMP2B	=	Charged multivesicular body protein 2B
CHOP	=	C/EBP homologous protein
CNS	=	Central nervous system
COX2	=	Cyclooxygenase 2
CREB	=	cAMP response element-binding protein
CSF	=	Cerebrospinal fluid
Ddit3	=	DNA damage-inducible transcript 3
eIF2α	=	Eukaryotic translation initiation factor 2α
ER	=	Endoplasmic reticulum
ERAD	=	ER-associated degradation
ERK	=	Extracellular signal-regulated kinase
ERp57	=	ER protein 57
ERSE	=	ER stress response element
FALS	=	Familial ALS
FTLD	=	Frontotemporal lobar degeneration
GM130	=	cis-Golgi matrix protein 130
GRASP55	=	Golgi reassembly stacking protein 55
GRP78	=	Glucose-regulated protein 78
GRP94	=	Glucose-regulated protein 94
GA	=	Golgi apparatus
GADD34	=	Growth arrest and DNA damage-inducible protein 34

GADD153 = Growth arrest and DNA damage-inducible protein 153

Hsp70 = Heat shock protein 70

IBMPFD = Inclusion body myopathy associated with Paget disease of bone and frontotemporal dementia

iNOS = Inducible nitric oxide synthetase

IRE1 = Inositol requiring kinase 1

JNK = c-jun N-terminal kinase

KA = Kainic acid

KIF3B = Kinesin family member 3B

LDCV = Large-dense core vesicle

MND = Motor neuron disease

MSP = Major sperm protein

NF-κB = Nuclear factor-kappa B

OASIS = Old astrocyte specifically induced = substance

p38 = p38 mitogen-activated protein kinase

p75 = p75 neurotrophin receptor

p115 = Vesicle docking protein 115

PCD = Programmed cell death

PDI = Protein disulfide isomerase

PERK = PRKR-like endoplasmic reticulum kinase

PKC = Protein kinase C

PLC = Phospholipase C

pmn = progressive motor neuronopathy

PP1 = Protein serine/threonine phosphatase 1

PUMA = p53-upregulated modulator of apoptosis

ROS = Reactive oxygen species

S1P = Site 1 protease

S2P = Site 2 protease

SALS = Sporadic ALS

SNAP25 = Synaptosome-associated protein 25

SNARE = N-ethylmaleimide-sensitive factor attachment protein receptor

SOD1 = Superoxide dismutase 1

TBCE = Tubulin folding cofactor E

TDP-43 = Tar DNA binding protein 43

Tisp40 = Transcript induced in spermiogenesis 40

TNF = Tumour necrosis factor

TRAF2 = TNF receptor-associated factor 2

UPR = Unfolded protein response

VAMP = Vesicle-associated membrane protein

VAPB = Vesicle-associated membrane protein/synaptobrevin-associated membrane protein B

VCP = Valsolin containing protein

Vps54 = Vacuolar protein sorting factor 54

WT = Wild-type

XBP1 = X box-binding protein 1

XBP1-s = X box-binding protein 1 spliced

XIAP = X-linked inhibitor of apoptosis

ACKNOWLEDGMENTS

This work was supported by the Australian National Health and Medical Research Council (NHMRC) Program Grant 236805, Project Grant 454749 and CJ Martin Fellowship 359269 (BJT), American ALS Association and a Motor Neuron Disease Research Institute of Australia Fellowship (JDA), MND Research Institute of Australia Henry H Roth Charitable Foundation Grant for MND Research, Bethlehem Griffiths Research Council, and an Australian Rotary Health Research Fund scholarship (AKW).

REFERENCES

1. Arai T, Hasegawa M, Akiyama H, *et al.* TDP-43 is a component of ubiquitin-positive tau-negative inclusions in frontotemporal lobar degeneration and amyotrophic lateral sclerosis. Biochem Biophys Res Commun 2006; 351(3):602-11.

2. Neumann M, Sampathu DM, Kwong LK, *et al.* Ubiquitinated TDP-43 in frontotemporal lobar degeneration and amyotrophic lateral sclerosis. Science 2006; 314(5796):130-3.

3. Wood JD, Beaujeux TP, Shaw PJ. Protein aggregation in motor neurone disorders. Neuropathol Appl Neurobiol 2003; 29(6):529-45.

4. Rosen DR. Mutations in Cu/Zn superoxide dismutase gene are associated with familial amyotrophic lateral sclerosis. Nature 1993; 364(6435):362.

5. Yang Y, Hentati A, Deng HX, *et al.* The gene encoding alsin, a protein with three guanine-nucleotide exchange factor domains, is mutated in a form of recessive amyotrophic lateral sclerosis. Nat Genet 2001; 29(2):160-5.

6. Nishimura AL, Mitne-Neto M, Silva HC, *et al.* A mutation in the vesicle-trafficking protein VAPB causes late-onset spinal muscular atrophy and amyotrophic lateral sclerosis. Am J Hum Genet 2004; 75(5):822-31.

7. Gitcho MA, Baloh RH, Chakraverty S, *et al.* TDP-43 A315T mutation in familial motor neuron disease. Ann Neurol 2008; 63(4):535-8.

8. Cleveland DW, Rothstein JD. From Charcot to Lou Gehrig: deciphering selective motor neuron death in ALS. Nat Rev Neurosci 2001; 2(11):806-19.

9. Bruijn LI, Miller TM, Cleveland DW. Unraveling the mechanisms involved in motor neuron degeneration in ALS. Annu Rev Neurosci 2004; 27:723-49.

10. Selverstone Valentine J, Doucette PA, Zittin Potter S. Copper-zinc superoxide dismutase and amyotrophic lateral sclerosis. Annu Rev Biochem 2005; 74:563-93.

11.   Potter SZ, Valentine JS. The perplexing role of copper-zinc superoxide dismutase in amyotrophic lateral sclerosis (Lou Gehrig's disease). J Biol Inorg Chem 2003; 8(4):373-80.

12.   Gurney ME, Pu H, Chiu AY, *et al.* Motor neuron degeneration in mice that express a human Cu,Zn superoxide dismutase mutation. Science 1994; 264(5166):1772-5.

13.   Turner BJ, Talbot K. Transgenics, toxicity and therapeutics in rodent models of mutant SOD1-mediated familial ALS. Prog Neurobiol 2008; 85(1):94-134.

14.   Johnston JA, Dalton MJ, Gurney ME, Kopito RR. Formation of high molecular weight complexes of mutant Cu, Zn-superoxide dismutase in a mouse model for familial amyotrophic lateral sclerosis. Proc Natl Acad Sci U S A 2000; 97(23):12571-6.

15.   Atkin JD, Farg MA, Turner BJ, *et al.* Induction of the unfolded protein response in familial amyotrophic lateral sclerosis and association of protein-disulfide isomerase with superoxide dismutase 1. J Biol Chem 2006; 281(40):30152-65.

16.   Atkin JD, Farg MA, Walker AK, McLean C, Tomas D, Horne MK. Endoplasmic reticulum stress and induction of the unfolded protein response in human sporadic amyotrophic lateral sclerosis. Neurobiol Dis 2008; 30(3):400-7.

17.   Ilieva EV, Ayala V, Jove M, *et al.* Oxidative and endoplasmic reticulum stress interplay in sporadic amyotrophic lateral sclerosis. Brain 2007; 130(Pt 12):3111-23.

18.   Schroder M, Kaufman RJ. The mammalian unfolded protein response. Annu Rev Biochem 2005; 74:739-89.

19.   Wickner W, Schekman R. Protein translocation across biological membranes. Science 2005; 310(5753):1452-6.

20.   Schroder M. Endoplasmic reticulum stress responses. Cell Mol Life Sci 2008; 65(6):862-94.

21.   Romisch K. Endoplasmic reticulum-associated degradation. Annu Rev Cell Dev Biol 2005; 21:435-56.

22.   Schafer FQ, Buettner GR. Redox environment of the cell as viewed through the redox state of the glutathione disulfide/glutathione couple. Free Radic Biol Med 2001; 30(11):1191-212.

23.   Wu J, Kaufman RJ. From acute ER stress to physiological roles of the Unfolded Protein Response. Cell Death Differ 2006; 13(3):374-84.

24.   Rutkowski DT, Kaufman RJ. A trip to the ER: coping with stress. Trends Cell Biol 2004; 14(1):20-8.

25.   Gass JN, Gifford NM, Brewer JW. Activation of an unfolded protein response during differentiation of antibody-secreting B cells. J Biol Chem 2002; 277(50):49047-54.

26.   Yang X, Matsuda K, Bialek P, *et al.* ATF4 is a substrate of RSK2 and an essential regulator of osteoblast biology; implication for Coffin-Lowry Syndrome. Cell 2004; 117(3):387-98.

27.   Ron D, Walter P. Signal integration in the endoplasmic reticulum unfolded protein response. Nat Rev Mol Cell Biol 2007; 8(7):519-29.

28.   Travers KJ, Patil CK, Wodicka L, Lockhart DJ, Weissman JS, Walter P. Functional and genomic analyses reveal an essential coordination between the unfolded protein response and ER-associated degradation. Cell 2000; 101(3):249-58.

29.   Breckenridge DG, Germain M, Mathai JP, Nguyen M, Shore GC. Regulation of apoptosis by endoplasmic reticulum pathways. Oncogene 2003; 22(53):8608-18.

30.   Urano F, Wang X, Bertolotti A, *et al.* Coupling of stress in the ER to activation of JNK protein kinases by transmembrane protein kinase IRE1. Science 2000; 287(5453):664-6.

31.   Ma K, Vattem KM, Wek RC. Dimerization and release of molecular chaperone inhibition facilitate activation of eukaryotic initiation factor-2 kinase in response to endoplasmic reticulum stress. J Biol Chem 2002; 277(21):18728-35.

32.   Shen J, Snapp EL, Lippincott-Schwartz J, Prywes R. Stable binding of ATF6 to BiP in the endoplasmic reticulum stress response. Mol Cell Biol 2005; 25(3):921-32.

33.   Liu CY, Xu Z, Kaufman RJ. Structure and intermolecular interactions of the luminal dimerization domain of human IRE1alpha. J Biol Chem 2003; 278(20):17680-7.

34.   Bernales S, Papa FR, Walter P. Intracellular signaling by the unfolded protein response. Annu Rev Cell Dev Biol 2006; 22:487-508.

35.   Kimata Y, Ishiwata-Kimata Y, Ito T, *et al.* Two regulatory steps of ER-stress sensor Ire1 involving its cluster formation and interaction with unfolded proteins. J Cell Biol 2007; 179(1):75-86.

36.   Harding HP, Zhang Y, Ron D. Protein translation and folding are coupled by an endoplasmic-reticulum-resident kinase. Nature 1999; 397(6716):271-4.

37.   Harding HP, Zhang Y, Bertolotti A, Zeng H, Ron D. Perk is essential for translational regulation and cell survival during the unfolded protein response. Mol Cell 2000; 5(5):897-904.

38.   Lu PD, Harding HP, Ron D. Translation reinitiation at alternative open reading frames regulates gene expression in an integrated stress response. J Cell Biol 2004; 167(1):27-33.

39.   Tirasophon W, Welihinda AA, Kaufman RJ. A stress response pathway from the endoplasmic reticulum to the nucleus requires a novel bifunctional protein kinase/endoribonuclease (Ire1p) in mammalian cells. Genes Dev 1998; 12(12):1812-24.

40.   Yoshida H, Matsui T, Yamamoto A, Okada T, Mori K. XBP1 mRNA is induced by ATF6 and spliced by IRE1 in response to ER stress to produce a highly active transcription factor. Cell 2001; 107(7):881-91.

41.   Calfon M, Zeng H, Urano F, *et al.* IRE1 couples endoplasmic reticulum load to secretory capacity by processing the XBP-1 mRNA. Nature 2002; 415(6867):92-6.

42.   Lee K, Tirasophon W, Shen X, *et al.* IRE1-mediated unconventional mRNA splicing and S2P-mediated ATF6 cleavage merge to regulate XBP1 in signaling the unfolded protein response. Genes Dev 2002; 16(4):452-66.

43.   Kondo S, Murakami T, Tatsumi K, *et al.* OASIS, a CREB/ATF-family member, modulates UPR signalling in astrocytes. Nat Cell Biol 2005; 7(2):186-94.

44.   Omori Y, Imai J, Watanabe M, *et al.* CREB-H: a novel mammalian transcription factor belonging to the CREB/ATF family and functioning via the box-B element with a liver-specific expression. Nucleic Acids Res 2001; 29(10):2154-62.

45.   Nagamori I, Yabuta N, Fujii T, *et al.* Tisp40, a spermatid specific bZip transcription factor, functions by binding to the unfolded protein response element via the Rip pathway. Genes Cells 2005; 10(6):575-94.

46.   Kondo S, Saito A, Hino S, *et al.* BBF2H7, a novel transmembrane bZIP transcription factor, is a new type of endoplasmic reticulum stress transducer. Mol Cell Biol 2007; 27(5):1716-29.

47.   Ferri KF, Kroemer G. Organelle-specific initiation of cell death pathways. Nat Cell Biol 2001; 3(11):E255-63.

48.   Rao RV, Niazi K, Mollahan P, *et al.* Coupling endoplasmic reticulum stress to the cell-death program: a novel HSP90-independent role for the small chaperone protein p23. Cell Death Differ 2006; 13(3):415-25.

49.   Hetz C, Bernasconi P, Fisher J, *et al.* Proapoptotic BAX and BAK modulate the unfolded protein response by a direct interaction with IRE1alpha. Science 2006; 312(5773):572-6.

50.   Yoshida H, Okada T, Haze K, *et al.* ATF6 activated by proteolysis binds in the presence of NF-Y (CBF) directly to the cis-acting element responsible for the mammalian unfolded protein response. Mol Cell Biol 2000; 20(18):6755-67.

51.   McCullough KD, Martindale JL, Klotz LO, Aw TY, Holbrook NJ. Gadd153 sensitizes cells to endoplasmic reticulum stress by down-regulating Bcl2 and perturbing the cellular redox state. Mol Cell Biol 2001; 21(4):1249-59.

52.   Oyadomari S, Mori M. Roles of CHOP/GADD153 in endoplasmic reticulum stress. Cell Death Differ 2004; 11(4):381-9.

53.   Ma Y, Brewer JW, Diehl JA, Hendershot LM. Two distinct stress signaling pathways converge upon the CHOP promoter during the mammalian unfolded protein response. J Mol Biol 2002; 318(5):1351-65.

54.   Rutkowski DT, Arnold SM, Miller CN, *et al.* Adaptation to ER stress is mediated by differential stabilities of pro-survival and pro-apoptotic mRNAs and proteins. PLoS Biol 2006; 4(11):e374.

55.   Lin JH, Li H, Yasumura D, *et al.* IRE1 signaling affects cell fate during the unfolded protein response. Science 2007; 318(5852):944-9.

56.   Fischer H, Koenig U, Eckhart L, Tschachler E. Human caspase 12 has acquired deleterious mutations. Biochem Biophys Res Commun 2002; 293(2):722-6.

57.   Saleh M, Vaillancourt JP, Graham RK, *et al.* Differential modulation of endotoxin responsiveness by human caspase-12 polymorphisms. Nature 2004; 429(6987):75-9.

58.   Hitomi J, Katayama T, Eguchi Y, *et al.* Involvement of caspase-4 in endoplasmic reticulum stress-induced apoptosis and Abeta-induced cell death. J Cell Biol 2004; 165(3):347-56.

59.   Obeng EA, Boise LH. Caspase-12 and caspase-4 are not required for caspase-dependent endoplasmic reticulum stress-induced apoptosis. J Biol Chem 2005; 280(33):29578-87.

60.   Puthalakath H, O'Reilly LA, Gunn P, *et al.* ER stress triggers apoptosis by activating BH3-only protein Bim. Cell 2007; 129(7):1337-49.

61.   Reimertz C, Kogel D, Rami A, Chittenden T, Prehn JH. Gene expression during ER stress-induced apoptosis in neurons: induction of the BH3-only protein Bbc3/PUMA and activation of the mitochondrial apoptosis pathway. J Cell Biol 2003; 162(4):587-97.

62.   Vila M, Przedborski S. Targeting programmed cell death in neurodegenerative diseases. Nat Rev Neurosci 2003; 4(5):365-75.

63.   Raoul C, Estevez AG, Nishimune H, *et al.* Motoneuron death triggered by a specific pathway downstream of Fas. potentiation by ALS-linked SOD1 mutations. Neuron 2002; 35(6):1067-83.

64.   Lowry KS, Murray SS, McLean CA, *et al.* A potential role for the p75 low-affinity neurotrophin receptor in spinal motor neuron degeneration in murine and human amyotrophic lateral sclerosis. Amyotroph Lateral Scler Other Motor Neuron Disord 2001; 2(3):127-34.

65.   Hensley K, Floyd RA, Gordon B, *et al.* Temporal patterns of cytokine and apoptosis-related gene expression in spinal cords of the G93A-SOD1 mouse model of amyotrophic lateral sclerosis. J Neurochem 2002; 82(2):365-74.

66.   Vukosavic S, Dubois-Dauphin M, Romero N, Przedborski S. Bax and Bcl-2 interaction in a transgenic mouse model of familial amyotrophic lateral sclerosis. J Neurochem 1999; 73(6):2460-8.

67.   Pasinelli P, Houseweart MK, Brown RH, Jr., Cleveland DW. Caspase-1 and -3 are sequentially activated in motor neuron death in Cu,Zn superoxide dismutase-mediated familial amyotrophic lateral sclerosis. Proc Natl Acad Sci U S A 2000; 97(25):13901-6.

68.   Guegan C, Vila M, Rosoklija G, Hays AP, Przedborski S. Recruitment of the mitochondrial-dependent apoptotic pathway in amyotrophic lateral sclerosis. J Neurosci 2001; 21(17):6569-76.

69.   Guegan C, Vila M, Teismann P, *et al.* Instrumental activation of bid by caspase-1 in a transgenic mouse model of ALS. Mol Cell Neurosci 2002; 20(4):553-62.

70.   Gould TW, Buss RR, Vinsant S, *et al.* Complete dissociation of motor neuron death from motor dysfunction by Bax deletion in a mouse model of ALS. J Neurosci 2006; 26(34):8774-86.

71.   Hetz C, Thielen P, Fisher J, *et al.* The proapoptotic BCL-2 family member BIM mediates motoneuron loss in a model of amyotrophic lateral sclerosis. Cell Death Differ 2007; 14(7):1386-9.

72.   Wootz H, Hansson I, Korhonen L, Napankangas U, Lindholm D. Caspase-12 cleavage and increased oxidative stress during motoneuron degeneration in transgenic mouse model of ALS. Biochem Biophys Res Commun 2004; 322(1):281-6.

73.   Kabuta T, Suzuki Y, Wada K. Degradation of amyotrophic lateral sclerosis-linked mutant Cu,Zn-superoxide dismutase proteins by macroautophagy and the proteasome. J Biol Chem 2006; 281(41):30524-33.

74.   Kieran D, Woods I, Villunger A, Strasser A, Prehn JH. Deletion of the BH3-only protein puma protects motoneurons from ER stress-induced apoptosis and delays motoneuron loss in ALS mice. Proc Natl Acad Sci U S A 2007; 104(51):20606-11.

75.   Tobisawa S, Hozumi Y, Arawaka S, *et al.* Mutant SOD1 linked to familial amyotrophic lateral sclerosis, but not wild-type SOD1, induces ER stress in COS7 cells and transgenic mice. Biochem Biophys Res Commun 2003; 303(2):496-503.

76.   Vlug AS, Teuling E, Haasdijk ED, French P, Hoogenraad CC, Jaarsma D. ATF3 expression precedes death of spinal motoneurons in amyotrophic lateral sclerosis-SOD1 transgenic mice and correlates with c-Jun phosphorylation, CHOP expression, somato-dendritic ubiquitination and Golgi fragmentation. Eur J Neurosci 2005; 22(8):1881-94.

77.   Wate R, Ito H, Zhang JH, Ohnishi S, Nakano S, Kusaka H. Expression of an endoplasmic reticulum-resident chaperone, glucose-regulated stress protein 78, in the spinal cord of a mouse model of amyotrophic lateral sclerosis. Acta Neuropathol (Berl) 2005; 110(6):557-62.

78.   Kikuchi H, Almer G, Yamashita S, *et al.* Spinal cord endoplasmic reticulum stress associated with a microsomal accumulation of mutant superoxide dismutase-1 in an ALS model. Proc Natl Acad Sci U S A 2006; 103(15):6025-30.

79.   Lobsiger CS, Boillee S, Cleveland DW. Toxicity from different SOD1 mutants dysregulates the complement system and the neuronal regenerative response in ALS

motor neurons. Proc Natl Acad Sci U S A 2007; 104(18):7319-26.

80.   Ferraiuolo L, Heath PR, Holden H, Kasher P, Kirby J, Shaw PJ. Microarray analysis of the cellular pathways involved in the adaptation to and progression of motor neuron injury in the SOD1 G93A mouse model of familial ALS. J Neurosci 2007; 27(34):9201-19.

81.   Yamagishi S, Koyama Y, Katayama T, *et al.* An In Vitro Model for Lewy Body-Like Hyaline Inclusion/Astrocytic Hyaline Inclusion: Induction by ER Stress with an ALS-Linked SOD1 Mutation. PLoS ONE 2007; 2(10):e1030.

82.   Oh YK, Shin KS, Yuan J, Kang SJ. Superoxide dismutase 1 mutants related to amyotrophic lateral sclerosis induce endoplasmic stress in neuro2a cells. J Neurochem 2008; 104(4):993-1005.

83.   Kanekura K, Nishimoto I, Aiso S, Matsuoka M. Characterization of amyotrophic lateral sclerosis-linked P56S mutation of vesicle-associated membrane protein-associated protein B (VAPB/ALS8). J Biol Chem 2006; 281(40):30223-33.

84.   Teuling E, Ahmed S, Haasdijk E, *et al.* Motor neuron disease-associated mutant vesicle-associated membrane protein-associated protein (VAP) B recruits wild-type VAPs into endoplasmic reticulum-derived tubular aggregates. J Neurosci 2007; 27(36):9801-15.

85.   Gkogkas C, Middleton S, Kremer AM, *et al.* VAPB interacts with and modulates the activity of ATF6. Hum Mol Genet 2008; 17(11):1517-26.

86.   Parkinson N, Ince PG, Smith MO, *et al.* ALS phenotypes with mutations in CHMP2B (charged multivesicular body protein 2B). Neurology 2006; 67(6):1074-7.

87.   Kanekura K, Hashimoto Y, Kita Y, *et al.* A Rac1/phosphatidylinositol 3-kinase/Akt3 anti-apoptotic pathway, triggered by AlsinLF, the product of the ALS2 gene, antagonizes Cu/Zn-superoxide dismutase (SOD1) mutant-induced motoneuronal cell death. J Biol Chem 2005; 280(6):4532-43.

88.   Hadano S, Hand CK, Osuga H, *et al.* A gene encoding a putative GTPase regulator is mutated in familial amyotrophic lateral sclerosis 2. Nat Genet 2001; 29(2):166-73.

89.   Kirby J, Menzies FM, Cookson MR, Bushby K, Shaw PJ. Differential gene expression in a cell culture model of SOD1-related familial motor neurone disease. Hum Mol Genet 2002; 11(17):2061-75.

90.   Schaefer MK, Schmalbruch H, Buhler E, *et al.* Progressive motor neuronopathy: a critical role of the tubulin chaperone TBCE in axonal tubulin routing from the Golgi apparatus. J Neurosci 2007; 27(33):8779-89.

91.   Zhao L, Longo-Guess C, Harris BS, Lee JW, Ackerman SL. Protein accumulation and neurodegeneration in the woozy mutant mouse is caused by disruption of SIL1, a cochaperone of BiP. Nat Genet 2005; 37(9):974-9.

92.   Schmitt-John T, Drepper C, Mussmann A, *et al.* Mutation of Vps54 causes motor neuron disease and defective spermiogenesis in the wobbler mouse. Nat Genet 2005; 37(11):1213-5.

93.   Ito D, Suzuki N. Molecular pathogenesis of seipin/BSCL2-related motor neuron diseases. Ann Neurol 2007; 61(3):237-50.

94.   Ito D, Suzuki N. Seipinopathy: a novel endoplasmic reticulum stress-associated disease. Brain 2008;

95.   McCracken AA, Brodsky JL. Assembly of ER-associated protein degradation in vitro: dependence on cytosol, calnexin, and ATP. J Cell Biol 1996; 132(3):291-8.

96.   Nakatsukasa K, Brodsky JL. The recognition and retrotranslocation of misfolded proteins from the endoplasmic reticulum. Traffic 2008; 9(6):861-70.

97.   Menendez-Benito V, Verhoef LG, Masucci MG, Dantuma NP. Endoplasmic reticulum stress compromises the ubiquitin-proteasome system. Hum Mol Genet 2005; 14(19):2787-99.

98.   Rabinovich E, Kerem A, Frohlich KU, Diamant N, Bar-Nun S. AAA-ATPase p97/Cdc48p, a cytosolic chaperone required for endoplasmic reticulum-associated protein degradation. Mol Cell Biol 2002; 22(2):626-34.

99.   Watts GD, Wymer J, Kovach MJ, *et al.* Inclusion body myopathy associated with Paget disease of bone and frontotemporal dementia is caused by mutant valosin-containing protein. Nat Genet 2004; 36(4):377-81.

100. Ju JS, Miller SE, Hanson PI, Weihl CC. Impaired protein aggregate handling and clearance underlie the pathogenesis of p97/VCP associated disease. J Biol Chem 2008; 283(44):30289-99.

101. Neumann M, Mackenzie IR, Cairns NJ, *et al.* TDP-43 in the ubiquitin pathology of frontotemporal dementia with VCP gene mutations. J Neuropathol Exp Neurol 2007; 66(2):152-7.

102. Talbot K, Ansorge O. Recent advances in the genetics of amyotrophic lateral sclerosis and frontotemporal dementia: common pathways in neurodegenerative disease. Hum Mol Genet 2006; 15 Spec No 2:R182-7.

103. Kwong LK, Uryu K, Trojanowski JQ, Lee VM. TDP-43 proteinopathies: neurodegenerative protein misfolding diseases without amyloidosis. Neurosignals 2008; 16(1):41-51.

104. Ye Y, Shibata Y, Yun C, Ron D, Rapoport TA. A membrane protein complex mediates retro-translocation from the ER lumen into the cytosol. Nature 2004; 429(6994):841-7.

105. Nishitoh H, Kadowaki H, Nagai A, *et al.* ALS-linked mutant SOD1 induces ER stress- and ASK1-dependent motor neuron death by targeting Derlin-1. Genes Dev 2008; 22(11):1451-64.

106. Maiuri MC, Zalckvar E, Kimchi A, Kroemer G. Self-eating and self-killing: crosstalk between autophagy and apoptosis. Nat Rev Mol Cell Biol 2007; 8(9):741-52.

107. Matus S, Lisbona F, Torres M, Leon C, Thielen P, Hetz C. The stress rheostat: an interplay between the unfolded protein response (UPR) and autophagy in neurodegeneration. Curr Mol Med 2008; 8(3):157-72.

108. Ogata M, Hino S, Saito A, *et al.* Autophagy is activated for cell survival after endoplasmic reticulum stress. Mol Cell Biol 2006; 26(24):9220-31.

109. Yorimitsu T, Nair U, Yang Z, Klionsky DJ. Endoplasmic reticulum stress triggers autophagy. J Biol Chem 2006; 281(40):30299-304.

110. Hoyer-Hansen M, Jaattela M. Connecting endoplasmic reticulum stress to autophagy by unfolded protein response and calcium. Cell Death Differ 2007; 14(9):1576-82.

111. Matsumoto N, Ezaki J, Komatsu M, *et al.* Comprehensive proteomics analysis of autophagy-deficient mouse liver. Biochem Biophys Res Commun 2008; 368(3):643-9.

112. Li J, Ni M, Lee B, Barron E, Hinton DR, Lee AS. The unfolded protein response regulator GRP78/BiP is required for endoplasmic reticulum integrity and stress-induced autophagy in mammalian cells. Cell Death Differ 2008; 15(9):1460-71.

113. Ding WX, Ni HM, Gao W, *et al.* Differential effects of endoplasmic reticulum stress-induced autophagy on cell survival. J Biol Chem 2007; 282(7):4702-10.

114. Corona JC, Tovar-y-Romo LB, Tapia R. Glutamate excitotoxicity and therapeutic targets for amyotrophic lateral sclerosis. Expert Opin Ther Targets 2007; 11(11):1415-28.

115. Tarabal O, Caldero J, Casas C, Oppenheim RW, Esquerda JE. Protein retention in the endoplasmic reticulum, blockade of programmed cell death and autophagy selectively occur in spinal cord motoneurons after glutamate receptor-mediated injury. Mol Cell Neurosci 2005; 29(2):283-98.

116. Sokka AL, Putkonen N, Mudo G, et al. Endoplasmic reticulum stress inhibition protects against excitotoxic neuronal injury in the rat brain. J Neurosci 2007; 27(4):901-8.

117. Yang DD, Kuan CY, Whitmarsh AJ, et al. Absence of excitotoxicity-induced apoptosis in the hippocampus of mice lacking the Jnk3 gene. Nature 1997; 389(6653):865-70.

118. Yu Z, Luo H, Fu W, Mattson MP. The endoplasmic reticulum stress-responsive protein GRP78 protects neurons against excitotoxicity and apoptosis: suppression of oxidative stress and stabilization of calcium homeostasis. Exp Neurol 1999; 155(2):302-14.

119. Haynes CM, Titus EA, Cooper AA. Degradation of misfolded proteins prevents ER-derived oxidative stress and cell death. Mol Cell 2004; 15(5):767-76.

120. Atlante A, Calissano P, Bobba A, Giannattasio S, Marra E, Passarella S. Glutamate neurotoxicity, oxidative stress and mitochondria. FEBS Lett 2001; 497(1):1-5.

121. Ferrari DM, Soling HD. The protein disulphide-isomerase family: unravelling a string of folds. Biochem J 1999; 339 (Pt 1):1-10.

122. Wilkinson B, Gilbert HF. Protein disulfide isomerase. Biochim Biophys Acta 2004; 1699(1-2):35-44.

123. Tian G, Xiang S, Noiva R, Lennarz WJ, Schindelin H. The crystal structure of yeast protein disulfide isomerase suggests cooperativity between its active sites. Cell 2006; 124(1):61-73.

124. Massignan T, Casoni F, Basso M, et al. Proteomic analysis of spinal cord of presymptomatic amyotrophic lateral sclerosis G93A SOD1 mouse. Biochem Biophys Res Commun 2007; 353(3):719-25.

125. Tsuda H, Han SM, Yang Y, et al. The amyotrophic lateral sclerosis 8 protein VAPB is cleaved, secreted, and acts as a ligand for Eph receptors. Cell 2008; 133(6):963-77.

126. Turner BJ, Atkin JD, Farg MA, et al. Impaired extracellular secretion of mutant superoxide dismutase 1 associates with neurotoxicity in familial amyotrophic lateral sclerosis. J Neurosci 2005; 25(1):108-17.

127. Uehara T, Nakamura T, Yao D, et al. S-nitrosylated protein-disulphide isomerase links protein misfolding to neurodegeneration. Nature 2006; 441(7092):513-7.

128. Matsumoto G, Stojanovic A, Holmberg CI, Kim S, Morimoto RI. Structural properties and neuronal toxicity of amyotrophic lateral sclerosis-associated Cu/Zn superoxide dismutase 1 aggregates. J Cell Biol 2005; 171(1):75-85.

129. Furukawa Y, Fu R, Deng HX, Siddique T, O'Halloran TV. Disulfide cross-linked protein represents a significant fraction of ALS-associated Cu, Zn-superoxide dismutase aggregates in spinal cords of model mice. Proc Natl Acad Sci U S A 2006; 103(18):7148-53.

130. Jonsson PA, Graffmo KS, Andersen PM, et al. Disulphide-reduced superoxide dismutase-1 in CNS of transgenic amyotrophic lateral sclerosis models. Brain 2006; 129:451-64.

131. Cozzolino M, Amori I, Pesaresi MG, Ferri A, Nencini M, Carri MT. Cysteine 111 affects aggregation and cytotoxicity of mutant Cu,Zn-superoxide dismutase associated with familial amyotrophic lateral sclerosis. J Biol Chem 2008; 283(2):866-74.

132. Fujiwara N, Nakano M, Kato S, et al. Oxidative modification to cysteine sulfonic acid of Cys111 in human copper-zinc superoxide dismutase. J Biol Chem 2007; 282(49):35933-44.

133. Niwa J, Yamada S, Ishigaki S, et al. Disulfide bond mediates aggregation, toxicity, and ubiquitylation of familial amyotrophic lateral sclerosis-linked mutant SOD1. J Biol Chem 2007; 282(38):28087-95.

134. Karch CM, Borchelt DR. A limited role for disulfide cross-linking in the aggregation of mutant SOD1 linked to familial amyotrophic lateral sclerosis. J Biol Chem 2008; 283(20):13528-37.

135. Deng HX, Shi Y, Furukawa Y, et al. Conversion to the amyotrophic lateral sclerosis phenotype is associated with intermolecular linked insoluble aggregates of SOD1 in mitochondria. Proc Natl Acad Sci U S A 2006; 103(18):7142-7.

136. Ray SS, Nowak RJ, Strokovich K, Brown RH, Jr., Walz T, Lansbury PT, Jr. An intersubunit disulfide bond prevents in vitro aggregation of a superoxide dismutase-1 mutant linked to familial amyotrophic lateral sclerosis. Biochemistry 2004; 43(17):4899-905.

137. Ray SS, Nowak RJ, Brown RH, Jr., Lansbury PT, Jr. Small-molecule-mediated stabilization of familial amyotrophic lateral sclerosis-linked superoxide dismutase mutants against unfolding and aggregation. Proc Natl Acad Sci U S A 2005; 102(10):3639-44.

138. Fan J, Hu Z, Zeng L, et al. Golgi apparatus and neurodegenerative diseases. Int J Dev Neurosci 2008; 26(6):523-34.

139. Gonatas NK, Stieber A, Gonatas JO. Fragmentation of the Golgi apparatus in neurodegenerative diseases and cell death. J Neurol Sci 2006; 246(1-2):21-30.

140. Mourelatos Z, Adler H, Hirano A, Donnenfeld H, Gonatas JO, Gonatas NK. Fragmentation of the Golgi apparatus of motor neurons in amyotrophic lateral sclerosis revealed by organelle-specific antibodies. Proc Natl Acad Sci U S A 1990; 87(11):4393-5.

141. Gonatas NK, Stieber A, Mourelatos Z, et al. Fragmentation of the Golgi apparatus of motor neurons in amyotrophic lateral sclerosis. Am J Pathol 1992; 140(3):731-7.

142. Mourelatos Z, Hirano A, Rosenquist AC, Gonatas NK. Fragmentation of the Golgi apparatus of motor neurons in amyotrophic lateral sclerosis (ALS). Clinical studies in ALS of Guam and experimental studies in deafferented neurons and in beta,beta'-iminodipropionitrile axonopathy. Am J Pathol 1994; 144(6):1288-300.

143. Fujita Y, Okamoto K, Sakurai A, et al. The Golgi apparatus is fragmented in spinal cord motor neurons of amyotrophic lateral sclerosis with basophilic inclusions. Acta Neuropathol (Berl) 2002; 103(3):243-7.

144. Fujita Y, Okamoto K. Golgi apparatus of the motor neurons in patients with amyotrophic lateral sclerosis and in mice models of amyotrophic lateral sclerosis. Neuropathology 2005; 25(4):388-94.

145. Fujita Y, Okamoto K, Sakurai A, Gonatas NK, Hirano A. Fragmentation of the Golgi apparatus of the anterior horn cells in patients with familial amyotrophic lateral sclerosis with SOD1 mutations and posterior column involvement. J Neurol Sci 2000; 174(2):137-40.

146. Fujita Y, Mizuno Y, Takatama M, Okamoto K. Anterior horn cells with abnormal TDP-43

immunoreactivities show fragmentation of the Golgi apparatus in ALS. J Neurol Sci 2008; 269(1-2):30-4.

147.   Gomes C, Palma AS, Almeida R, *et al.* Establishment of a cell model of ALS disease: Golgi apparatus disruption occurs independently from apoptosis. Biotechnol Lett 2008; 30(4):603-10.

148.   Stieber A, Gonatas JO, Moore JS, *et al.* Disruption of the structure of the Golgi apparatus and the function of the secretory pathway by mutants G93A and G85R of Cu, Zn superoxide dismutase (SOD1) of familial amyotrophic lateral sclerosis. J Neurol Sci 2004; 219(1-2):45-53.

149.   Turner BJ, Atkin JD. ER stress and UPR in familial amyotrophic lateral sclerosis. Curr Mol Med 2006; 6(1):79-86.

150.   Ligon LA, LaMonte BH, Wallace KE, Weber N, Kalb RG, Holzbaur EL. Mutant superoxide dismutase disrupts cytoplasmic dynein in motor neurons. Neuroreport 2005; 16(6):533-6.

151.   Millecamps S, Gentil BJ, Gros-Louis F, Rouleau G, Julien JP. Alsin is partially associated with centrosome in human cells. Biochim Biophys Acta 2005; 1745(1):84-100.

152.   Ramamohan PY, Gourie-Devi M, Nalini A, *et al.* Cerebrospinal fluid from amyotrophic lateral sclerosis patients causes fragmentation of the Golgi apparatus in the neonatal rat spinal cord. Amyotroph Lateral Scler 2007; 8(2):79-82.

153.   Mourelatos Z, Gonatas NK, Stieber A, Gurney ME, Dal Canto MC. The Golgi apparatus of spinal cord motor neurons in transgenic mice expressing mutant Cu,Zn superoxide dismutase becomes fragmented in early, preclinical stages of the disease. Proc Natl Acad Sci U S A 1996; 93(11):5472-7.

154.   Stieber A, Gonatas JO, Collard J, *et al.* The neuronal Golgi apparatus is fragmented in transgenic mice expressing a mutant human SOD1, but not in mice expressing the human NF-H gene. J Neurol Sci 2000; 173(1):63-72.

155.   Stieber A, Gonatas JO, Gonatas NK. Aggregation of ubiquitin and a mutant ALS-linked SOD1 protein correlate with disease progression and fragmentation of the Golgi apparatus. J Neurol Sci 2000; 173(1):53-62.

156.   Stieber A, Gonatas JO, Gonatas NK. Aggregates of mutant protein appear progressively in dendrites, in periaxonal processes of oligodendrocytes, and in neuronal and astrocytic perikarya of mice expressing the SOD1(G93A) mutation of familial amyotrophic lateral sclerosis. J Neurol Sci 2000; 177(2):114-23.

157.   Nakagomi S, Barsoum MJ, Bossy-Wetzel E, Sutterlin C, Malhotra V, Lipton SA. A Golgi fragmentation pathway in neurodegeneration. Neurobiol Dis 2007;

158.   Zhang F, Strom AL, Fukada K, Lee S, Hayward LJ, Zhu H. Interaction between familial amyotrophic lateral sclerosis (ALS)-linked SOD1 mutants and the dynein complex. J Biol Chem 2007; 282(22):16691-9.

159.   Strom AL, Shi P, Zhang F, *et al.* Interaction of amyotrophic lateral sclerosis (ALS)-related mutant copper-zinc superoxide dismutase with the dynein-dynactin complex contributes to inclusion formation. J Biol Chem 2008; 283(33):22795-805.

160.   Garcia-Mata R, Bebok Z, Sorscher EJ, Sztul ES. Characterization and dynamics of aggresome formation by a cytosolic GFP-chimera. J Cell Biol 1999; 146(6):1239-54.

161.   Teuling E, van Dis V, Wulf PS, *et al.* A novel mouse model with impaired dynein/dynactin function develops amyotrophic lateral sclerosis (ALS)-like features in motor neurons and improves lifespan in

SOD1-ALS mice. Hum Mol Genet 2008; 17(18):2849-62.

162.   Strey CW, Spellman D, Stieber A, *et al.* Dysregulation of stathmin, a microtubule-destabilizing protein, and up-regulation of Hsp25, Hsp27, and the antioxidant peroxiredoxin 6 in a mouse model of familial amyotrophic lateral sclerosis. Am J Pathol 2004; 165(5):1701-18.

163.   Jahn R, Scheller RH. SNAREs--engines for membrane fusion. Nat Rev Mol Cell Biol 2006; 7(9):631-43.

164.   Rizo J, Chen X, Arac D. Unraveling the mechanisms of synaptotagmin and SNARE function in neurotransmitter release. Trends Cell Biol 2006; 16(7):339-50.

165.   Schiffer D, Cordera S, Giordana MT, Attanasio A, Pezzulo T. Synaptic vesicle proteins, synaptophysin and chromogranin A in amyotrophic lateral sclerosis. J Neurol Sci 1995; 129 Suppl:68-74.

166.   Ikemoto A, Nakamura S, Akiguchi I, Hirano A. Differential expression between synaptic vesicle proteins and presynaptic plasma membrane proteins in the anterior horn of amyotrophic lateral sclerosis. Acta Neuropathol 2002; 103(2):179-87.

167.   Brockington A, Wharton SB, Fernando M, *et al.* Expression of vascular endothelial growth factor and its receptors in the central nervous system in amyotrophic lateral sclerosis. J Neuropathol Exp Neurol 2006; 65(1):26-36.

168.   Sasaki S, Maruyama S. Synapse loss in anterior horn neurons in amyotrophic lateral sclerosis. Acta Neuropathol 1994; 88(3):222-7.

169.   Ikemoto A, Hirano A. Comparative immunohistochemical study on synaptophysin expression in the anterior horn of post-poliomyelitis and sporadic amyotrophic lateral sclerosis. Acta Neuropathol 1996; 92(5):473-8.

170.   Schrott-Fischer A, Bitsche M, Humpel C, *et al.* Chromogranin peptides in amyotrophic lateral sclerosis. Regul Pept 2009; 152(1-3):13-21.

171.   Devos D, Moreau C, Lassalle P, *et al.* Low levels of the vascular endothelial growth factor in CSF from early ALS patients. Neurology 2004; 62(11):2127-9.

172.   Morselli LL, Bongioanni P, Genovesi M, *et al.* Growth hormone secretion is impaired in amyotrophic lateral sclerosis. Clin Endocrinol (Oxf) 2006; 65(3):385-8.

173.   Kawajiri M, Mogi M, Higaki N, *et al.* Reduced angiotensin II levels in the cerebrospinal fluid of patients with amyotrophic lateral sclerosis. Acta Neurol Scand 2008;

174.   Zhao Z, Lange DJ, Ho L, *et al.* Vgf is a novel biomarker associated with muscle weakness in amyotrophic lateral sclerosis (ALS), with a potential role in disease pathogenesis. Int J Med Sci 2008; 5(2):92-9.

175.   Jacobsson J, Jonsson PA, Andersen PM, Forsgren L, Marklund SL. Superoxide dismutase in CSF from amyotrophic lateral sclerosis patients with and without CuZn-superoxide dismutase mutations. Brain 2001; 124(Pt 7):1461-6.

176.   Frutiger K, Lukas TJ, Gorrie G, Ajroud-Driss S, Siddique T. Gender difference in levels of Cu/Zn superoxide dismutase (SOD1) in cerebrospinal fluid of patients with amyotrophic lateral sclerosis. Amyotroph Lateral Scler 2008; 9(3):184-7.

177.   Zelko IN, Mariani TJ, Folz RJ. Superoxide dismutase multigene family: a comparison of the CuZn-SOD (SOD1), Mn-SOD (SOD2), and EC-SOD (SOD3) gene structures, evolution, and expression. Free Radic Biol Med 2002; 33(3):337-49.

178. Crapo JD, Oury T, Rabouille C, Slot JW, Chang LY. Copper,zinc superoxide dismutase is primarily a cytosolic protein in human cells. Proc Natl Acad Sci U S A 1992; 89(21):10405-9.

179. Sturtz LA, Diekert K, Jensen LT, Lill R, Culotta VC. A fraction of yeast Cu,Zn-superoxide dismutase and its metallochaperone, CCS, localize to the intermembrane space of mitochondria. A physiological role for SOD1 in guarding against mitochondrial oxidative damage. J Biol Chem 2001; 276(41):38084-9.

180. Urushitani M, Sik A, Sakurai T, Nukina N, Takahashi R, Julien JP. Chromogranin-mediated secretion of mutant superoxide dismutase proteins linked to amyotrophic lateral sclerosis. Nat Neurosci 2006; 9(1):108-18.

181. Mondola P, Annella T, Santillo M, Santangelo F. Evidence for secretion of cytosolic CuZn superoxide dismutase by Hep G2 cells and human fibroblasts. Int J Biochem Cell Biol 1996; 28(6):677-81.

182. Mondola P, Annella T, Seru R, *et al.* Secretion and increase of intracellular CuZn superoxide dismutase content in human neuroblastoma SK-N-BE cells subjected to oxidative stress. Brain Res Bull 1998; 45(5):517-20.

183. Mondola P, Ruggiero G, Seru R, *et al.* The Cu,Zn superoxide dismutase in neuroblastoma SK-N-BE cells is exported by a microvesicles dependent pathway. Brain Res Mol Brain Res 2003; 110(1):45-51.

184. Nickel W. Unconventional secretory routes: direct protein export across the plasma membrane of mammalian cells. Traffic 2005; 6(8):607-14.

185. Gomes C, Keller S, Altevogt P, Costa J. Evidence for secretion of Cu,Zn superoxide dismutase via exosomes from a cell model of amyotrophic lateral sclerosis. Neurosci Lett 2007; 428(1):43-6.

186. Urushitani M, Ezzi SA, Matsuo A, Tooyama I, Julien JP. The endoplasmic reticulum-Golgi pathway is a target for translocation and aggregation of mutant superoxide dismutase linked to ALS. Faseb J 2008; 22(7):2476-87.

187. Santillo M, Secondo A, Seru R, *et al.* Evidence of calcium- and SNARE-dependent release of CuZn superoxide dismutase from rat pituitary GH3 cells and synaptosomes in response to depolarization. J Neurochem 2007; 102(3):679-85.

188. Cimini V, Ruggiero G, Buonomo T, *et al.* CuZn-superoxide dismutase in human thymus: immunocytochemical localisation and secretion in thymus-derived epithelial and fibroblast cell lines. Histochem Cell Biol 2002; 118(2):163-9.

189. Lafon-Cazal M, Adjali O, Galeotti N, *et al.* Proteomic analysis of astrocytic secretion in the mouse. Comparison with the cerebrospinal fluid proteome. J Biol Chem 2003; 278(27):24438-48.

190. Mondola P, Bifulco M, Seru R, Annella T, Ciriolo MR, Santillo M. Presence of CuZn superoxide dismutase in human serum lipoproteins. FEBS Lett 2000; 467(1):57-60.

191. Kyle ME, Nakae D, Sakaida I, Miccadei S, Farber JL. Endocytosis of superoxide dismutase is required in order for the enzyme to protect hepatocytes from the cytotoxicity of hydrogen peroxide. J Biol Chem 1988; 263(8):3784-9.

192. Dini L, Rotilio G. Electron microscopic evidence for endocytosis of superoxide dismutase by hepatocytes using protein-gold adducts. Biochem Biophys Res Commun 1989; 162(3):940-4.

193. Dini L, Rossi L, Lentini A, De Martino A, Rotilio G. Immunocytochemical study of binding and internalization of carrier-free Cu, Zn Superoxide dismutase by cultured rat hepatocytes. Cell Mol Biol 1995; 41(8):1051-9.

194. Dini L, Falasca L, Rossi L, Rotilio G. In vivo uptake of Cu, Zn superoxide dismutase. Morphological evidence for preferential endocytosis and accumulation by sinusoidal liver cells. Cell Mol Biol 1996; 42(2):269-77.

195. Filipe P, Emerit I, Vassy J, Levy A, Huang V, Freitas J. Cellular penetration of fluorescently labeled superoxide dismutases of various origins. Mol Med 1999; 5(8):517-25.

196. Waelti ER, Barton M. Rapid endocytosis of copper-zinc superoxide dismutase into human endothelial cells: role for its vascular activity. Pharmacology 2006; 78(4):198-201.

197. Mondola P, Santillo M, Seru R, *et al.* Cu,Zn superoxide dismutase increases intracellular calcium levels via a phospholipase C-protein kinase C pathway in SK-N-BE neuroblastoma cells. Biochem Biophys Res Commun 2004; 324(2):887-92.

198. Secondo A, De Mizio M, Zirpoli L, Santillo M, Mondola P. The Cu-Zn superoxide dismutase (SOD1) inhibits ERK phosphorylation by muscarinic receptor modulation in rat pituitary GH3 cells. Biochem Biophys Res Commun 2008; 376(1):143-7.

199. Fitzgerald M, Nairn P, Bartlett CA, Chung RS, West AK, Beazley LD. Metallothionein-IIA promotes neurite growth via the megalin receptor. Exp Brain Res 2007; 183(2):171-80.

200. Ambjorn M, Asmussen JW, Lindstam M, *et al.* Metallothionein and a peptide modeled after metallothionein, EmtinB, induce neuronal differentiation and survival through binding to receptors of the low-density lipoprotein receptor family. J Neurochem 2008; 104(1):21-37.

201. Chung RS, Penkowa M, Dittmann J, *et al.* Redefining the role of metallothionein within the injured brain: extracellular metallothioneins play an important role in the astrocyte-neuron response to injury. J Biol Chem 2008; 283(22):15349-58.

202. Kang J, Rivest S. MyD88-deficient bone marrow cells accelerate onset and reduce survival in a mouse model of amyotrophic lateral sclerosis. J Cell Biol 2007; 179(6):1219-30.

203. Son M, Fathallah-Shaykh HM, Elliott JL. Survival in a transgenic model of FALS is independent of iNOS expression. Ann Neurol 2001; 50(2):273.

204. Gowing G, Dequen F, Soucy G, Julien JP. Absence of tumor necrosis factor-alpha does not affect motor neuron disease caused by superoxide dismutase 1 mutations. J Neurosci 2006; 26(44):11397-402.

205. Urushitani M, Ezzi SA, Julien JP. Therapeutic effects of immunization with mutant superoxide dismutase in mice models of amyotrophic lateral sclerosis. Proc Natl Acad Sci U S A 2007; 104(7):2495-500.

206. Ezzi SA, Urushitani M, Julien JP. Wild-type superoxide dismutase acquires binding and toxic properties of ALS-linked mutant forms through oxidation. J Neurochem 2007; 102(1):170-8.

207. Prosser DC, Tran D, Gougeon PY, Verly C, Ngsee JK. FFAT rescues VAPA-mediated inhibition of ER-to-Golgi transport and VAPB-mediated ER aggregation. J Cell Sci 2008; 121(Pt 18):3052-61.

CHAPTER 5

ER Stress Signaling Network in Pancreatic β-Cells

Sonya G. Fonseca and Fumihiko Urano*

University of Massachusetts Medical School, Worcester, MA 01605, USA

Abstract: Pancreatic β-cells are specialized to control blood glucose levels by producing and secreting the hormone insulin. Increasing evidence indicates that the endoplasmic reticulum (ER) stress signaling network has an important function in maintaining β-cell homeostasis. Thus, dysfunction of ER stress signaling has harmful effects on β-cell function, leading to β-cell dysfunction and death in type 1 and type 2 diabetes. In this article, we will summarize the role of ER stress signaling in pancreatic β-cells.

INTRODUCTION

Pancreatic β-cells are specialized to control blood glucose levels by producing and secreting the hormone insulin. These cells, with their high insulin client load, have been found to be very sensitive to endoplasmic reticulum (ER) stress. Characteristic features of these cells include a highly developed ER, as well as high expression levels of the key ER stress pathway regulators, inositol requiring 1 (IRE1) and PKR-like ER kinase (PERK). The ability of β-cells to adapt to ER stress is particularly important, as any disparity between insulin translation and the folding capacity of the ER negatively impacts their homeostasis. Proper activation of ER stress signaling, therefore, is crucial to β-cell survival. Hypo- and hyper-activation of this signaling pathway can lead to β-cell dysfunction and apoptosis, leading ultimately to diabetes. It is important, for that reason, to understand the molecular mechanisms which lead to ER stress-mediated β-cell apoptosis and diabetes, and dissect the function of the ER stress signaling network in these cells.

ER STRESS SIGNALING PATH-WAYS

ER stress signaling, also referred to as the Unfolded Protein Response (UPR), has an important function in β-cells and is an adaptive response that mitigates ER stress [1]. There are four distinct responses of the UPR: 1) upregulation of molecular chaperones to increase the folding activity and reduce protein aggregation, 2) translational attenuation to reduce ER workload and prevent further accumulation of unfolded proteins, 3) ER -associated protein degradation (ERAD) to promote clearance of unfolded proteins, and 4) apoptosis when function is extensively impaired [2, 3]. The UPR, an adaptive response, must maintain a balance between its downstream targets which are anti-apoptotic and those which are pro-apoptotic Fig. (**1**).

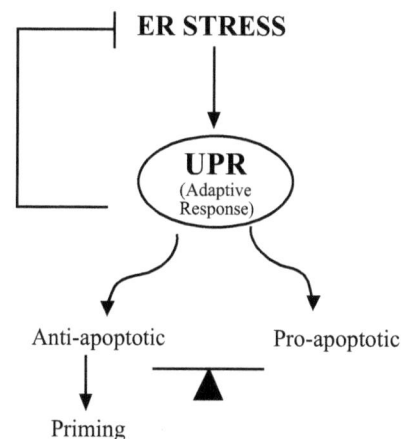

Fig. (1). ER Homeostasis. ER stress elicits an adaptive, protective response, the UPR. The UPR must maintain a balance between its downstream targets which are anti-apoptotic and those which are pro-apoptotic in order for the cell to maintain ER homeostasis.

When the cell encounters ER stress and the UPR is properly balanced, the cell is then primed for a future insult. However, when activation is tipped in the favor of pro-apoptotic components due to UPR dysfunction, the cell undergoes irreversible dysfunction which leads to cell death. There are three master regulators of this signaling pathway: inositol requiring 1 (IRE1), PKR-like kinase (PERK), and activating transcription factor 6 (ATF6) Fig. (**2**). The signaling from downstream effectors of these pathways merges in the nucleus to activate UPR target gene transcription.

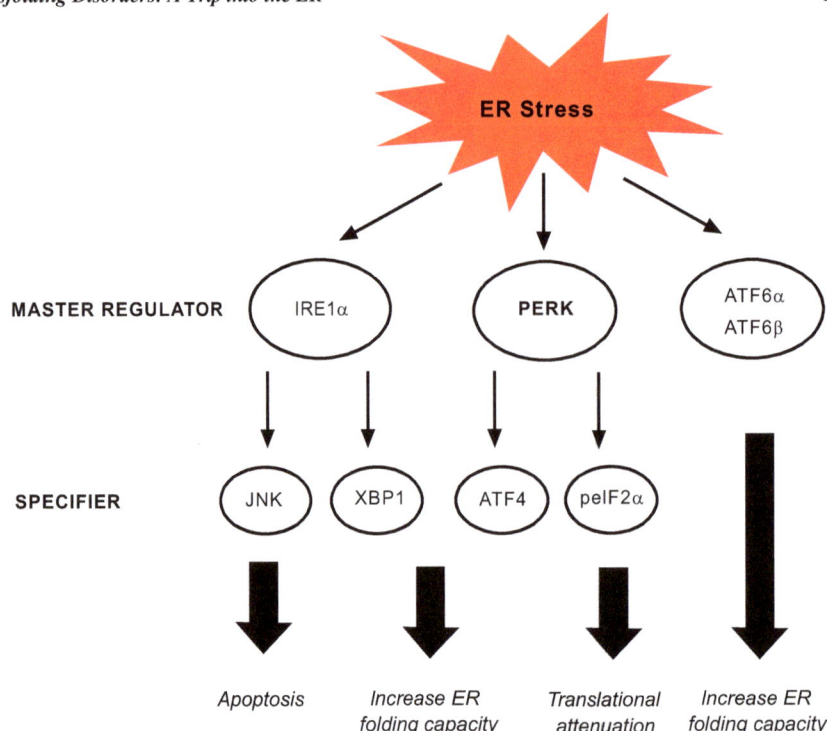

Fig. (2). The ER Stress Signaling Networks. There are three master regulators of ER stress signaling: IRE1, PERK, and ATF6. Each regulator has unique signaling specifiers that elicit an adaptive response to stress.

IRE1, a central regulator of the UPR, is a type I ER transmembrane kinase. Its N-terminal luminal domain acts as a sensor for ER stress signaling [4]. Upon sensing the presence of unfolded or misfolded proteins, IRE1 dimerizes and autophosphorylates to become active. Activated IRE1 splices X-box binding protein 1 (XBP1) Mrna [5-7]. Spliced XBP1 mRNA encodes a basic leucine zipper transcription factor that upregulates UPR target genes, including genes that function in ERAD such as ER-degradation-enhancing-α-mannidose-like protein (EDEM) [8], as well genes that function in folding proteins such as protein disulfide isomerase (PDI) [9]. Chronic stress leads to the recruitment of TNF-receptor-associated factor 2 (TRAF2) by IRE1 and the activation of apoptosis-signaling-kinase 1 (ASK1). Activated ASK1 activates c-Jun N-terminal protein kinase (JNK) and leads to apoptosis [10-12].

PERK, a second regulator of the UPR, is responsible for regulating protein synthesis during ER stress [13, 14]. It is also a type I ER transmembrane kinase. Like IRE1, its N-terminal luminal domain is sensitive to ER stress. When activated by ER stress, PERK oligomerizes, autophosphorylates and then directly phosphorylates Ser51 on the α subunit of eukaryotic initiation factor 2 (eIF2α) [13]. This in turn inhibits protein translation by reducing the formation of ribosomal initiation complexes and

recognition of AUG initiation codons. This reduction in ER workload protects cells from ER stress-mediated apoptosis [14]. Ironically, the translation of activating transcription factor 4 (ATF4), a b-ZIP transcription factor, is preferentially activated with phosphorylation of eIF2α and induces transcription of UPR target genes [15].

A third regulator of ER stress signaling and mediator of transcriptional induction, ATF6, is a type II ER transmembrane transcription factor [16]. Upon sensing stress in its N-terminal luminal domain, ATF6 transits to the Golgi where it is cleaved by S1 and S2 proteases, generating an activated b-ZIP factor [17]. This processed form of ATF6 translocates to the nucleus to activate UPR target genes [18, 19].

ER STRESS IN PANCREATIC β-CELLS

Insulin is secreted from β-cells from a readily available pool in response to acute hyperglycemia. This response activates insulin biosynthesis. This process begins as the transcription of a precursor of insulin, preproinsulin, is activated. Preproinsulin is synthesized in the cytoplasm and cotranslationally translocated to the ER through the Sec61 translocator complex via an interaction between its signal peptide and a signal-recognition particle

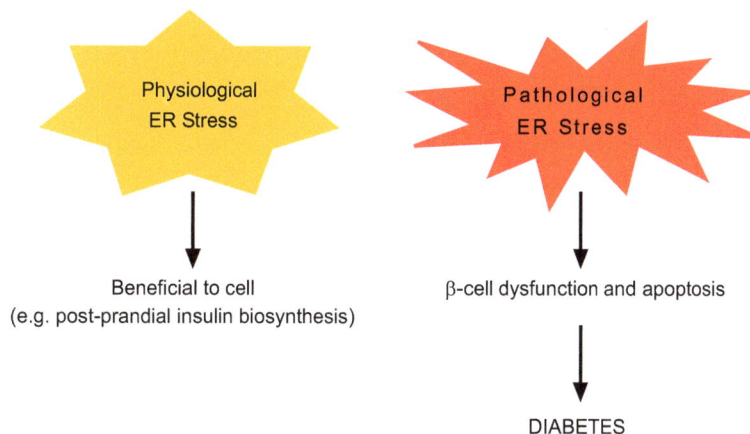

Fig. (3). Types of ER Stress in β-cells. There are two types of ER stress: physiological and pathological. Physiological ER stress is beneficial to the cell and promotes insulin biosynthesis, while pathological stress, which occurs when excessive stress on the ER cannot be resolved, can lead to β-cell dysfunction and diabetes.

(SRP) on the ER membrane. The signal peptide is cleaved in the ER to generate proinsulin. Proinsulin undergoes precise folding in the lumen of the ER, whereby three disulfide bonds are formed which is catalyzed by the ER resident proteins endoplasmic oxidoreductin 1 (ERO1) and protein disulfide isomerase (PDI). Once proinsulin is properly folded, it is translocated to the Golgi apparatus and packaged into secretory granules. Here, proinsulin is processed to mature insulin which is then released from the granule in response to elevation in blood glucose levels [20, 21].

β-cells are exposed to frequent energy fluctuations (i.e. intermittent changes in blood glucose levels), and therefore require precise and proper folding of

proinsulin to respond to such variations. Any imbalance between the load of insulin translation placed on the ER and folding capacity of the ER leads to a disruption in β-cell homeostasis and ER stress. Physiological ER stress in the β-cell (i.e. acute post-prandial ER stress) is beneficial and leads to the activation of insulin biosynthesis [22] Fig. (3).

Pathological ER stress can also occur in these cells, for example when they are exposed to chronic and prolonged hyperglycemia. This leads to β-cell dysfunction and death, and ultimately a diabetic phenotype Fig. (3). Other causes of ER stress in β-cells include exposure to free fatty acids, hyperinsulinemia, glucose deprivation, IAPP

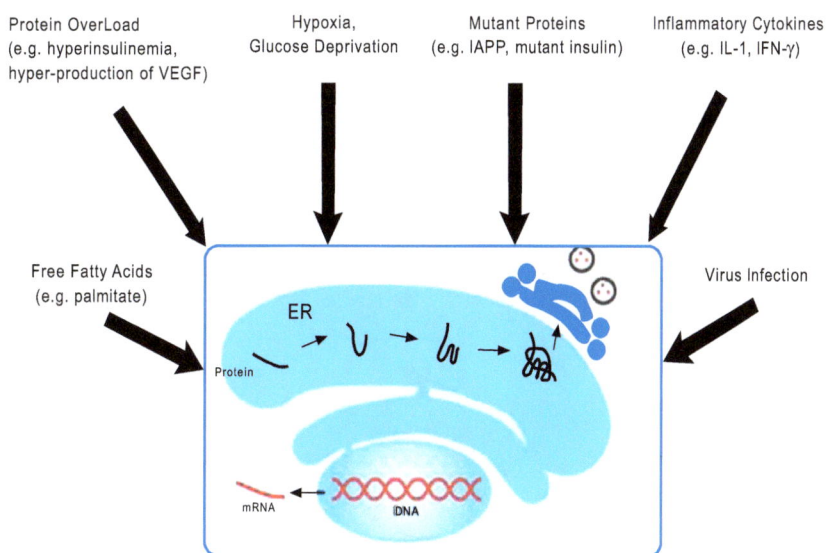

Fig. (4). Causes of ER Stress in β-cells. There are multiple factors which can lead to ER stress in the β-cell, leading to cell dysfunction and death. Exposure to free fatty acids, hyperinsulinemia, and inflammatory cytokines are just a few examples of ER stress-inducing agents.

expression, and exposure to inflammatory cytokines such as IL-1β and IFN-γ [23] Fig. (**4**).

The IRE1-XBP1 signaling pathway, in addition to upregulating genes important for protein degradation and is also important for ER expansion [24], which is particularly important for the differentiation of antibody-secreting plasma cells [25], as well as other secretory cells such as pancreatic β-cells. In mammalian cells, there are two forms of IRE1: IRE1α and IRE1β. IRE1β is only expressed in intestinal epithelial cells, whose deletion leads to high levels of ER stress and colitis [26]. IRE1α is ubiquitously expressed, with high expression found in the pancreas and placenta [27]. β-cells also have a baseline activation of IRE1α, as measured by its phosphorylation, and IRE1 signaling has a key role in insulin biosynthesis. Acute hyperglycemia leads to activation of IRE1α and upregulation of insulin biosynthesis, while disruption of this signaling molecule leads to a suppression of proinsulin biosynthesis. This signaling pathway is also referred to as SCAEF or "Stimulus-Coupling Adaptation to ER Folding" because under conditions of acute hyperglycemia, the known downstream targets of IRE1α, XBP1 and JNK, are not activated [22]. While the downstream targets of SCAEF have yet to be identified, the ER-resident oxidoreductase ERO1α, which functions in proinsulin folding, is upregulated.

PERK, one of the three ER stress sensors of the cell, is also highly expressed in pancreatic islets [28, 29]. Activation of PERK (i.e. its autophosphorylation) is part of the anti-apopototic branch of ER stress signaling; attenuation of

general protein translation has a protective effect by reducing ER workload [14]. While IRE1 is a positive regulator or insulin biosynthesis, PERK is a negative regulator. In PERK knockout mouse islets, insulin biosynthesis from acute hyperglycemia is enhanced compared to control littermates [28].

Recently it has been shown that ATF6 may have a function in regulating insulin. Under ER stress, ATF6 is activated, leading to a decrease in insulin gene expression [30]. This suggests that ATF6 has dual functions: positively regulating ER chaperones and negatively regulating insulin promoter activity.

Disruption of ER homeostasis in β-cells can lead to apoptosis, when this disruption is severe and/or prolonged. There are at least three pathways involved in this event which can lead to the activation of caspase-3: transcriptional activation of C/EBP homologous protein (CHOP) [31], activation of c-Jun NH$_2$-terminal kinase (JNK) [10], and activation of ER-associated caspase-12 [32]. The mechanisms underlying the downstream targets of ER stress-mediated JNK activation have yet to be defined, however, proteins of the BCL-2 family are involved. JNK phosphorylation of Bcl-2 and Bcl-X$_L$ leads to inhibition of their anti-apoptotic functions [33-36]. While the molecular mechanisms by which CHOP induces ER stress-mediated apoptosis are also unclear, CHOP-induced gene expression of carbonic anhydrase IV [37], Bcl-2 [38], death receptor 5 (DR5) [39], tribbles-realted protein 3 (TRB3) [40], and Bcl-X$_L$ [38] may be involved. The roles of the IRE1-JNK, CHOP, and caspase-12 pathways in ER stress-

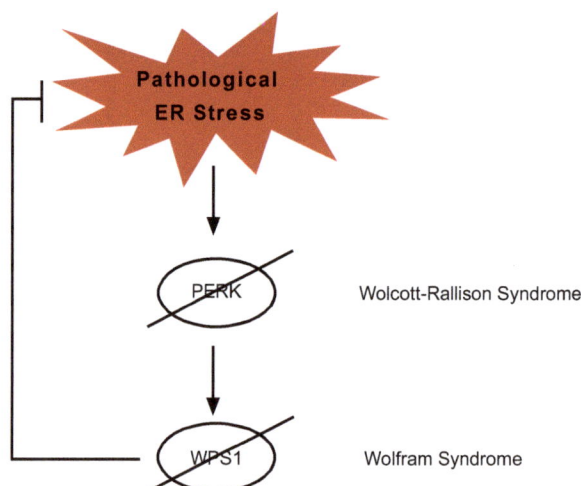

Fig. (5). Mutations in ER Stress Signaling Regulators Lead to High ER Stress and Diabetes. Mutations in the ER stress regulator, PERK, leads to a genetic form of diabetes called Wolcott-Rallison syndrome, while a mutation in one of its downstream specifier, WFS1, leads to a rare form of juvenile diabetes, Wolfram syndrome.

mediated β-cell death has not been extensively studied nor well defined.

GENETIC FORMS OF ER STRESS-MEDIATED DIABETES

Wolcott-rallison Syndrome

The relationship between ER stress and diabetes was first revealed in a rare autosomal recessive form of juvenile diabetes, Wolcott-Rallison syndrome. In 1972, Wolcott and Rallison described two brothers and a sister with infancy-onset diabetes mellitus and multiple epiphyseal dysplasia [41]. In this syndrome, mutations have been reported in the *EIF2AK3* gene encoding PERK, one of the most important upstream components of ER stress signaling [42] Fig. (**2**). Because these mutations are within the catalytic domain of PERK, it is highly likely that they cause loss of function of the kinase activity of PERK and lead to decreased phosphorylation of eIF2α, a substrate of PERK. When a high workload is placed on the ER, eIF2α phosphorylation is essential to mitigate ER stress and thereby promote cell survival [14]. Therefore, the loss of function of PERK and decreased eIF2α phosphorylation could directly lead to β-cell death Fig. (**5**).

Indeed, PERK knockout mice develop diabetes due to β-cell apoptosis caused by a high level of ER stress in the pancreatic islets [28]. In addition, when mutant mice having a heterozygous mutation

in the phosphorylation site of eIF2α are fed a high-fat diet, they become obese and, due to β-cell dysfunction, diabetic [43]. These observations strongly suggest that β-cell death in patients with Wolcott-Rallison syndrome is caused by a high level of ER stress and a defect in the UPR (i.e., PERK signaling).

The negative regulator of PERK signaling, P58[IPK], also functions in maintaining ER homeostasis in pancreatic β cells. P58[IPK] is an important component of a negative feedback loop used by these cells to inhibit eIF2-α signaling and attenuate the UPR [44]. P58[IPK] knockout mice show a gradual onset of glucosuria and hyperglycemia associated with increased apoptosis of islet cells [45]. P58[IPK] may participate in the pathogenesis of human diabetes.

Wolfram Syndrome

Wolfram syndrome (WFS), a rare autosomal recessive disorder characterized by diabetes mellitus and optical atrophy, was first described by Wolfram and Wagener in 1938 [46]. Diabetes presents in patients in the first decade of life, while optical atrophy follows in the second decade. While diabetes mellitus and optical atrophy are the only necessary symptoms to diagnose this syndrome, a significant portion of WFS patients exhibit symptoms of diabetes insipidus and auditory nerve deafness. Thus, this syndrome is also referred to as the diabetes insipidus, diabetes mellitus, optic atrophy, and deafness (DIDMOAD)

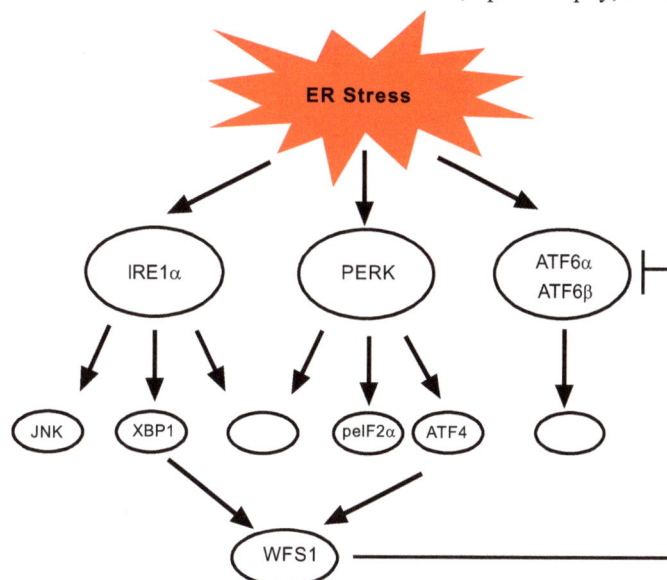

Fig. (6). WFS1 Negatively Regulates ER Stress Signaling. WFS1 is a downstream specifier of the IRE1 and PERK signaling pathways. WFS1 is induced by ER stress and negatively regulates the third regulator of ER stress signaling, ATF6.

syndrome [47, 48]. Postmortem studies reveal a non-autoimmune-linked selective loss of pancreatic β-cells [49]. The nuclear gene responsible for this syndrome was identified by two separate groups in 1998 and named WFS1 [50, 51]. WFS1 protein is a transmembrane protein localized to the ER. While ubiquitously expressed, WFS1 is highly expressed in the pancreas; it is specifically restricted to the β-cells of the pancreas [50, 51].

WFS1 was recently found to be a component of ER stress signaling. WFS1 mRNA and protein are induced by ER stress and its expression is regulated by the IRE1 and PERK pathways [52] Fig. (**6**).

Inactivation of WFS1 in β-cells causes a high level of ER stress, with upregulation of the stress markers BiP, ERO1α, spliced XBP-1, and CHOP. WFS1 knockout mice also develop diabetes due to β-cell apoptosis. These suggest that the pathogenesis of WFS involves chronic ER stress in β-cells due to a loss-of-function of WFS1 [52] Fig. (**5**). The precise molecular mechanisms by which WFS1 mutations cause β-cell death, however, are unknown.

A clue to how WFS1 functions in ER stress signaling has recently been found. WFS1 negatively regulates the ER stress transcription factor ATF6. WFS1, which has a distant homology to Sel1/Hrd3 – a protein that stabilizes the E3 ligase Hrd1 and enhances its function, also stabilizes Hrd1. Through HRD1 stabilization, WFS1 enhances ATF6 degradation under non-stress conditions (Fonseca SG and Urano F, manuscript in review). This in turn prevents premature activation of the ATF6 pathway, thus having a protective effect for the cell – hyperactivation of ER stress signaling is detrimental to ER homeostasis and to the cell as a whole.

In addition to functioning as a negative regulator of ER stress signaling, WFS1 may also have a function in insulin biosynthesis and secretion in β-cells. WFS1 has been found to be upregulated during insulin secretion [52].

Permanent Neonatal Diabetes

Neonatal diabetes is defined as insulin-requiring hyperglycemia within the first month of life. This is typically associated with slowed intrauterine growth and is a rare disorder. Permanent neonatal diabetes, considered a genetic disorder, can be caused by several types of mutations, including mutations in insulin promoter factor 1 (IPF-1), and results in lifelong dependence on insulin injections. It has been recently shown, however, that mutations in the human insulin gene can also cause this disorder [53]. This is an autosomal dominant disorder, with mutations primarily occurring in critical regions of preproinsulin. This presumably leads to the improper folding of insulin and triggers the ER stress signaling pathway. Severe ER stress occurs, leading to β-cell apoptosis.

In the mouse models of this disease, the Akita and Munich mice, mice have a dominant missense mutation in the Ins2 gene. In the Akita mouse, there is a cysteine^{96}-to-tyrosine substitution. These mutations lead to disruption of disulphide formation between the A and B chain of proinsulin, causing insulin to misfold and accumulate in the ER [54]. This accumulation of misfolded insulin leads to severe ER stress, β-cell apoptosis and ultimately diabetes [55].

ER Stress and Type 1 Diabetes

Increasing evidence supports the role of ER-stress mediated β-cell death in the pathogenesis of type 1A diabetes (i.e. autoimmune diabetes). The baseline of ER stress in β-cells is higher than that of other cell types due to their exposure to frequent energy fluctuations and high client load, insulin. It is therefore possible that any additional ER stress applied to these cells by genetic or environmental factors can lead to cell death. β-cells that undergo apoptosis as a consequence of this additional, unresolved ER stress contain misfolded proteins that can act as "neo-autoantigens" – dendritic cells in the islets engulf ER stress-induced apoptotic β-cells and stimulate the maturation of β-cell-reactive T cells that mediate autoimmune destruction of remaining β-cells [56].

There are various insults to the β-cell that can lead to unresolved ER stress, triggering an apoptotic cascade and leading to production of "neo-autoantigens." These include viral infection, other environmental factors, as well as nitric oxide (NO) Fig. (**7**).

NO plays an important role in β-cell apoptosis in type 1 diabetes [57]. Inflammatory cytokines such as γ-interferon (IFN-γ) and intereukin-1β (IL-1β) in β-cells induce the production of NO, which leads to β-cell failure and consequently cell death. There is evidence that this process is mediated by ER stress [58]. Production of NO leads to the attenuation of sarcoendoplasmic reticulum pump Ca^{2+} ATPase 2b (SERCA2b) and consequently the reduction of Ca^{2+} in the ER. This depletion of Ca^{2+} leads to severe ER stress and the induction of the proapoptotic transcription factor CHOP [59, 60] Fig. (**7**). It has been shown that CHOP is induced by an NO donor, *S*-nitroso-N-acetyl-$_{D,L}$-penicillamine (SNAP), and pancreatic islets from CHOP knockout mice are resistant to NO-induced apoptosis [58].

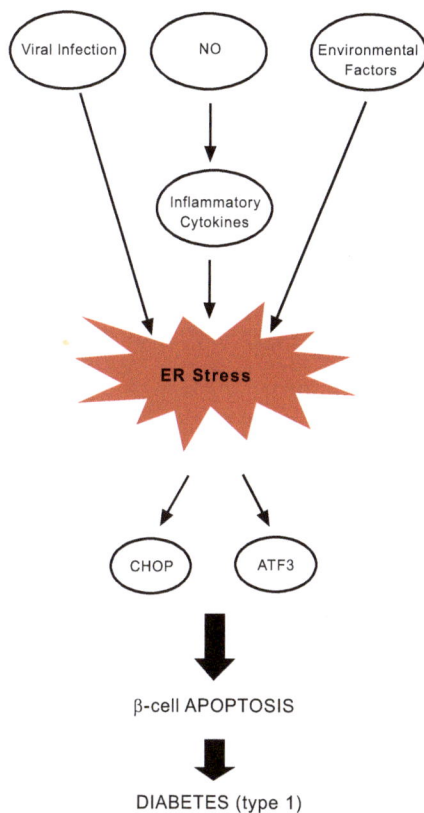

Fig. (7). ER Stress-Mediated Type 1 Diabetes. There is evidence of ER stress-mediated β-cell death leading to type 1 diabetes. Factors which cause ER stress and are linked to type 1 diabetes are viral infections, nitric oxide (NO) production, as well as other environmental factors. High levels of ER stress lead to the production of misfolded proteins which can act as "neo-autoantigens." ER stress-mediated apoptosis can also lead to the production of "neo-autoantigens" and type 1 diabetes. Activating transcription factor 3 (ATF3), a proapoptotic transcription factor of the ATF/CREB family, may also contribute to ER stress-mediated β-cell apoptosis in type 1 diabetes Fig. (**7**). ATF3 is induced by proinflammatory cytokines and NO.

ATF3 knockout mouse islets are partially protected from NO- and cytokine-induced β-cell apoptosis, while overexpression of this transcription factor in mouse islets leads to β-cell dysfunction [61].

ER Stress in Type 2 Diabetes

One of the contributing factors to the pathogenesis of type 2 diabetes is the reduction of β-cell mass [62]. Resistance to insulin action in peripheral tissues (i.e. adipose, muscle, and liver) is one of the primary presenting features of type 2 diabetes. This insulin resistance leads to the hyperproduction of insulin (i.e. hyperinsulinemia) in the β-cell. This increase in insulin biosynthesis overwhelms the folding capacity of the ER, leading to chronic activation of ER stress signaling pathways. This chronic, hyperactivation of ER stress signaling can lead to β-cell dysfunction and apoptosis Fig. (**8**).

There are several components of ER stress signaling in the β-cell that contribute to β-cell apoptosis: IRE1-JNK, CHOP, and GSK3β. The IRE1 pathway has an important function in β-cells. Transient increases in insulin biosynthesis lead to IRE1 activation [22] and therefore prolonged increases in insulin biosynthesis, which occurs in type 2 diabetes, may lead to β-cell death – during chronic ER stress, IRE1 activates JNK and elicits apoptosis [10, 11]. CHOP is also an important player of ER stress-mediated β-cell death and may promote the progression of type 2 diabetes [55, 58]. A third signaling component, glycogen synthase kinase 3β (GSK3β), also plays a role in β-cell death caused by ER stress. GSK3β is a substrate of the survival kinase, Akt [63], and it has been demonstrated that attenuation of Akt phosphorylation mediates dephosphorylation of GSK3β, leading to ER stress-mediated β-cell apoptosis [64].

Insulin resistance leads to β-cell exhaustion, glucotoxicity, and hyperinsulinemia, which places a huge strain on the β-cell's ER. This, however, is not the only source of stress for the ER. It has been recently shown that free fatty acids (FFAs) also induce β-cell apoptosis [65-67]. Treatment of β-cell lines with palmitate increases levels of ER stress markers, such as ATF4 and spliced XBP-1. Circulating FFAs lead to β-cell lipotoxicity and consequently excessive ER stress.

Recent studies show an involvement of ER stress in insulin resistance of liver, muscle, and adipose tissues. IRE1-JNK signaling plays an important role in the insulin-resistant liver tissue of type 2

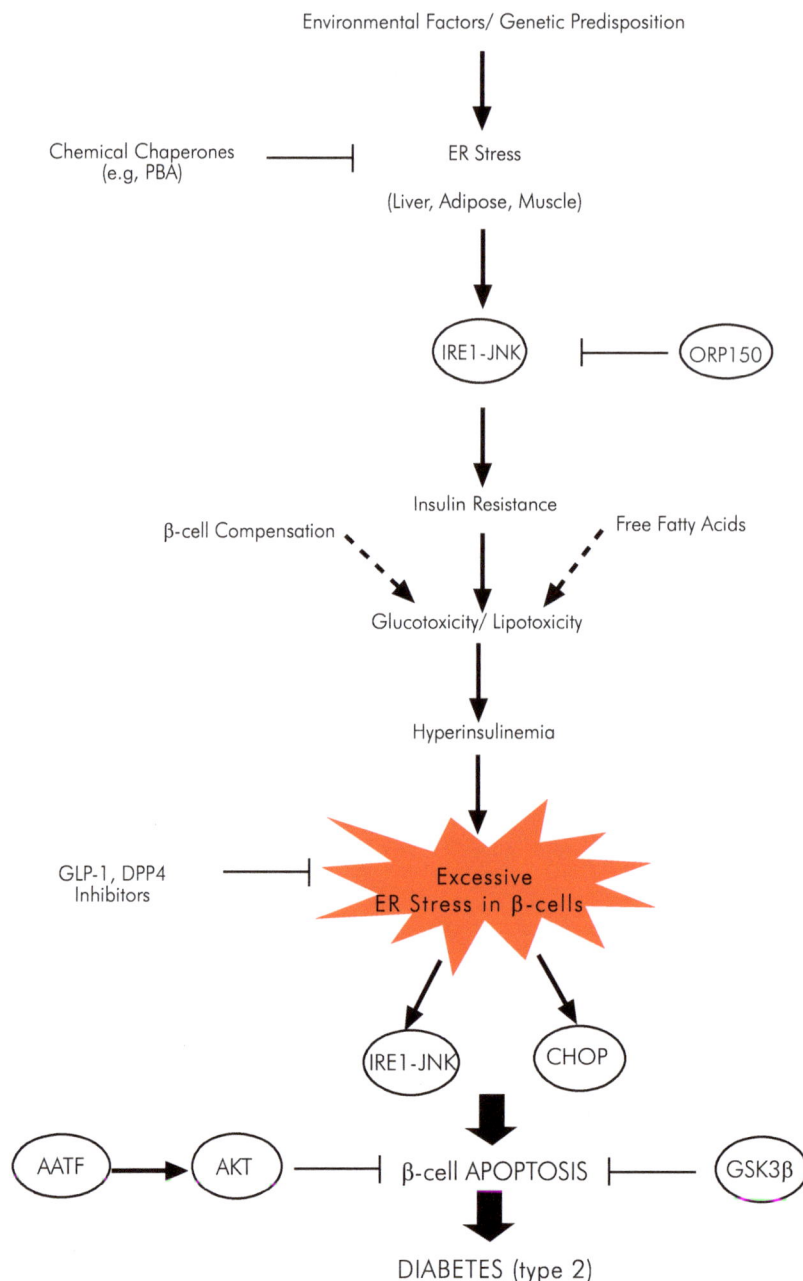

Fig. (8). ER Stress and Type 2 Diabetes. Severe and chronic ER stress in peripheral tissues such as adipose, liver, and muscle, can cause insulin resistance via the IRE1-JNK pathway. Insulin resistance can lead to glucotoxicity and lipotoxicity, causing hyperinsulinemia and placing excessive ER stress on the β-cell. This excessive stress leads to JNK and CHOP activation, leading to β-cell apoptosis and type 2 diabetes. There are several components of this cascade that can be targeted by small molecules and drugs. Chemical chaperones, such as PBA, can target the upstream portion of this cascade, while modulation of the anti-apoptotic factor AATF, can prevent β-cell apoptosis.

diabetes patients. Obesity leads to hyperactivation of JNK signaling via severe ER stress, leading to serine phosphorylation of insulin receptor substrate-1 (IRS-1), which inhibits insulin action [68]. Like β-cells, hepatocytes have a high baseline ER stress level (Ghosh R and Urano F, unpublished observation), and therefore may be

sensitive to additional ER stress. It has been shown that high ER stress in liver cells can be resolved via overexpression of the ER-resident chaperone oxygen-regulated protein 150 (ORP150), while suppression of this chaperone in mice inhibits insulin sensitivity [32].

FUTURE DIRECTION

Our understanding of ER stress signaling in β-cells is far from complete. This is because interactions of the three pathways regulated by three master regulators have not been studied extensively. Systems approaches using genomics, transcriptomics, and proteomics are necessary to the complete understanding of ER stress signaling. However, based on the information that we have today, predictions can be made about the future of research in ER stress signaling in β-cell biology and diabetes.

Interactions between ER Stress Signaling Pathways and Other Signaling Pathways

Increasing evidence suggests that there exist crosstalk between ER stress signaling and other signaling pathways, such as mTOR signaling and insulin receptor signaling pathways. The complete understanding of this crosstalk will lead to a discovery of an unexpected link between ER stress and biological outcomes, such as cell proliferation and regulation of glucose metabolism.

Discovery of Endogenous Molecules and Chemical Compounds That can Modulate ER Stress and Thereby Combat ER Stress-Mediated β-Cell Death

It has been shown that mild activation of ER stress signaling or specific activation of proapoptotic components of ER stress signaling has a beneficial effect on β-cell function and survival [22, 69]. Glucagon-like peptide 1 (GLP-1) is a gut-derived peptide secreted from intestinal L-cells after a meal and has numerous physiological actions, including enhancement of β-cell growth and survival. Interestingly, GLP-1 is a physiological activator of ER stress signaling. Activation of GLP-1 signaling improves β-cell function and survival through the activation of the PERK-ATF-4 pathway. We predict that other endogenous factors like GLP-1 or chemical compounds that can activate ER stress signaling will be discovered and will be used to increase the viability of β-cells.

Using SNPs of ER Stress Response Genes for Prevention of Diabetes

Genomewide association studies have identified numerous single nucleotide polymorphisms (SNPs) associated with increased risk for type-2 diabetes.

WFS1 is one of such genes. In the future, human genetics will identify more ER stress-related genes as markers of susceptibility to type 1 and type 2 diabetes. These markers will be potentially useful in targeting patients who would benefit from screening for early detection of diabetes.

To understand the transition from the latent to the overt diabetes state, we need to define the dynamics of β-cell function at the system level. Recent evidence strongly suggests that a level of ER stress that exceeds the anti-ER stress capacity of β-cells has an important function in β-cell dysfunction and death during the progression of type1 and type 2 diabetes, as well as genetic forms of diabetes such as Wolfram syndrome. A complete understanding of the states of protein homeostasis regulated by ER stress signaling pathways will have a direct impact on future therapies for diabetes.

ACKNOWLEDGEMENTS

Research in the laboratory of F. Urano is supported by an NIH R01DK067493 grant, a grant from the Diabetes and Endocrinology Research Center at the University of Massachusetts Medical School (DK032520), a Juvenile Diabetes Research Foundation Regular Research Grant (1-2008-593), a grant from the Worcester Foundation for Biomedical Research, and an Iacocca Foundation/Juvenile Diabetes Research Foundation joint Grant.

REFERENCES

1. Fonseca, S.G., Lipson, K.L. & Urano, F. Endoplasmic reticulum stress signaling in pancreatic beta-cells. Antioxidants & redox signaling **9**, 2335-2344 (2007).

2. Ron, D. & Walter, P. Signal integration in the endoplasmic reticulum unfolded protein response. Nature reviews **8**, 519-529 (2007).

3. Rutkowski, D.T. & Kaufman, R.J. That which does not kill me makes me stronger: adapting to chronic ER stress. Trends Biochem Sci **32**, 469-476 (2007).

4. Urano, F., Bertolotti, A. & Ron, D. IRE1 and efferent signaling from the endoplasmic reticulum. Journal of cell science **113**, 3697-3702 (2000).

5. Yoshida, H., Matsui, T., Yamamoto, A., Okada, T. & Mori, K. XBP1 mRNA is induced by ATF6 and spliced by IRE1 in response to ER stress to produce a highly active transcription factor. Cell **107**, 881-891 (2001).

6. Shen, X., et al. Complementary signaling pathways regulate the unfolded protein response and are required for C. elegans development. Cell **107**, 893-903 (2001).

7. Calfon, M., et al. IRE1 couples endoplasmic reticulum load to secretory capacity by processing the XBP-1 mRNA. Nature **415**, 92-96 (2002).

8. Yoshida, H., et al. A time-dependent phase shift in the mammalian unfolded protein response. Dev Cell **4**, 265-271 (2003).

9.   Lee, A.H., Iwakoshi, N.N. & Glimcher, L.H. XBP-1 regulates a subset of endoplasmic reticulum resident chaperone genes in the unfolded protein response. Mol Cell Biol **23**, 7448-7459 (2003).

10. Urano, F., *et al.* Coupling of stress in the ER to activation of JNK protein kinases by transmembrane protein kinase IRE1. Science (New York, N.Y **287**, 664-666 (2000).

11. Nishitoh, H., *et al.* ASK1 is essential for endoplasmic reticulum stress-induced neuronal cell death triggered by expanded polyglutamine repeats. Genes Dev **16**, 1345-1355 (2002).

12. Nishitoh, H., *et al.* ASK1 is essential for JNK/SAPK activation by TRAF2. Molecular Cell **2**, 389-395 (1998).

13. Harding, H.P., Zhang, Y. & Ron, D. Protein translation and folding are coupled by an endoplasmic-reticulum-resident kinase. Nature **397**, 271-274 (1999).

14. Harding, H.P., Zhang, Y., Bertolotti, A., Zeng, H. & Ron, D. Perk is essential for translational regulation and cell survival during the unfolded protein response. Mol Cell **5**, 897-904 (2000).

15. Harding, H.P., *et al.* Regulated translation initiation controls stress-induced gene expression in mammalian cells. Mol Cell **6**, 1099-1108 (2000).

16. Yoshida, H., Haze, K., Yanagi, H., Yura, T. & Mori, K. Identification of the cis-acting endoplasmic reticulum stress response element responsible for transcriptional induction of mammalian glucose-regulated proteins. Involvement of basic leucine zipper transcription factors. The Journal of biological chemistry **273**, 33741-33749 (1998).

17. Ye, J., *et al.* ER stress induces cleavage of membrane-bound ATF6 by the same proteases that process SREBPs. Mol Cell **6**, 1355-1364 (2000).

18. Yoshida, H., *et al.* ATF6 activated by proteolysis binds in the presence of NF-Y (CBF) directly to the cis-acting element responsible for the mammalian unfolded protein response. Mol Cell Biol **20**, 6755-6767 (2000).

19. Haze, K., Yoshida, H., Yanagi, H., Yura, T. & Mori, K. Mammalian transcription factor ATF6 is synthesized as a transmembrane protein and activated by proteolysis in response to endoplasmic reticulum stress. Mol Biol Cell **10**, 3787-3799 (1999).

20. Rhodes, C.J. Processing of the insulin molecule. in Diabetes Mellitus (eds. LeRoith, D., Taylor, S.I. & Olefsky, J.M.) 27-50 (Lippincott Williams & Wilkins, Philadelphia, PA, 2004).

21. Rhodes, C.J., Shoelson, S. & Halban, P.A. Insulin Biosynthesis, Processing, and Chemistry. in Joslin's Diabetes Mellitus (eds. Kahn, C.R., et al.) 65-82 (Joslin Diabetes Center, Boston, 2005).

22. Lipson, K.L., *et al.* Regulation of insulin biosynthesis in pancreatic beta cells by an endoplasmic reticulum-resident protein kinase IRE1. Cell Metab **4**, 245-254 (2006).

23. Eizirik, D.L., Cardozo, A.K. & Cnop, M. The role for endoplasmic reticulum stress in diabetes mellitus. Endocrine reviews **29**, 42-61 (2008).

24. Sriburi, R., Jackowski, S., Mori, K. & Brewer, J.W. XBP1: a link between the unfolded protein response, lipid biosynthesis, and biogenesis of the endoplasmic reticulum. J Cell Biol **167**, 35-41 (2004).

25. Shaffer, A.L., *et al.* XBP1, downstream of Blimp-1, expands the secretory apparatus and other organelles, and increases protein synthesis in plasma cell differentiation. Immunity **21**, 81-93 (2004).

26. Bertolotti, A., *et al.* Increased sensitivity to dextran sodium sulfate colitis in IRE1beta-deficient mice. Journal of Clinical Investigation **107**, 585-593 (2001).

27. Tirasophon, W., Welihinda, A.A. & Kaufman, R.J. A stress response pathway from the endoplasmic reticulum to the nucleus requires a novel bifunctional protein kinase/endoribonuclease (Ire1p) in mammalian cells. Genes Dev **12**, 1812-1824 (1998).

28. Harding, H.P., *et al.* Diabetes mellitus and exocrine pancreatic dysfunction in perk-/- mice reveals a role for translational control in secretory cell survival. Molecular Cell **7**, 1153-1163 (2001).

29. Shi, Y., *et al.* Identification and characterization of pancreatic eukaryotic initiation factor 2 alpha-subunit kinase, PEK, involved in translational control. Mol Cell Biol **18**, 7499-7509 (1998).

30. Seo, H.Y., *et al.* Endoplasmic reticulum stress-induced activation of activating transcription factor 6 decreases insulin gene expression via up-regulation of orphan nuclear receptor small heterodimer partner. Endocrinology **149**, 3832-3841 (2008).

31. Ron, D. & Habener, J.F. CHOP, a novel developmentally regulated nuclear protein that dimerizes with transcription factors C/EBP and LAP and functions as a dominant-negative inhibitor of gene transcription. Genes Dev **6**, 439-453 (1992).

32. Nakagawa, T., *et al.* Caspase-12 mediates endoplasmic-reticulum-specific apoptosis and cytotoxicity by amyloid-beta. Nature **403**, 98-103 (2000).

33. Fan, M., *et al.* Vinblastine-induced phosphorylation of Bcl-2 and Bcl-XL is mediated by JNK and occurs in parallel with inactivation of the Raf-1/MEK/ERK cascade. The Journal of biological chemistry **275**, 29980-29985 (2000).

34. Kharbanda, S., *et al.* Translocation of SAPK/JNK to mitochondria and interaction with Bcl-x(L) in response to DNA damage. The Journal of biological chemistry **275**, 322-327 (2000).

35. Maundrell, K., *et al.* Bcl-2 undergoes phosphorylation by c-Jun N-terminal kinase/stress-activated protein kinases in the presence of the constitutively active GTP-binding protein Rac1. The Journal of biological chemistry **272**, 25238-25242 (1997).

36. Yamamoto, K., Ichijo, H. & Korsmeyer, S.J. BCL-2 is phosphorylated and inactivated by an ASK1/Jun N-terminal protein kinase pathway normally activated at G(2)/M. Mol Cell Biol **19**, 8469-8478 (1999).

37. Sok, J., *et al.* CHOP-Dependent stress-inducible expression of a novel form of carbonic anhydrase VI. Mol Cell Biol **19**, 495-504 (1999).

38. McCullough, K.D., Martindale, J.L., Klotz, L.O., Aw, T.Y. & Holbrook, N.J. Gadd153 sensitizes cells to endoplasmic reticulum stress by down-regulating Bcl2 and perturbing the cellular redox state. Mol Cell Biol **21**, 1249-1259 (2001).

39. Yamaguchi, H. & Wang, H.G. CHOP is involved in endoplasmic reticulum stress-induced apoptosis by enhancing DR5 expression in human carcinoma cells. The Journal of biological chemistry **279**, 45495-45502 (2004).

40. Ohoka, N., Yoshii, S., Hattori, T., Onozaki, K. & Hayashi, H. TRB3, a novel ER stress-inducible gene, is induced via ATF4-CHOP pathway and is involved in cell death. Embo J **24**, 1243-1255 (2005).

41. Wolcott, C.D. & Rallison, M.L. Infancy-onset diabetes mellitus and multiple epiphyseal dysplasia. J Pediatr **80**, 292-297 (1972).

42. Delepine, M., *et al.* EIF2AK3, encoding translation initiation factor 2-alpha kinase 3, is mutated in patients

with Wolcott-Rallison syndrome. Nature Genetics **25**, 406-409 (2000).

43. Scheuner, D., *et al.* Control of mRNA translation preserves endoplasmic reticulum function in beta cells and maintains glucose homeostasis. Nat Med **11**, 757-764 (2005).

44. Yan, W., *et al.* Control of PERK eIF2alpha kinase activity by the endoplasmic reticulum stress-induced molecular chaperone P58IPK. Proceedings of the National Academy of Sciences of the United States of America **99**, 15920-15925 (2002).

45. Ladiges, W.C., *et al.* Pancreatic beta-cell failure and diabetes in mice with a deletion mutation of the endoplasmic reticulum molecular chaperone gene P58IPK. Diabetes **54**, 1074-1081 (2005).

46. Wolfram, D.J. & Wagener, H.P. Diabetes mellitus and simple optic atrophy among siblings: report of four cases. May Clin Proc **1**, 715-718 (1938).

47. Barrett, T.G. & Bundey, S.E. Wolfram (DIDMOAD) syndrome. J Med Genet **34**, 838-841 (1997).

48. Rando, T.A., Horton, J.C. & Layzer, R.B. Wolfram syndrome: evidence of a diffuse neurodegenerative disease by magnetic resonance imaging. Neurology **42**, 1220-1224 (1992).

49. Karasik, A., *et al.* Genetically programmed selective islet beta-cell loss in diabetic subjects with Wolfram's syndrome. Diabetes Care **12**, 135-138 (1989).

50. Inoue, H., *et al.* A gene encoding a transmembrane protein is mutated in patients with diabetes mellitus and optic atrophy (Wolfram syndrome). Nature Genetics **20**, 143-148 (1998).

51. Strom, T.M., *et al.* Diabetes insipidus, diabetes mellitus, optic atrophy and deafness (DIDMOAD) caused by mutations in a novel gene (wolframin) coding for a predicted transmembrane protein. Hum Mol Genet **7**, 2021-2028 (1998).

52. Fonseca, S.G., *et al.* WFS1 Is a Novel Component of the Unfolded Protein Response and Maintains Homeostasis of the Endoplasmic Reticulum in Pancreatic {beta}-Cells. The Journal of biological chemistry **280**, 39609-39615 (2005).

53. Stoy, J., *et al.* Insulin gene mutations as a cause of permanent neonatal diabetes. Proceedings of the National Academy of Sciences of the United States of America **104**, 15040-15044 (2007).

54. Wang, J., *et al.* A mutation in the insulin 2 gene induces diabetes with severe pancreatic beta-cell dysfunction in the Mody mouse. Journal of Clinical Investigation **103**, 27-37 (1999).

55. Oyadomari, S., *et al.* Targeted disruption of the Chop gene delays endoplasmic reticulum stress-mediated diabetes. Journal of Clinical Investigation **109**, 525-532 (2002).

56. Casciola-Rosen, L.A., Anhalt, G.J. & Rosen, A. DNA-dependent protein kinase is one of a subset of autoantigens specifically cleaved early during apoptosis. J Exp Med **182**, 1625-1634 (1995).

57. Eizirik, D.L., Flodstrom, M., Karlsen, A.E. & Welsh, N. The harmony of the spheres: inducible nitric oxide synthase and related genes in pancreatic beta cells. Diabetologia **39**, 875-890 (1996).

58. Oyadomari, S., *et al.* Nitric oxide-induced apoptosis in pancreatic beta cells is mediated by the endoplasmic reticulum stress pathway. Proceedings of the National Academy of Sciences of the United States of America **98**, 10845-10850 (2001).

59. Cardozo, A.K., *et al.* A comprehensive analysis of cytokine-induced and nuclear factor-kappa B-dependent genes in primary rat pancreatic beta-cells. The Journal of biological chemistry **276**, 48879-48886 (2001).

60. Cardozo, A.K., *et al.* Cytokines downregulate the sarcoendoplasmic reticulum pump Ca2+ ATPase 2b and deplete endoplasmic reticulum Ca2+, leading to induction of endoplasmic reticulum stress in pancreatic beta-cells. Diabetes **54**, 452-461 (2005).

61. Hartman, M.G., *et al.* Role for activating transcription factor 3 in stress-induced beta-cell apoptosis. Mol Cell Biol **24**, 5721-5732 (2004).

62. Butler, A.E., *et al.* Beta-cell deficit and increased beta-cell apoptosis in humans with type 2 diabetes. Diabetes **52**, 102-110 (2003).

63. Cross, D.A., Alessi, D.R., Cohen, P., Andjelkovich, M. & Hemmings, B.A. Inhibition of glycogen synthase kinase-3 by insulin mediated by protein kinase B. Nature **378**, 785-789 (1995).

64. Srinivasan, S., *et al.* Endoplasmic reticulum stress-induced apoptosis is partly mediated by reduced insulin signaling through phosphatidylinositol 3-kinase/Akt and increased glycogen synthase kinase-3beta in mouse insulinoma cells. Diabetes **54**, 968-975 (2005).

65. Cnop, M., *et al.* Selective inhibition of eukaryotic translation initiation factor 2 alpha dephosphorylation potentiates fatty acid-induced endoplasmic reticulum stress and causes pancreatic beta-cell dysfunction and apoptosis. The Journal of biological chemistry **282**, 3989-3997 (2007).

66. Karaskov, E., *et al.* Chronic palmitate but not oleate exposure induces endoplasmic reticulum stress, which may contribute to INS-1 pancreatic beta-cell apoptosis. Endocrinology **147**, 3398-3407 (2006).

67. Kharroubi, I., *et al.* Free fatty acids and cytokines induce pancreatic beta-cell apoptosis by different mechanisms: role of nuclear factor-kappaB and endoplasmic reticulum stress. Endocrinology **145**, 5087-5096 (2004).

68. Ozcan, U., *et al.* Endoplasmic reticulum stress links obesity, insulin action, and type 2 diabetes. Science (New York, N.Y **306**, 457-461 (2004).

69. Han, D., *et al.* A kinase inhibitor activates the IRE1alpha RNase to confer cytoprotection against ER stress. Biochem Biophys Res Commun **365**, 777-783 (2008).

CHAPTER 6

Heritable Neurodevelopmental Disorders and Endoplasmic Reticulum Stress

Takashi Momoi and Eriko Fujita

Divisions of Development and Differentiation, Department of Human Inherited Metabolic Disease, National Institute of Neuroscience, 4-1-1 Ogawahigashi-machi, Kodaira, Tokyo 187-8502, Japan

Address correspondence to: Dr. Takashi Momoi, Divisions of Development and Differentiation, Department of Human Inherited Metabolic Disease, National Institute of Neuroscience, 4-1-1 Ogawahigashi-machi, Kodaira, Tokyo 187-8502, Japan; Tel: 81-42-341-2711 (ext.5273); Email: momoi@ncnp.go.jp

Abstract: The molecular pathogenesis of heritable neurodevelopmental disorders, including autism spectrum disorder (ASD) and speech-language disorder, is not well understood; although, several mutations in genes encoding neuroligin and FOXP2 have been identified. Here, we evaluate the relationship between the protein quality control system of the endoplasmic reticulum (ER) and the molecular pathogenesis of these disorders.

1. INTRODUCTION

The endoplasmic reticulum (ER) quality-control system recognizes and removes nascent proteins that fail to fold or assemble properly; ER stress response is part of this system. The relationship between ER stress and neurodegenerative disorders, including polyglutamine disorder and Parkinson disorder, have been well studied [1,2]; while the relationship between ER stress and developmental disorders has not been sufficiently examined.

2. AUTISM SPECTRUM DISORDER

Autism spectrum disorder (ASD) is a neural developmental disorder characterized by impaired social interactions, communication impairment, and restricted and repetitive behaviors [3]. The molecular pathogenesis of ASD is still unknown; although recently, mutations have been shown in genes encoding neuroligin 3 (NLGN3), NLGN4, and SHANK3 [4,5]. Mutations in NLGNs and SHANK do not frequently occur in ASD, yet understanding the precise role of NLGNs in synapse function may shed light on the development of this wide spectrum of diseases. The NLGNs are postsynaptic cell adhesion proteins capable of interacting with neurexins (Nrxs) [6,7].

SHANK3, a protein of the postsynaptic density (PSD) of excitatory synapses, may function as a master scaffold by forming large sheets that serve as a platform for construction of the PSD complex [8]. Mutations in synaptic cell adhesion molecules and the scaffold protein suggest impaired synaptic function is closely associated with the pathogenesis of ASD.

An interaction between NLGNs and Nrxs forms a functional synapse by assembling highly ordered complexes composed of ion channel, receptor, neurotransmitter storage, and cell adhesion via scaffolding protein (including PSD-95) at the complementary presynaptic and postsynaptic sites. PSD-95 modulates targeting of NLGNs to excitatory synapses via their intracellular PDZ-binding motif [9]. The NLGN-Nrx trans-synaptic adhesion system is a major determinant of synaptic balance between excitatory and inhibitory synapse via assembling PSD-95. One particular NLGN-3 mutation (R451C), identified in a set of twins with autism, resulted in enhanced inhibition and impaired social interaction in mice [10]. This suggests impaired NLGN-mediated modulation of excitatory versus inhibitory synapse function is a cause of ASD. However, it is still unclear how the NLGN-3 mutation (R451C) could modulate the change of this balance. We will focus on the relationship between the protein quality control

Claudio Hetz (Ed.)

system of the ER in NLGL-3 (R451C) mutants and the pathogenesis of ASD.

3. PROTEIN QUALITY CONTROL SYSTEM IN ER

The relationship between intracellular aggregation of misfolded and malfolded proteins and endoplasmic reticulum (ER) stress has been intensively studied. The misfolded and malfolded proteins activate stress-signaling pathways, called unfolded protein response (UPR), via ER stress-sensor proteins such as PERK (protein kinase regulated by RNA (PKR)-like ER kinase), activating transcription factor 6 (ATF6), and inositol requiring kinase (IREs) [11-14]. Up-regulated Bip, an ER chaperone, helps to refold the proteins into normal folded protein structure. The excess misfolded or malfolded proteins, which are not refolded by chaperones, are extracted and retrotranslocated to the cytoplasm where they are degraded by the ubiquitin/proteasome system

(UPS) [1] of the ER-associated degradation (ERAD) system. If insufficiently degraded, misfolded or malfolded proteins accumulate in the ER and are assumed to activate the ER stress-mediated cell death pathway [2]. The structure, localization, and solubility of the improperly folded proteins determine the degradation system utilized. Some misfolded proteins, such as the 1-antitrypsin z mutant, can polymerize within the ER and may not be retro-transported out [13]. They then form inclusion bodies in the ER, like Russell's body [14].

Mutations in the dysferlin gene have been found in patients with the muscle diseases, limb girdle muscular dystrophy/Miyoshi myopathy (LGMD2B/MM). Some novel variants of LGMD2B/MM have shown patchy sarcolemmal immunostaining or intracellular aggregates of dysferlin in the muscle fibers of patients. A relationship between ER stress and mutant (L1341P)-dysferlin aggregates has been also

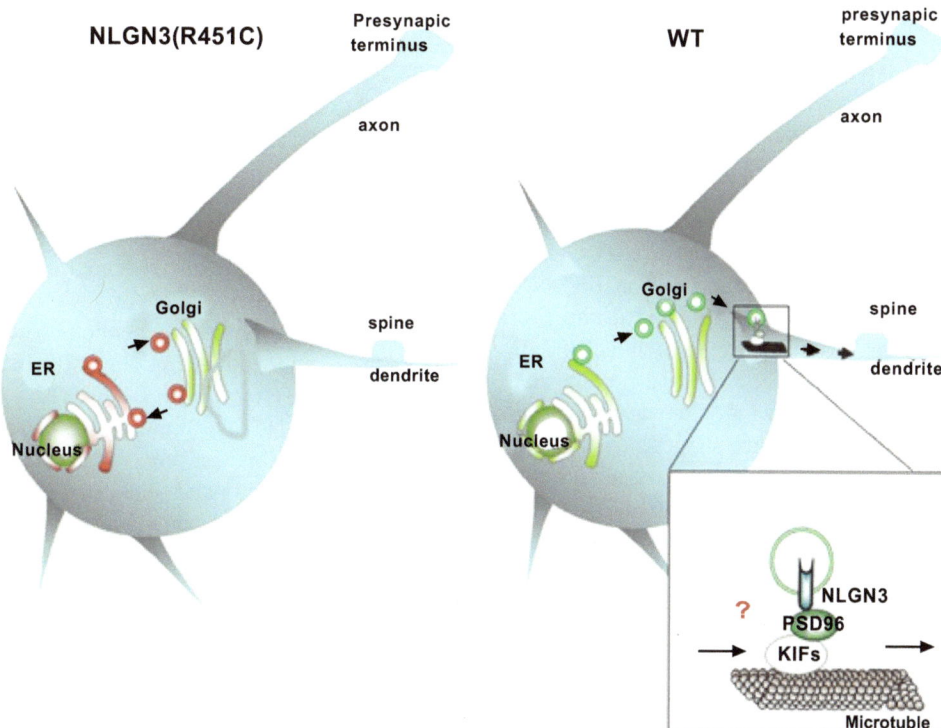

Fig. (1). Retention of mutated NLGN3 (R451C) in the ER.
NLGNs are synaptic cell adhesion molecules located at the postsynaptic membrane. PSD-95 controls the trafficking of NLGNs to the postsynaptic membrane. The mutated NLGN (R451C) is largely retained in the ER, with little of the nascent protein reaching its cell membrane location. Residual protein that reaches the cell surface has an altered affinity for β-Nrx. The mutated NLGN may be checked by the protein quality control system of the ER and their expression and degradation could be regulated by ER stress.

suggested [15]. The aggregated proteins are subjected to clearance by autophagy [16]. This autophagy/lysosomal degradation system (ERAD-II), regulated by ER stress, is an alternative to the UPS-dependent ERAD system (ERAD-I).

4. RETENTION OF MUTATED NEURO-LIGINS IN THE ER AND PATHOGE-NESIS OF AUTISM SPECTRUM DISOR-DER

Recently, high resolution crystal structures of the extracellular domains of a NLGN showed mutations, including R451C, are not located within the binding interface but rather between the dimerization interface and the AChE active site [17]. Mutations found in ASD, including R451C, do not directly interfere with the binding of NLGNs to Nrxs. The mutations seem to cause defects in NLGN folding or affect its dimerization, altering the processing and indirectly resulting in altered binding to Nrxs. Thus, crystal structure analysis of NLGN-3 may provide a new understanding of mutations linked to ASD. In addition to impairment of binding activity, the conformational alteration of mutated NLGNs may be directly related to the pathogenesis of ASD. This may explain why NLGN-3-KO mice and NLGN-3 (R451C)-KI mice have different impaired social behavior.

On the other hand, a cell biological study has shown the R451C NLGN mutation gives rise to an altered cellular phenotype. As shown in Fig. (1), the mutated NLGN is largely retained in the ER, with little of the nascent protein reaching its cell membrane location [18]. The residual protein that reaches the cell surface has an altered affinity for β-Nrx. Accumulated evidence suggests the R451C NLGN retained in the ER is checked under the quality control system. However, the ER stress effect has not been examined as developmental disorders are not progressive like neurodegenerative disease. NGLNs are type II membrane proteins with structures similar to dysferlin. It is possible the mutated NLGN (R451C) generates ER stress if excess mutated molecules are not retrotransported into the cytoplasm.

5. FOXP2 MUTATION IN SPEECH-LANGUAGE DISORDER

Another example of a developmental disorder related to ER stress is speech-language disorder.

The phenotype of speech-language disorder segregates as an autosomal dominant trait. Half of the members of the KE family, affected by speech-language disorder, have severe articulation difficulties accompanied by verbal and orofacial impairment. Mutation of the forkhead box P2 (FOXP2) gene was determined to be the responsible genetic factor [19-21]; a missense mutation (R553H) in the forkhead domain of FOXP2 co-segregates with the disorder in this family.

FOXP2 contains a forkhead domain with a winged-helix DNA binding domain [22], a glutamine-rich region (polyQ tract), zinc finger, and a leucine zipper motif for homo- and hetero-dimerization to FOXP1, 2, and 4 family members. The familial FOXP2 mutated protein (R553H) exhibits reduced DNA binding and defects in nuclear localization *in vitro* [23,24], suggesting loss of transcriptional activity causes lack of expression of the genes required for synaptic function, neural circuit, and the region for speech-language ability.

An animal model is necessary for the analysis of the speech learning disorder at the molecular level. FOXP2 was highly conserved during evolution and the human FOXP2 protein differs by only 2 amino acids with its mouse homologue. In addition, one glutamine from the human protein is absent in the polyQ tract in the mouse FOXP2 [25]. Infant rodents emit ultrasonic vocalizations (USVs), whistle-like sounds with frequencies between 40-100 kHz, which play an important communicative role in mother-offspring interactions when isolated from the mother and littermates [26]. Homozygous knock-in (KI) mice for FOXP2 (R552H), corresponding to the human FOXP2 (R553H) mutation, exhibit severe USV and motor impairment at postnatal day 10 (p10), achieve crisis stage for survival three weeks after birth, and finally die. Whereas, heterozygous FOXP2 (R552H)-KI mice exhibit modest impairment of USVs, a slight defect of motor ability, and can survive [27,28].

In contrast with heterozygous mice, the homozygous FOXP2 (R552H)-KI mice show reduced weight, immature development of cerebellum with incompletely folded folia, and Purkinje cells with poor dendritic arbors. In homozygous FOXP2 (R552H)-KI mice, some of the FOXP2 (R552H) protein aggregates in the nuclei, compromising the function of the Purkinje

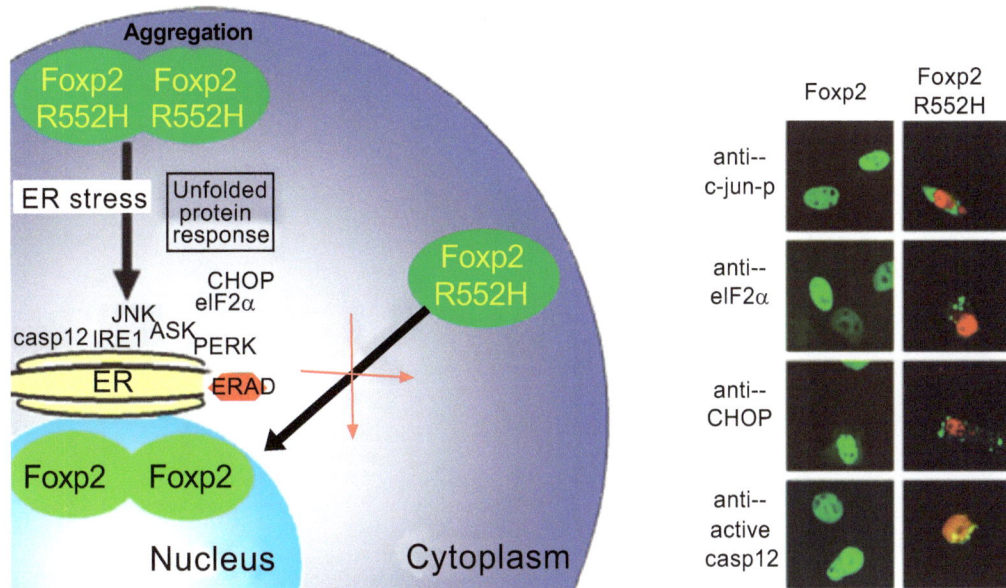

Fig. (2). ER stress of FOXP2 (R553H) and FOXP2 (R552H).
Ectopically expressed human FOXP2 (R553H) and mouse FOXP2 (R552H) exhibit defects in nuclear localization *in vitro* [24]; they are localized in the cytoplasm and nuclei of COS cells and aggregate there in a time-dependent manner. Cells expressing FOXP2 (R552H) aggregates show increased ER stress makers including c-Jun phosphorylation (c-Jun-p), eIF2α-phosphorylation (eIF2α-p), up-regulation of CHOP, and activation of caspase-12 (anti-m12D341 reactivity) [27]. This may be due to the similar molecular mechanism by which polyQ aggregates induce ER stress.

cells and cerebral neurons, resulting in their death [27]. Ectopically expressed FOXP2 (R552H) exhibits defects in nuclear localization *in vitro* [24]; they are localized in the cytoplasm and nuclei of COS cells and aggregate there in a time-dependent manner. Cells expressing FOXP2 (R552H) aggregates show increased ER stress markers including c-Jun phosphorylation (c-Jun-p), eIF2α-phosphorylation (eIF2α-p), up-regulation of CHOP, and activation of caspase-12 (anti-m12D341 reactivity) (Fig. (2)) [27].

Thus, in the mouse model, cytoplasmic and/or nuclear aggregates of ectopically expressed FOXP2 (R552H) induce ER stress in cells. The polyQ aggregates stimulate ER stress signals and induce ER stress-mediated cell death, presumably by the accumulation of unfolded proteins in the ER due to inhibition of ERAD and retrotranslocation [29]. Therefore, it is likely that human FOXP2 (R553H), containing the polyQ tract, also brings about ER stress.

It is presently not clear whether or not immature development of the cerebellum, including Purkinje cells with poor development of dendrites, is associated with speech-language ability. Speech-language disorder shows autosomal dominant inheritance and all the affected members of the KE family with speech-language disorders are heterozygous.

6.CONCLUSION

In contrast with neurodegenerative disorders, ASD and speech-language disorder are not progressive. In view of this, it is unlikely ER stress-mediated neuronal cell death is related to the pathogenesis of these developmental disorders. However, expression of essential factors of synaptic function may be affected by ER stress induced by mutated proteins associated with these disorders. The relationship between ER stress and the pathogenesis of developmental disorders will be further examined by the mouse model.

7. ABBREVIATIONS

ATF6	=	Activating transction factor 6
ASD	=	AUTISM spectrum disorder
c-Jun-p	=	c-Jun phosphorylation
eIF2α-p	=	eIF2α-phosphorylation
ER	=	Endoplasmic reticulum
ERAD	=	ER-associated degradation
ERAD-I	=	Ubiquitine/proteasome system-dependent ERAD system

ERAD-II   = Autophagy/lysosomal
                  degradation system

FOXP2   = Forkhead box P2

IREs   = Inositol requiring kinase

LGMD2B/MM = Limb girdle muscular
                  dystrophy /Miyoshi myopathy

NLGN   = Neuroligin

Nrxs   = Neurexins

PERK   = Protein kinase regulated by
                  RNA (PKR)-like ER kinase

PSD   = Postsynaptic density

UPR   = Unfolded protein response

UPS   = Ubiquitin/ proteasome system

USVs   = Ultrasonic vocalizations

7. ACKNOLDGEMENT

We thank Dr. Yuko Tanabe for valuable discussion and the preparation of Figures.

8. REFERENCES

1.   Kopito RR, Ron D. Conformational disease. Nat Cell Biol 2000;2(11):207-209.
2.   Momoi T. Conformational diseases and ER stress-mediated cell death: apoptotic cell death and autophagic cell death. Curr Mol Med 2006;6(1):111-118.
3.   Pickett J, London E. The neuropathology of autism. J Neuropathol Exp Neurol 2005;64(11):925-935.
4.   Jamain S, Quach H, Betancur C, Råstam M, Colineaux C, Gillberg IC, Soderstrom H, Giros B, Leboyer M, Gillberg C, Bourgeron T. Nat Genet 2003;34(1):27-29.
5.   Durand CM, Betancur C, Boeckers TM, Bockmann J, Chaste P, Fauchereau F, Nygren G, Rastam M, Gillberg IC, Anckarsäter H, Sponheim E, Goubran-Botros H, Delorme R, Chabane N, Mouren-Simeoni MC, de Mas P, Bieth E, Rogé B, Héron D, Burglen L, Gillberg C, Leboyer M, Bourgeron T. Mutations in the gene encoding the synaptic scaffolding protein SHANK3 are associated with autism spectrum disorders. Nat Genet 2007;39(1):25-27.
6.   Scheiffele P, Fan J, Choih J, Fetter R, Serafini T. Neuroligin expressed in nonneuronal cells triggers presynaptic development in contacting axons. Cell. 2000;101(6):657-669.
7.   Graf ER, Zhang X, Jin SX, Linhoff MW, Craig AM. Neurexins induce differentiation of GABA and glutamate postsynaptic specializations via neuroligins. Cell 2004;119(7):1013-1026.
8.   Moessner R, Marshall CR, Sutcliffe JS, Skaug J, Pinto D, Vincent J, Zwaigenbaum L, Fernandez B, Roberts W, Szatmari P, Scherer SW. Contribution of SHANK3

mutations to autism spectrum disorder. Am J Hum Genet 2007;81(6):1289-1297.
9.   Levinson JN, El-Husseini A. Building excitatory and inhibitory synapses: balancing neuroligin partnerships. Neuron 2005;48(2):171-174.
10.   Tabuchi K, Blundell J, Etherton MR, Hammer RE, Liu X, Powell CM, Südhof TC. A neuroligin-3 mutation implicated in autism increases inhibitory synaptic transmission in mice. Science 2007;318(5847):71-76.
11.   Kopito RR. ER quality control: the cytoplasmic connection. Cell 1997;88(4):427-430.
12.   Ron D. Translational control in the endoplasmic reticulum stress response. J Clin Invest 2002;110(10):1383-1388.
13.   Ye Y, Shibata Y, Yun C, Ron D, Rapoport TA. A membrane protein complex mediates retro-translocation from the ER lumen into the cytosol. Nature 2004;429(6994):841-847.
14.   Sitia R, Braakman I. Quality control in the endoplasmic reticulum protein factory. Nature 2003;426(6968):891-894.
15.   Wenzel K, Carl M, Perrot A, Zabojszcza J, Assadi M, Ebeling M, Geier C, Robinson PN, Kress W, Osterziel KJ, Spuler S. Novel sequence variants in dysferlin-deficient muscular dystrophy leading to mRNA decay and possible C2-domain misfolding. Hum Mutat 2006;27(6):599-600.
16.   Fujita E, Kouroku Y, Isoai A, Kumagai H, Misutani A, Matsuda C, Hayashi YK, Momoi T. Two endoplasmic reticulum-associated degradation (ERAD) systems for the novel variant of the mutant dysferlin: ubiquitin/proteasome ERAD(I) and autophagy/lysosome ERAD(II). Hum Mol Genet 2007;16(6):618-629.
17.   Fabrichny IP, Leone P, Sulzenbacher G, Comoletti D, Miller MT, Taylor P, Bourne Y, Marchot P. Structural analysis of the synaptic protein neuroligin and its beta-neurexin complex: determinants for folding and cell adhesion. Neuron 2007;56(6):979-991.
18.   Comoletti D, De Jaco A, Jennings LL, Flynn RE, Gaietta G, Tsigelny I, Ellisman MH, Taylor P. : The Arg451Cys-neuroligin-3 mutation associated with autism reveals a defect in protein processing. J Neurosci 2004;24(20):4889-4893.
19.   Fisher SE, Vargha-Khadem F, Watkins KE, Monaco AP, Pembrey ME. Localisation of a gene implicated in a severe speech and language disorder. Nat Genet 1998;18(2):168-170.
20.   Lai CS, Fisher SE, Hurst JA, Vargha-Khadem F, Monaco AP. A forkhead-domain gene is mutated in a severe speech and language disorder. Nature 2001;413(6855):519-523.
21.   Vargha-Khadem F, Gadian DG, Copp A, Mishkin M. FOXP2 and the neuroanatomy of speech and language. Nat Rev Neurosci 2005;6(2):131-138.
22.   Shu W, Yang H, Zhang L, Lu MM, Morrisey EE. Characterization of a new subfamily of winged-helix/forkhead (Fox) genes that are expressed in the lung and act as transcriptional repressors. J Biol Chem 2001;276(29):27488-27497.
23.   Vernes SC, Nicod J, Elahi FM, Coventry JA, Kenny N, Coupe AM, Bird LE, Davies KE, Fisher SE. Functional genetic analysis of mutations implicated in a human speech and language disorder. Hum Mol Genet 2006;15(21):3154-3167.
24.   Mizutani A, Matsuzaki A, Momoi MY, Fujita E, Tanabe Y, Momoi T. Intracellular distribution of a speech/language disorder associated FOXP2 mutant. Biochem Biophys Res Commun 2007;353(4):869-874.
25.   Enard W, Przeworski M, Fisher SE, Lai CS, Wiebe V, Kitano T, Monaco AP, Pääbo S. Molecular evolution

of FOXP2, a gene involved in speech and language. Nature 2002;418(6900):869-872.

26.   Branchi I, Santucci D, Alleva E. Ultrasonic vocalisation emitted by infant rodents: a tool for assessment of neurobehavioural development. Behav Brain Res 2001;125(1-2):49-56.

27.   Fujita E, Tanabe Y, Shiota A, Ueda M, Suwa K, Momoi MY, Momoi T. Ultrasonic vocalization impairment of Foxp2 (R552H) knockin mice related to speech-language disorder and abnormality of Purkinje cells. Proc Natl Acad Sci U S A 2008;105(8):3117-3122.

28.   Groszer M, Keays DA, Deacon RM, de Bono JP, Prasad-Mulcare S, Gaub S, Baum MG, French CA, Nicod J, Coventry JA, Enard W, Fray M, Brown SD, Nolan PM, Pääbo S, Channon KM, Costa RM, Eilers J, Ehret G, Rawlins JN, Fisher SE. Impaired synaptic plasticity and motor learning in mice with a point mutation implicated in human speech deficits. Curr Biol 2008;18(5):354-362.

29.   Kouroku Y, Fujita E, Jimbo A, Kikuchi T, Yamagata T, Momoi MY, Kominami E, Kuida K, Sakamaki K, Yonehara S, Momoi T. Polyglutamine aggregates stimulate ER stress signals and caspase-12 activation. Hum Mol Genet 2002;11(13):1505-1515.

CHAPTER 7

ER Quality Control, ER Stress-Induced Apoptosis, and Neurodegenerative Diseases

Hideki Nishitoh, Hisae Kadowaki, Kohsuke Takeda and Hidenori Ichijo*

Cell Signaling, Graduate School of Pharmaceutical Sciences, The University of Tokyo, 7-3-1 Hongo, Bunkyo-ku, Tokyo 113-0033, Japan

Abstract: The endoplasmic reticulum (ER) is the intracellular organelle in which newly synthesized secretory and transmembrane proteins achieve proper structure as a result of post-translational modification, folding, and oligomerization. However, many of these proteins are malfolded (unfolded or misfolded) as a result of various intracellular or extracellular stimuli. ER stress is caused by disturbances of ER function with the accumulation of malfolded proteins and alterations in calcium homeostasis. To restore ER function, cells possess a highly specific ER quality control system to increase the capacity of protein folding and to reduce the amount of malfolded proteins in the ER. In case of prolonged ER stress or malfunction of the ER quality control system, apoptosis signaling is activated. ER stress-induced apoptosis has recently been implicated in human neurodegenerative diseases such as Alzheimer disease, Parkinson disease, polyglutamine diseases, and amyotrophic lateral sclerosis. This review summarizes the molecular mechanisms of the ER quality control system and ER stress-induced apoptosis and the possible roles of ER stress in neurodegenerative diseases.

INTRODUCTION

Multiple physiological or pathophysiological conditions including glucose starvation, misglycosylation of glycoproteins, calcium deprivation from the endoplasmic reticulum (ER) lumen, elevated protein synthesis and secretion, and failure of protein folding, transport, or degradation trigger ER stress. In response to such conditions, cells react to ER dysfunction through adaptive pathways known as the ER stress response, which is mediated by three types of ER transmembrane receptors: pancreatic ER kinase (PKR)-like ER kinase (PERK), activating transcription factor 6 (ATF6), and inositol-requiring enzyme 1 (IRE1), Fig. (**1**). Under non-stressed conditions, all three ER stress receptors are maintained in inactive state through their association with the ER chaperone, BiP (also known as GRP78). Upon accumulation of malfolded proteins, BiP dissociates from receptors, leading to their activation with triggering of the ER stress response [1], Fig. (**1**). The ER stress response is a pro-survival response to reduce the accumulation of malfolded proteins and restore ER function [2]. The ER stress response consists of three major pathways: (1) translational attenuation to modulate ER protein synthesis; (2) gene expression to induce ER luminal chaperones and other components to increase capacity for protein folding [unfolded protein response (UPR)]; and (3) ER-associated degradation (ERAD) to remove malfolded proteins from the ER, Fig. (**1**). However, if ER stress persists or is aggravated, ER stress signaling appears to be switched from pro-survival to pro-apoptosis. ER stress-induced apoptosis has recently been implicated in various neurodegenerative diseases, including brain ischemia, Alzheimer disease, Parkinson disease, polyglutamine (polyQ) diseases, and amyotrophic lateral sclerosis (ALS) [3]. One common feature of some neurodegenerative disorders is that the accumulation of disease-specific malfolded proteins triggers neuronal cell death. Although it has generally been thought that activity of the ubiquitin proteasome system (UPS) is mitigated by the accumulation of malfolded proteins in these diseases, the causal relationship between this event and neuronal cell death remains unclear. Recent studies have shown that the ER stress caused by accumulation of malfolded proteins is a key mechanism of neuronal cell death in polyQ diseases, familial Parkinson disease, and familial ALS, Fig. (**3**).

Understanding of the molecular mechanisms of ER quality control system and ER stress-induced cell death may provide insights into potential targets for treatment of diseases. We describe here the molecular mechanisms of the ER quality control system and ER stress-induced apoptosis and the causal relationships between ER stress and neurodegenerative diseases.

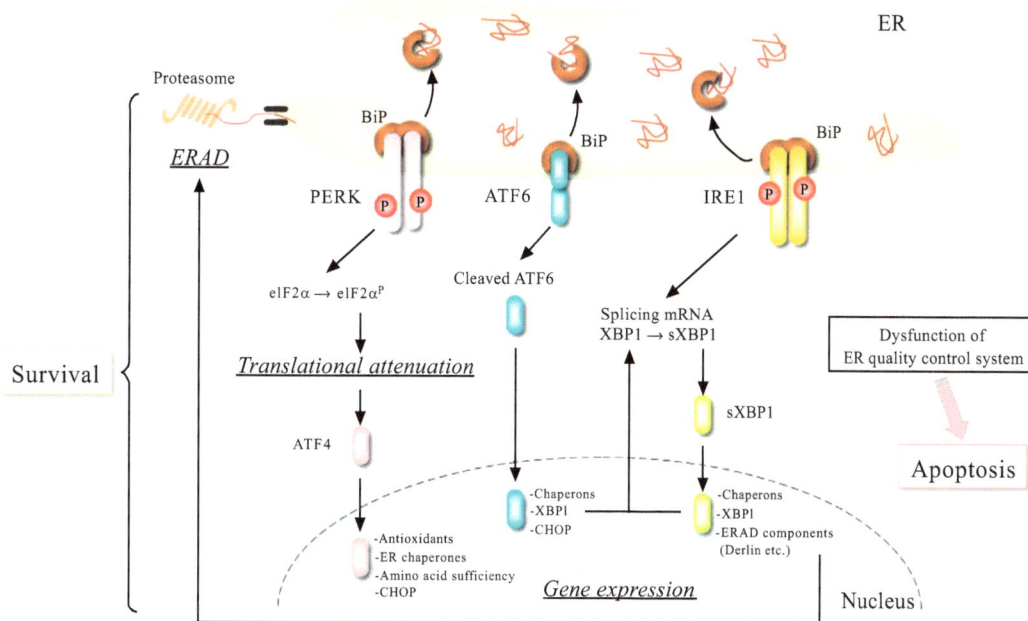

Fig. (1). During ER stress, BiP dissociates from three ER stress receptors, PERK, ATF6, and IRE1, permitting their activation. Activated PERK blocks general protein synthesis by phosphorylation of eIF2α. This phosphorylation enables translation of ATF4. ATF4 translocates to the nucleus and induces the transcription of genes required for ER quality control. ATF6 is activated by cleavage after transport to the Golgi. Activated ATF6 is also a transcription factor and regulates the expression of ER chaperones and XBP1. XBP1 must undergo mRNA splicing for its transcriptional activation, which is carried out by activated IRE1. Spliced XBP1 protein (sXBP1) translocates to the nucleus and controls the transcription of chaperones and genes involved in ERAD.

ER QUALITY CONTROL SYSTEM

I. Translational Attenuation

During ER stress, since newly synthesized chaperones through the UPR cannot immediately be produced, the protein folding capacity of the ER is initially limited. To avoid further accumulation of malfolded proteins in the ER before folding capacity can be increased, the rate of ER protein synthesis must be decreased through a more rapid, transcription-independent mechanism. PERK is a type I transmembrane Ser/Thr kinase receptor. Activation of PERK through its oligomerization and trans-phosphorylation results in phosphorylation of eukaryotic initiation factor 2α (eIF2α), leading to translational attenuation [4], Fig. (**1**). When eIF2α is phosphorylated, formation of the ternary translation initiation complex eIF2/GTP/Met-tRNA is prevented, leading to attenuation of translation in general. Whereas phosphorylation of eIF2α by PERK leads to attenuation of global mRNA translation, phosphorylated eIF2α selectively stimulates translation of a specific subset of mRNAs, including activating transcription factor 4 (ATF4) mRNA, in response to ER stress, Fig. (**1**).

ii. Gene Expression

Upon ER stress, ATF4 subsequently activates transcription of ER stress-responsive genes involved in ER protein maturation, anti-oxidative activity [e.g., ER oxidase 1α (ERO1α)], transcription [e.g. C/EBP homologous protein (CHOP)], and amino acid metabolism, Fig. (**1**). ATF6 is a basic leucine zipper (bZIP)-containing transcription factor, which includes a transmembrane domain and is activated by limited proteolysis after its translocation from the ER to the Golgi apparatus. Cleaved and activated ATF6 translocates into the nucleus and regulates the gene expression of ER chaperones and transcription factor [X box-binding protein 1 (XBP1)]. To achieve its active form, XBP1 must undergo mRNA splicing, which is carried out by IRE1, Fig. (**1**). IRE1 is a type I transmembrane Ser/Thr kinase that also has site-specific endoribonuclease (RNase) activity [5,6]. The RNase activity is fully activated after autophosphorylation then splices target mRNAs including XBP1. Spliced XBP1 protein (sXBP1) translocates into the nucleus and controls the transcription of ER chaperone genes, as well as genes involved in ERAD, Fig. (**1**).

These concerted activities restore ER function by enhancing folding capacity and initiating degradation of misfolded proteins.

III. ERAD

Some ER proteins fail to fold correctly by any refolding mechanisms. These malfolded ER proteins must be disposed by ERAD. In ERAD, malfolded proteins in the ER membrane or lumen are actively retro-translocated into the cytosol, where they are degraded by UPS. ERAD consists of three steps: the recognition and targeting of ERAD substrates to the retro-translocation apparatus, its transport across the ER membrane to the cytosol, and its degradation [7-9], Fig. (**2**). The components that mediate each step are not fully understood. The recognition and targeting of malfolded proteins are mediated by protein glycosylation and chaperones in the ER lumen. ER resident chaperones such as BiP and Hsp40 have been shown to prevent soluble substrate aggregation prior to degradation [10]. Protein disulfide isomerase (PDI) has also been shown to

play an important role prior to substrate retro-translocation [11]. In some cases, glycosylation of malfolded proteins is also required for recognition by the ERAD machinery such as ER degradation enhancing α-mannosidase-like protein (EDEM) [12]. A recent study showed that the ER-resident protein ERdj5 has a reductase activity, cleaves the disulfide bonds of malfolded proteins, and accelerates ERAD activity through its associations with EDEM and BiP [13], Fig. (**2**).

Although the identity of the retro-translocon channel and the mechanism by which ERAD substrates cross the ER membrane have remained unclear, several lines of evidence support a role for the original Sec61 translocon complex or a new retro-translocon complex containing p97 (a member of the AAA ATPase family) [14,15], Fig. (**2**). Both genetic and biochemical evidence suggests that several ERAD substrates require the Sec61 channel, which also mediates the entry of nascent polypeptides into the lumen from ribosomes [16,17], suggesting that the channel may act bidirectionally [18]. However, the impairment of ERAD in Sec61-deleted cells may

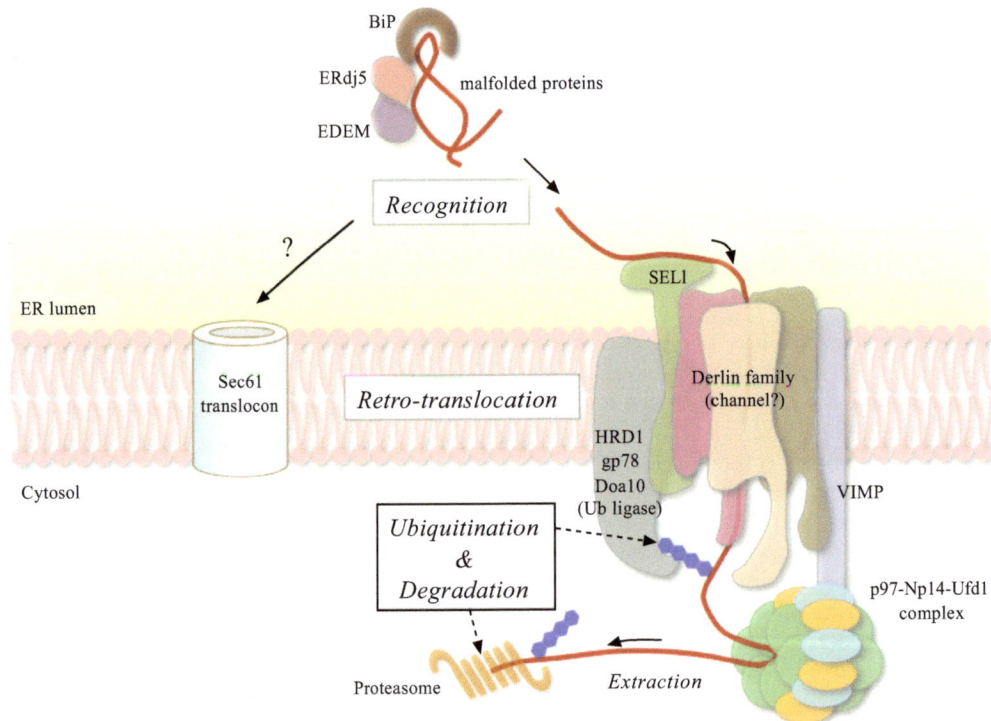

Fig. (2). Malfolded proteins are recognized by ER luminal machinery, including BiP, EDEM, and ERdj5, which present terminally malfolded proteins to a putative retro-translocon channel, which may include Derlin family proteins and that facilitates their retro-translocation from the ER. Cytoplasmically exposed lysine residues are ubiquitinated by E3 ubiquitin ligases, including HRD1, gp78, and Doa10. Retro-translocated and ubiquitinated substrates are extracted by the p97-Npl4-Ufd1 complex, which associates with the ER membrane in ATP-dependent fashion. Finally, membrane-extracted substrates are conveyed to the proteasome.

be an indirect effect of the disruption of ER homeostasis by impairment of translocation of ER proteins, rather than a direct effect on the retro-translocon channel. In addition, the retro-translocation of an ERAD substrate, pro-α factor, was unaffected by inhibition of Sec61 function using anti-Sec61 antibody in an in vitro ERAD experiment [15]. This finding suggests that some ERAD substrates may cross the ER membrane through an unknown retro-translocon channel other than Sec61.

On the other hand, the delivery of ubiquitinated substrates to the proteasome depends on p97 ATPase activity [14]. p97 associates with Npl4 and Ufd1, which bind ubiquitinated proteins. The p97-Npl4-Ufd1 complex contributes to extraction of malfolded proteins to the cytosol in ATP-dependent fashion, Fig. (**2**). This motor activity depends on binding of this complex to ERAD substrates in the retro-translocation pathway, and also requires the interaction of this complex with the cytosolic side of the retro-translocon. Derlin-1 has been identified as a p97-interacting ER membrane protein complex and is a multi-spanning membrane protein that is required for retro-translocation [19,20]. Recently, two other Derlin-1-like proteins, designated Derlin-2 and Derlin-3, have been identified [21]. Derlin family proteins are capable of homo- or hetero-oligomerizing with each other [22,23]. These interactions have lead to the proposal that Derlin family proteins may be components of the retro-translocon, Fig. (**2**). This hypothesis is supported by the finding of the in vitro ERAD experiment noted above that retro-translocation of pro-α factor was significantly inhibited by anti-Derlin-1 antibody [15]. Polyubiquitination of retro-translocated ERAD substrates is caused by E3 ubiquitin ligases. Transmembrane type E3 ubiquitin ligases have been implicated in ERAD, including HRD1, gp78, and Doa10, which have transmembrane segments and a cytosolic E3 ligase domain. These E3 ligases associate with p97, SEL1, and Derlin-1, and are essential for the ubiquitination of retro-translocated substrates [22]. The SEL1-Derlin family-p97-E3 complex may thus unify mechanisms of substrate recognition in the ER lumen, retro-translocation, and extraction through the ER membrane, and ubiquitination of retro-translocated substrates in the cytosol, Fig. (**2**).

ER STRESS-INDUCED APOPTOSIS

If overloading of malfolded proteins in the ER is not resolved, prolonged ER stress response will result in apoptosis. Several studies have shown that several molecules, including transcription factors, caspase family proteins, Bcl-2 family proteins, and those of the MAP kinase cascade, are related to the ER stress-induced apoptosis pathway [24].

I. CHOP

CHOP was first reported as a molecule involved in ER stress-induced apoptosis [25]. The level of expression of CHOP is low under non-stressed conditions, but is markedly increased in response to ER stress, Fig. (**3**). Overexpression of CHOP promotes apoptosis in several cell lines [25-27], while deficiency of CHOP can protect cells from ER stress-induced apoptosis [25]. CHOP thus plays an important role in the induction of apoptosis. However, exactly how CHOP mediates ER stress-induces apoptosis remains unclear. CHOP inhibits the expression of Bcl-2 anti-apoptotic protein [28] and induces the expression of Bim, BH3-only pro-apoptotic proteins [29], and DR5, a member of the death receptor protein family [30,31]. Interestingly, CHOP also induces depletion of cellular glutathione and increase in reactive oxygen species (ROS) in the ER through induction of ERO1α expression [28,32]. ERO1α may thus be an important mediator of apoptosis downstream of CHOP.

II. Bcl-2 Family Proteins

ER stress-induced apoptosis is also regulated by well-known general apoptosis pathways such as the Bcl-2 family proteins and caspase pathways. Bcl-2 is known to reside in the ER membrane as well as the mitochondrial membrane [33]. While Bcl-2 family proteins are thought to act principally at the mitochondrial outer membrane, they also influence ER homeostasis and ER stress-induced apoptosis [34,35]. On the other hand, ER stress upregulates or activates several BH3-only pro-apoptotic proteins, including Bim [29,36], BIK [37,38], NOXA [39] and PUMA [40,41], Fig. (**3**). ER stress-induced apoptosis signal is thus linked to BH3-only family proteins. Other BH3-only family proteins, Bax and Bak, are normally located in the cytosol and translocate to the mitochondria in response to various apoptotic stimuli. MEFs from the double-knockout mice Bax-/- and Bak-/- were found to be remarkably resistant to ER stress [42,43]. Furthermore, a recent study showed that Bax and Bak function in the ER as an essential gateway for ER stress-induced apoptosis by maintaining the homeostasis of ER Ca2+ [44]. Thus, Bax and Bak are thus key molecules in the triggering and mediation of ER stress-induced apoptosis [45].

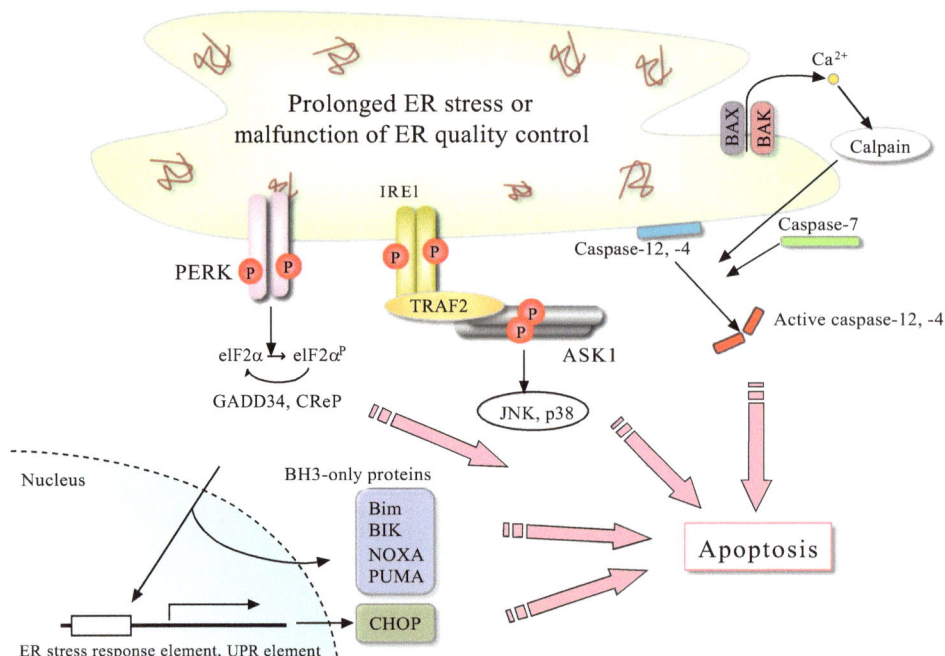

Fig. (3). Caspase-12 or -4 associates with the cytosolic face of the ER membrane and can be activated by ER stress in several fashions. Bax and Bak reside in the ER membrane and influence apoptosis through the regulation of calcium flux. BH3-only pro-apoptotic proteins, including Bim, BIK, NOXA, and PUMA, are upregulated by ER stress and mediate apoptosis. The GADD34- or CReP-phosphatase complex, which dephosphorylates eIF2α, might be related to ER stress-induced apoptosis. Upon ER stress, activated IRE1 recruits TRAF2 and ASK1 on the ER membrane and thus activates the ASK1-dependent apoptosis pathway. See text for details.

III. Caspase

Caspase pathways also play an important role in ER stress-induced apoptosis, Fig. (**3**). Caspase-12, a murine protein associated with the ER membrane, is activated by ER stress in several fashions [46]. For example, the cytosolic calcium-activated protease, calpain, cleaves and activates caspase-12 in response to Ca2+ flux from the ER [47]. Caspase-12 is also autocleaved and activated through interaction with an adaptor protein, TNF receptor-associated factor (TRAF) 2, and IRE1α [48]. It has also been shown that caspase-7 translocates to the ER and activates caspase-12 directly in response to some types of apoptotic stimuli [49,50]. Activated caspase-12 induces the cleavage and activation of the downstream caspase cascade, including caspase-9 [51,52]. Studies with caspase-12-/- mice have shown that caspase-12 is required for ER stress-induced apoptosis [46]. In addition, caspase-12 has been shown to be activated by amyloid ß peptide (Aß), which plays an important role in the development of Alzheimer disease [53], in primary neurons through calpain activation [47], and caspase-12-/- neurons are partially resistant to Aß-induced cell death [46]. However, the human CASPASE-12 gene is disrupted by a termination codon [54]. Human caspase-4, which is 48% homologous to murine caspase-12, has been identified as one of the functional counterparts of caspase-12. Human caspase-4 is localized to the ER membrane and is specifically activated by ER stress and required for apoptosis [55]. However, caspase-4 belongs to the group of pro-inflammatory caspases that induce the proteolytic activation of cytokines. Although siRNA knockdown of caspase-4 in human neuroblastoma cells reduces ER stress- and Aß-induced apoptosis in Hela cells, knockdown of caspase-4 has a marginal effect on ER stress-induced apoptosis [55]. These findings suggest that the relevance of caspase-4 to ER stress-induced apoptosis is cell- and tissue-specific. Identification of other functional human homologues of caspase-12 and determination of their physiological significance in ER stress-induced apoptosis remain to be performed.

IV. PERK- eIF2α

GADD34 and CReP, which are the eIF2α phosphatase cofactors, are also related to ER stress-induced apoptosis. During ER stress, GADD34-/- cells exhibit persistence of eIF2α phosphorylation

[56] and less accumulation of malfolded protei ns in the ER lumen [57]. These findings suggest that GADD34 may function as a pro-apoptotic factor. GADD34-/- mice are resistant to the toxic effects of ER stressors [32]. Similarly, siRNA knockdown of CReP protects cells from ER stress-induce apoptosis [58]. Since the sustained phosphorylation of eIF2α by constitutively active PERK inhibits ER stress-induced apoptosis [59], the cytoprotective effect of deficiency of GADD34 or CReP might be due to increased eIF2α phosphorylation. Indeed, a pharmacological inhibitor of eIF2α phosphatase, salubrinal, protects cells from ER stress-induced apoptosis [60].

V. MAP Kinase Pathway

The c-Jun amino-terminal kinase pathway (JNK) has been reported to be activated by ER stress through the interaction of TRAF2 with the cytosolic kinase domain of IRE1 [61]. Apoptosis signal-regulating kinase (ASK) 1 was shown to be required for TRAF2-dependent JNK activation in the TNF signaling pathway [62,63]. ASK1 is a ubiquitously expressed mitogen-activated protein kinase kinase kinase (MAPKKK) which activates both JNK and p38 pathways [64]. ASK1 rapidly associates with TRAF2 after stimulation by ER stressors and is activated in this fashion. ASK1-/- cells have been found to be resistant to ER stress-induced JNK activation and apoptosis. The IRE1-TRAF2-ASK1 axis has thus been shown to be important for ER stress-induced JNK activation and apoptosis [65], Fig. (**3**). Although the precise mechanism by which ASK1 executes apoptosis under ER stress is still controversial, several lines of evidence suggest that Bcl-2 family proteins and caspase pathways regulate ASK1-mediated apoptosis. ASK1-induced apoptosis has been found to be dependent on caspase-9 activation. ASK1-induced apoptosis was dependent on caspase-9 activation [66], suggesting that the ASK1-caspase-9 pro-apoptotic pathway might be crucial for ER stress-induced apoptosis. Furthermore, the ASK1-JNK pathway also induces the activation of pro-apoptotic Bcl-2 family proteins (e.g., Bim [67]), or the inhibition of anti-apoptotic Bcl-2 family proteins (e.g., BcL-2 [68] and Mcl-1 [69]) through their phosphorylation. Bcl-2 family proteins might thus contribute to ER stress-induced apoptosis in the presence of activation of ASK1. Since phosphorylation of CHOP by p38 increases its transcriptional and apoptotic activity [25,70], the IRE1-ASK1-p38 pathway may also enhance CHOP-mediated apoptosis during ER stress.

These various ER stress-induced apoptosis pathways have been implicated in a wide variety of human diseases and conditions, including hypoxia, ischemia/reperfusion injury, heart diseases, diabetes, and neurodegenerative diseases.

ER STRESS AND NEURO-DEGENERATIVE DISEASES

I. Brain Ischemia

Brain ischemia/reperfusion injury activates the PERK-eIF2α pathway and induces BiP, GRP94, and CHOP in rat and mouse hippocampus [71,72]. Moreover, NO, a known mediator of brain injury during stroke, induces the expression of CHOP in cultured neurons, Fig. (**4**). NOS inhibitors protect neurons from pathological effects of brain ischemia [73], and mice lacking the gene encoding iNOS display decreased sensitivity to brain ischemia [74]. Furthermore, ischemia-induced neuronal cell death was decreased in CHOP-/- mice, and primary hippocampal neurons from CHOP-/- mice were more resistant to hypoxia/reoxygenation-induced apoptosis than were those from wild-type mice [75]. These findings suggest that ischemia-induced neuronal cell death may be mediated at least in part through ER stress-induced CHOP induction.

II. Parkinson Disease

Several recent studies have suggested that loss of ERAD function plays a key role in some neurodegenerative disorders. A prominent example of this is Parkinson disease. Hereditary mutations in the ER-associated ubiquitin ligase Parkin are found in patients with familial Parkinson disease. Overexpression of wild-type Parkin suppresses the cell death induced by several ER stressors and by α-synuclein, the principal component of pathological Lewy bodies in Parkinson disease [76]. Parkin expression is induced by ER stress, suggesting that Parkin might play a role in adaptation to ER stress by degradation of ER luminal malfolded proteins. Parkin functions as an ubiquitin ligase in a complex with the carboxyl terminus of Hsc70-interacting protein (CHIP) [77]. A number of putative ERAD substrates for this complex have been suggested. One of them, the Pael receptor (Pael-R), a G protein-coupled orphan receptor, is abundantly expressed in dopaminergic neurons and tends to unfold even in physiological conditions [78]. Overexpression of Pael-R leads to ER stress-induced cell death, which can be prevented by coexpression of wild-type Parkin [78]. It is thus possible that excessive levels of unfolded Pael-R due to Parkin mutations lead to neuronal cell death as a result of ERAD dysfunction, Fig. (**4**).

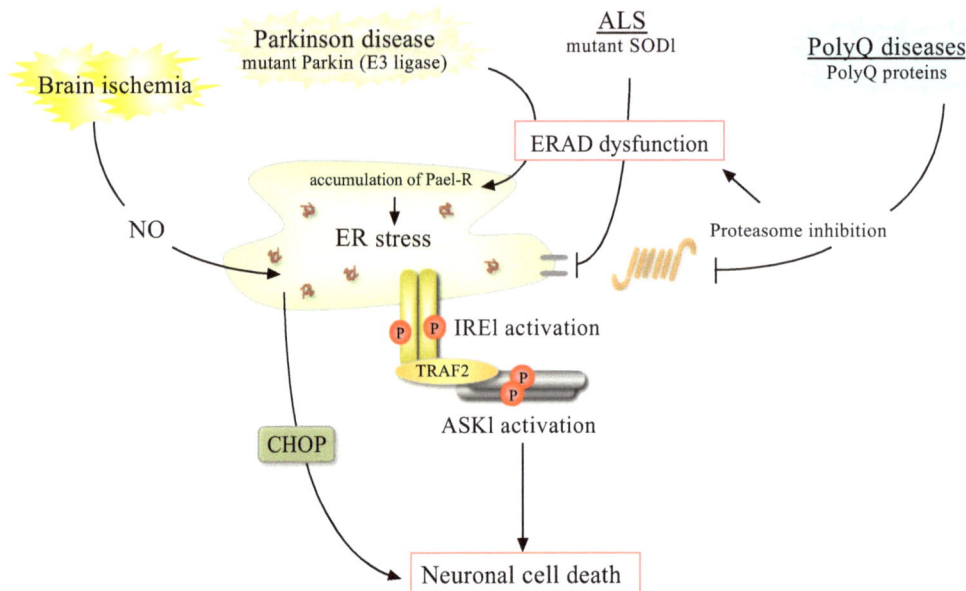

Fig. (4). Brain ischemia/reperfusion injury induces the expression of CHOP mediated by production of NO in neurons. Some cases of familial Parkinson disease are associated with Parkin mutations. Parkin functions as an ubiquitin ligase for ERAD. Accumulation of misfolded Pael-R, a putative ER substrate, by Parkin mutations leads to ER stress. In polyQ diseases, pathogenic polyQ proteins cause accumulation of malfolded proteins. This accumulation inhibits proteasome activity and thus triggers ER stress. In familial ALS, mutant SOD1 specifically binds to an ER membrane protein that plays a key role in ERAD. This interaction inhibits ERAD function and eventually causes ER stress. Deletion of the *ASK1* gene mitigates neuronal cell death by polyQ proteins and by mutant SOD1. The IRE1-TRAF2-ASK1 axis thus plays important roles in the pathogenesis of neurodegenerative diseases.

III. PolyQ diseases

The polyQ diseases are another example of loss of ERAD function. Expansion of CAG trinucleotide repeats that encode polyQ proteins is the underlying cause of at least nine inherited human neurodegenerative disorders, including Huntington's disease and Machado-Joseph disease [79,80]. PolyQ proteins accumulate as aggregates in the cytoplasm and/or in the nucleus and cause accumulation of malfolded proteins, inhibition of proteasome activity, and ER stress-mediated neuronal cell death, Fig. (4). Exactly how polyQ compromises ERAD function remains to be determined. However, findings indicating that a p97 complex interacts and co-localizes with polyQ [81,82], suggest that polyQ might thus target the ERAD complex directly. Furthermore, ASK1 has been shown to associate with TRAF2 via polyQ expression through activation of IRE1 and is activated in this fashion [65], Fig. (4). ASK1-/- cells are resistant to polyQ-induced JNK activation and neuronal cell death. A recent study provided significant evidence that sequence variations in the ASK1 gene are associated with the age at onset of Huntington's disease [83]. These findings suggest that the ER stress-ASK1 axis might play an important role in the pathogenesis of polyQ diseases, Fig. (4).

IV. ALS

ALS is the most frequent adult-onset motor neuron disease and is characterized by the selective loss of motor neurons, leading to muscle atrophy and paralysis and ultimately death. About 1-2% of all cases of ALS are caused by dominantly-inherited mutations of the SOD1 gene. It is thought that mutant SOD1 exhibits pathological effects in familial ALS [84]. ER stress signaling has been suggested to be involved in the pathogenesis of ALS [85-87]. Moreover, several groups have also reported that activation of the ASK1 cascade is associated with induction of motor neuron death by mutant SOD1 both in vitro [88] and in vivo [89-91]. Recently, we have shown that impairment of ERAD plays an important role in neuronal cell death in familial ALS. Mutant SOD1 specifically interacts with Derlin-1 and triggers ER stress through dysfunction of ERAD. Mutant SOD1-induced ER stress activates the ASK1-dependent cell death pathway. Perturbation of binding between mutant SOD1 and Derlin-1 suppresses mutant SOD1-induced ER stress, ASK1 activation, and motor neuron death. Moreover, deletion of ASK1 mitigates motor neuron loss and extends the life span of mutant SOD1 transgenic mice. These findings demonstrate that ER stress-induced ASK1 activation, which is triggered by the specific interaction of Derlin-1 with mutant

SOD1, is crucial for the progression of familial ALS [92], Fig. (**4**).

CONCLUDING REMARKS

The mammalian cell has evolved numerous signaling pathways to respond to ER stress. Although a number of these pathways remain unknown, it is becoming clear that the ER stress response and ER stress-induced apoptosis signaling pathways play roles in numerous neurodegenerative diseases. Understanding of the molecular mechanisms of the ER quality control system and ER stress-induced apoptosis will be required for the development of novel therapeutic targets.

ACKNOWLEDGEMENTS

We thank to all the members of the Laboratory of Cell Signaling for valuable discussion.

REFERENCES

1.   Bertolotti, A.; Zhang, Y.; Hendershot, L. M.; Harding, H. P.; Ron, D.; Nat. Cell Biol., 2000, 2, 326-332.
2.   Marciniak, S. J.; Ron, D.; Physiol. Rev., 2006, 86, 1133-1149.
3.   Sekine, Y.; Takeda, K.; Ichijo, H.; Curr. Mol. Med., 2006, 6, 87-97.
4.   Zhang, K.; Kaufman, R. J.; Neurology, 2006, 66, S102-109.
5.   Tirasophon, W.; Welihinda, A. A.; Kaufman, R. J.; Genes Dev., 1998, 12, 1812-1824.
6.   Wang, X. Z.; Harding, H. P.; Zhang, Y.; Jolicoeur, E. M.; Kuroda, M.; Ron, D.; EMBO J., 1998, 17, 5708-5717.
7.   Kopito, R. R.; Cell, 1997, 88, 427-430.
8.   Meusser, B.; Hirsch, C.; Jarosch, E.; Sommer, T.; Nat. Cell Biol., 2005, 7, 766-772.
9.   Tsai, B.; Ye, Y.; Rapoport, T. A.; Nat. Rev. Mol. Cell Biol., 2002, 3, 246-255.
10. Nishikawa, S. I.; Fewell, S. W.; Kato, Y.; Brodsky, J. L.; Endo, T.; J. Cell Biol., 2001, 153, 1061-1070.
11. Gillece, P.; Luz, J. M.; Lennarz, W. J.; de La Cruz, F. J.; Romisch, K.; J. Cell Biol., 1999, 147, 1443-1456.
12. Hosokawa, N.; Wada, I.; Hasegawa, K.; Yorihuzi, T.; Tremblay, L. O.; Herscovics, A.; Nagata, K.; EMBO Rep., 2001, 2, 415-422.
13. Ushioda, R.; Hoseki, J.; Araki, K.; Jansen, G.; Thomas, D. Y.; Nagata, K.; Science, 2008, 321, 569-572.
14. Ye, Y.; Meyer, H. H.; Rapoport, T. A.; Nature, 2001, 414, 652-656.
15. Wahlman, J.; DeMartino, G. N.; Skach, W. R.; Bulleid, N. J.; Brodsky, J. L.; Johnson, A. E.; Cell, 2007, 129, 943-955.
16. Rapoport, T. A.; Matlack, K. E.; Plath, K.; Misselwitz, B.; Staeck, O.; Biol. Chem., 1999, 380, 1143-1150.
17. Clemons, W. M., Jr.; Menetret, J. F.; Akey, C. W.; Rapoport, T. A.; Curr. Opin. Struct. Biol., 2004, 14, 390-396.
18. Zhou, M.; Schekman, R.; Mol. Cell, 1999, 4, 925-934.
19. Ye, Y.; Shibata, Y.; Yun, C.; Ron, D.; Rapoport, T. A.; Nature, 2004, 429, 841-847.
20. Lilley, B. N.; Ploegh, H. L.; Nature, 2004, 429, 834-840.
21. Oda, Y.; Okada, T.; Yoshida, H.; Kaufman, R. J.; Nagata, K.; Mori, K.; J. Cell Biol., 2006, 172, 383-393.
22. Lilley, B. N.; Ploegh, H. L.; Proc. Natl. Acad. Sci. USA, 2005, 102, 14296-14301.
23. Ye, Y.; Shibata, Y.; Kikkert, M.; van Voorden, S.; Wiertz, E.; Rapoport, T. A.; Proc. Natl. Acad. Sci. USA, 2005, 102, 14132-14138.
24. Kadowaki, H.; Nishitoh, H.; Ichijo, H.; J. Chem. Neuroanat., 2004, 28, 93-100.
25. Zinszner, H.; Kuroda, M.; Wang, X.; Batchvarova, N.; Lightfoot, R. T.; Remotti, H.; Stevens, J. L.; Ron, D.; Genes Dev., 1998, 12, 982-995.
26. Harding, H. P.; Zhang, Y.; Zeng, H.; Novoa, I.; Lu, P. D.; Calfon, M.; Sadri, N.; Yun, C.; Popko, B.; Paules, R.; Stojdl, D. F.; Bell, J. C.; Hettmann, T.; Leiden, J. M.; Ron, D.; Mol. Cell, 2003, 11, 619-633.
27. Matsumoto, M.; Minami, M.; Takeda, K.; Sakao, Y.; Akira, S.; FEBS Lett., 1996, 395, 143-147.
28. McCullough, K. D.; Martindale, J. L.; Klotz, L. O.; Aw, T. Y.; Holbrook, N. J.; Mol. Cell. Biol., 2001, 21, 1249-1259.
29. Puthalakath, H.; O'Reilly, L. A.; Gunn, P.; Lee, L.; Kelly, P. N.; Huntington, N. D.; Hughes, P. D.; Michalak, E. M.; McKimm-Breschkin, J.; Motoyama, N.; Gotoh, T.; Akira, S.; Bouillet, P.; Strasser, A.; Cell, 2007, 129, 1337-1349.
30. Yamaguchi, H.; Wang, H. G.; J. Biol. Chem., 2004, 279, 45495-45502.
31. Schneider, P.; Tschopp, J.; Pharm. Acta Helv., 2000, 74, 281-286.
32. Marciniak, S. J.; Yun, C. Y.; Oyadomari, S.; Novoa, I.; Zhang, Y.; Jungreis, R.; Nagata, K.; Harding, H. P.; Ron, D.; Genes Dev., 2004, 18, 3066-3077.
33. Krajewski, S.; Tanaka, S.; Takayama, S.; Schibler, M. J.; Fenton, W.; Reed, J. C.; Cancer Res., 1993, 53, 4701-4714.
34. Annis, M. G.; Yethon, J. A.; Leber, B.; Andrews, D. W.; Biochim. Biophys. Acta, 2004, 1644, 115-123.
35. Thomenius, M. J.; Distelhorst, C. W.; J. Cell Sci., 2003, 116, 4493-4499.
36. Morishima, N.; Nakanishi, K.; Tsuchiya, K.; Shibata, T.; Seiwa, E.; J. Biol. Chem., 2004, 279, 50375-50381.
37. Mathai, J. P.; Germain, M.; Marcellus, R. C.; Shore, G. C.; Oncogene, 2002, 21, 2534-2544.
38. Germain, M.; Mathai, J. P.; Shore, G. C.; J. Biol. Chem., 2002, 277, 18053-18060.
39. Li, J.; Lee, B.; Lee, A. S.; J. Biol. Chem., 2006, 281, 7260-7270.
40. Reimertz, C.; Kogel, D.; Rami, A.; Chittenden, T.; Prehn, J. H.; J. Cell Biol., 2003, 162, 587-597.
41. Luo, X.; He, Q.; Huang, Y.; Sheikh, M. S.; Cell Death Differ., 2005, 12, 1310-1318.
42. Zong, W. X.; Lindsten, T.; Ross, A. J.; MacGregor, G. R.; Thompson, C. B.; Genes Dev., 2001, 15, 1481-1486.
43. Wei, M. C.; Zong, W. X.; Cheng, E. H.; Lindsten, T.; Panoutsakopoulou, V.; Ross, A. J.; Roth, K. A.; MacGregor, G. R.; Thompson, C. B.; Korsmeyer, S. J.; Science, 2001, 292, 727-730.
44. Hetz, C.; Bernasconi, P.; Fisher, J.; Lee, A. H.; Bassik, M. C.; Antonsson, B.; Brandt, G. S.; Iwakoshi, N. N.; Schinzel, A.; Glimcher, L. H.; Korsmeyer, S. J.; Science, 2006, 312, 572-576.
45. Reed, J. C.; Cell Death Differ., 2006, 13, 1378-1386.
46. Nakagawa, T.; Zhu, H.; Morishima, N.; Li, E.; Xu, J.; Yankner, B. A.; Yuan, J.; Nature, 2000, 403, 98-103.
47. Nakagawa, T.; Yuan, J.; J. Cell Biol., 2000, 150, 887-894.

48. Yoneda, T.; Imaizumi, K.; Oono, K.; Yui, D.; Gomi, F.; Katayama, T.; Tohyama, M.; J. Biol. Chem., 2001, 276, 13935-13940.

49. Chandler, J. M.; Cohen, G. M.; MacFarlane, M.; J. Biol. Chem., 1998, 273, 10815-10818.

50. Rao, R. V.; Hermel, E.; Castro-Obregon, S.; del Rio, G.; Ellerby, L. M.; Ellerby, H. M.; Bredesen, D. E.; J. Biol. Chem., 2001, 276, 33869-33874.

51. Rao, R. V.; Castro-Obregon, S.; Frankowski, H.; Schuler, M.; Stoka, V.; del Rio, G.; Bredesen, D. E.; Ellerby, H. M.; J. Biol. Chem., 2002, 277, 21836-21842.

52. Morishima, N.; Nakanishi, K.; Takenouchi, H.; Shibata, T.; Yasuhiko, Y.; J. Biol. Chem., 2002, 277, 34287-34294.

53. Kadowaki, H.; Nishitoh, H.; Urano, F.; Sadamitsu, C.; Matsuzawa, A.; Takeda, K.; Masutani, H.; Yodoi, J.; Urano, Y.; Nagano, T.; Ichijo, H.; Cell Death Differ., 2005, 12, 19-24.

54. Fischer, H.; Koenig, U.; Eckhart, L.; Tschachler, E.; Biochem. Biophys. Res. Commun., 2002, 293, 722-726.

55. Hitomi, J.; Katayama, T.; Eguchi, Y.; Kudo, T.; Taniguchi, M.; Koyama, Y.; Manabe, T.; Yamagishi, S.; Bando, Y.; Imaizumi, K.; Tsujimoto, Y.; Tohyama, M.; J. Cell Biol., 2004, 165, 347-356.

56. Kojima, E.; Takeuchi, A.; Haneda, M.; Yagi, A.; Hasegawa, T.; Yamaki, K.; Takeda, K.; Akira, S.; Shimokata, K.; Isobe, K.; FASEB J., 2003, 17, 1573-1575.

57. Novoa, I.; Zeng, H.; Harding, H. P.; Ron, D.; J. Cell Biol., 2001, 153, 1011-1022.

58. Jousse, C.; Oyadomari, S.; Novoa, I.; Lu, P.; Zhang, Y.; Harding, H. P.; Ron, D.; J. Cell Biol., 2003, 163, 767-775.

59. Lu, P. D.; Jousse, C.; Marciniak, S. J.; Zhang, Y.; Novoa, I.; Scheuner, D.; Kaufman, R. J.; Ron, D.; Harding, H. P.; EMBO J., 2004, 23, 169-179.

60. Boyce, M.; Bryant, K. F.; Jousse, C.; Long, K.; Harding, H. P.; Scheuner, D.; Kaufman, R. J.; Ma, D.; Coen, D. M.; Ron, D.; Yuan, J.; Science, 2005, 307, 935-939.

61. Urano, F.; Wang, X.; Bertolotti, A.; Zhang, Y.; Chung, P.; Harding, H. P.; Ron, D.; Science, 2000, 287, 664-666.

62. Nishitoh, H.; Saitoh, M.; Mochida, Y.; Takeda, K.; Nakano, H.; Rothe, M.; Miyazono, K.; Ichijo, H.; Mol. Cell, 1998, 2, 389-395.

63. Liu, H.; Nishitoh, H.; Ichijo, H.; Kyriakis, J. M.; Mol. Cell. Biol., 2000, 20, 2198-2208.

64. Ichijo, H.; Nishida, E.; Irie, K.; ten Dijke, P.; Saitoh, M.; Moriguchi, T.; Takagi, M.; Matsumoto, K.; Miyazono, K.; Gotoh, Y.; Science, 1997, 275, 90-94.

65. Nishitoh, H.; Matsuzawa, A.; Tobiume, K.; Saegusa, K.; Takeda, K.; Inoue, K.; Hori, S.; Kakizuka, A.; Ichijo, H.; Genes Dev., 2002, 16, 1345-1355.

66. Hatai, T.; Matsuzawa, A.; Inoshita, S.; Mochida, Y.; Kuroda, T.; Sakamaki, K.; Kuida, K.; Yonehara, S.; Ichijo, H.; Takeda, K.; J. Biol. Chem., 2000, 275, 26576-26581.

67. Putcha, G. V.; Le, S.; Frank, S.; Besirli, C. G.; Clark, K.; Chu, B.; Alix, S.; Youle, R. J.; LaMarche, A.; Maroney, A. C.; Johnson, E. M., Jr.; Neuron, 2003, 38, 899-914.

68. Yamamoto, K.; Ichijo, H.; Korsmeyer, S. J.; Mol. Cell. Biol., 1999, 19, 8469-8478.

69. Inoshita, S.; Takeda, K.; Hatai, T.; Terada, Y.; Sano, M.; Hata, J.; Umezawa, A.; Ichijo, H.; J. Biol. Chem., 2002, 277, 43730-43734.

70. Wang, X. Z.; Ron, D.; Science, 1996, 272, 1347-1349.

71. Kumar, R.; Azam, S.; Sullivan, J. M.; Owen, C.; Cavener, D. R.; Zhang, P.; Ron, D.; Harding, H. P.; Chen, J. J.; Han, A.; White, B. C.; Krause, G. S.; DeGracia, D. J.; J. Neurochem., 2001, 77, 1418-1421.

72. Paschen, W.; Gissel, C.; Linden, T.; Althausen, S.; Doutheil, J.; Brain Res., 1998, 60, 115-122.

73. Kohno, K.; Higuchi, T.; Ohta, S.; Kohno, K.; Kumon, Y.; Sakaki, S.; Neurosci. Lett., 1997, 224, 17-20.

74. Iadecola, C.; Zhang, F.; Casey, R.; Nagayama, M.; Ross, M. E.; J. Neurosci., 1997, 17, 9157-9164.

75. Tajiri, S.; Oyadomari, S.; Yano, S.; Morioka, M.; Gotoh, T.; Hamada, J. I.; Ushio, Y.; Mori, M.; Cell Death Differ., 2004, 11, 403-415.

76. Takahashi, R.; Imai, Y.; Hattori, N.; Mizuno, Y.; Ann. N. Y. Acad. Sci., 2003, 991, 101-106.

77. Imai, Y.; Soda, M.; Hatakeyama, S.; Akagi, T.; Hashikawa, T.; Nakayama, K. I.; Takahashi, R.; Mol. Cell, 2002, 10, 55-67.

78. Imai, Y.; Soda, M.; Inoue, H.; Hattori, N.; Mizuno, Y.; Takahashi, R.; Cell, 2001, 105, 891-902.

79. Kakizuka, A.; Trends Genet., 1998, 14, 396-402.

80. Paulson, H. L.; Bonini, N. M.; Roth, K. A.; Proc. Natl. Acad. Sci. USA, 2000, 97, 12957-12958.

81. Higashiyama, H.; Hirose, F.; Yamaguchi, M.; Inoue, Y. H.; Fujikake, N.; Matsukage, A.; Kakizuka, A.; Cell Death Differ., 2002, 9, 264-273.

82. Hirabayashi, M.; Inoue, K.; Tanaka, K.; Nakadate, K.; Ohsawa, Y.; Kamei, Y.; Popiel, A. H.; Sinohara, A.; Iwamatsu, A.; Kimura, Y.; Uchiyama, Y.; Hori, S.; Kakizuka, A.; Cell Death Differ., 2001, 8, 977-984.

83. Arning, L.; Monte, D.; Hansen, W.; Wieczorek, S.; Jagiello, P.; Akkad, D. A.; Andrich, J.; Kraus, P. H.; Saft, C.; Epplen, J. T.; J. Mol. Med., 2008, 86, 485-490.

84. Julien, J. P.; Cell, 2001, 104, 581-591.

85. Atkin, J. D.; Farg, M. A.; Turner, B. J.; Tomas, D.; Lysaght, J. A.; Nunan, J.; Rembach, A.; Nagley, P.; Beart, P. M.; Cheema, S. S.; Horne, M. K.; J. Biol. Chem., 2006, 281, 30152-30165.

86. Kikuchi, H.; Almer, G.; Yamashita, S.; Guegan, C.; Nagai, M.; Xu, Z.; Sosunov, A. A.; McKhann, G. M. I.; Przedborski, S.; Proc. Natl. Acad. Sci. USA, 2006, 103, 6025-6030.

87. Tobisawa, S.; Hozumi, Y.; Arawaka, S.; Koyama, S.; Wada, M.; Nagai, M.; Aoki, M.; Itoyama, Y.; Goto, K.; Kato, T.; Biochem. Biophys. Res. Commun., 2003, 303, 496-503.

88. Raoul, C.; Estevez, A. G.; Nishimune, H.; Cleveland, D. W.; deLapeyriere, O.; Henderson, C. E.; Haase, G.; Pettmann, B.; Neuron, 2002, 35, 1067-1083.

89. Holasek, S. S.; Wengenack, T. M.; Kandimalla, K. K.; Montano, C.; Gregor, D. M.; Curran, G. L.; Poduslo, J. F.; Brain Res., 2005, 1045, 185-198.

90. Veglianese, P.; Lo Coco, D.; Bao Cutrona, M.; Magnoni, R.; Pennacchini, D.; Pozzi, B.; Gowing, G.; Julien, J. P.; Tortarolo, M.; Bendotti, C.; Mol. Cell Neurosci., 2006, 31, 218-231.

91. Wengenack, T. M.; Holasek, S. S.; Montano, C. M.; Gregor, D.; Curran, G. L.; Poduslo, J. F.; Brain Res., 2004, 1027, 73-86.

92. Nishitoh, H.; Kadowaki, H.; Nagai, A.; Maruyama, T.; Yokota, T.; Fukutomi, H.; Noguchi, T.; Matsuzawa, A.; Takeda, K.; Ichijo, H.; Genes Dev., 2008, 22, 1451-1464.

CHAPTER 8

Role of Alzheimer's β-Amyloid on *Wnt* Signaling

Nibaldo C. Inestrosa[*], Catalina Grabowski, Macarena Arrázola, Lorena Varela-Nallar and Enrique M. Toledo

Centro de Envejecimiento y Regeneración (CARE), Centro de Regulación Celular y Patología "Joaquín V. Luco" (CRCP), MIFAB, Facultad de Ciencias Biológicas, Pontificia Universidad Católica de Chile, Alameda 340, Santiago, Chile

Address correspondence to: Dr. Nibaldo C. Inestrosa Email: ninestrosa@bio.puc.cl

Abstract: Recent evidence supports a neuroprotective role for *Wnt* signaling in neurodegenerative disorders such as Alzheimer's Disease. In fact, a relationship between amyloid-β-peptide induced neurotoxicity and a decrease in the cytoplasmic levels of β-catenin has been observed. Apparently, Aβ binds to the extracellular cysteine-rich domain of the Frizzled receptor inhibiting *Wnt*/β-catenin signaling. These studies indicate that a sustained loss of *Wnt* signaling function may be involved in the Aβ-dependent neurodegeneration observed in Alzheimer's brain. So far, we have demonstrated that activation of *Wnt* signaling protects neurons against neurotoxic injuries, including both amyloid-β fibrils and Aβ oligomers by using either lithium, an inhibitor of the glycogen synthase kinase 3β, or different *Wnt* ligands. In particular, the activation of non-canonical *Wnt* signaling was able to protect postsynaptic regions and dendritic spines against Aβ oligomers. In conclusion, the activation of the *Wnt* signaling pathway could be proposed as a therapeutic target for the treatment of AD.

1. THE BASIC BIOLOGY OF *WNT* SIGNALING. IMPLICATION IN THE CENTRAL NERVOUS SYSTEM

Wnt ligands constitute a family of proteins, which are secreted as glycoproteins with a palmitoylation at a conserved C-terminal cysteine, a post-translational modification important for the actions of *Wnt-1*, *Wnt-3a* and *Wnt-5a* [1-3]. The process of palmitoylation consists in the addition of the fatty acid palmitate which increases the hydrophobic nature of *Wnt* ligands [2]. The *Wnt* ligands vary in length between 350 and 400 amino acids (aa) and show 20%-85% aa identity within the family. To date, 19 *Wnts* ligands have been characterized in the mouse genome. The classical view of the canonical *Wnt* signaling transduction pathway implies the presence of an extracellular secreted *Wnt* ligand, that interacts with the receptor protein Frizzled (Fz), which is a member of a family of seven-pass transmembrane proteins. The *Wnt*-Fz receptor complex forms a ternary cell surface complex with the co-receptor low density lipoprotein receptor related protein 5/6 (LRP5/6) receptor [4] and eventually with casein kinase-1 [5, 6]. This activates Dishevelled (*Dvl*) usually by phosphorylation, which in turn inactivates glycogen-synthase-kinase-3β (GSK-3β), a key

modulator of this pathway. *Wnt* signaling regulates GSK-3 activity by physically displacing complexed GSK-3 from a member of regulatory binding partners, consequently preventing the phosphorylation and degradation of β-catenin. In the absence of *Wnt*, β-catenin pool is maintained at low level through degradation, Fig. (**1**) [7, 8]. β-catenin is targeted for ubiquitination by the β-transducing repeat-containing protein (β-TrCP) and is then degraded by the proteasome. β-catenin is phosphorylated by the serine/threonine kinases casein kinase 1 (CK1) and GSK-3β. Phosphorylation of β-catenin occurs in a multiprotein complex (the destruction complex) [9], comprising axin, adenomatous polyposis coli (APC) and diversion. Upon receipt of a *Wnt* signal, Dvl prevents degradation of β-catenin through the recruitment of GSK-3 binding proteins (GBP)/Frat-1 which displace GSK-3β from the destruction complex. Stabilized β-catenin enters the nucleus and associates with T-cell factor/lymphoid enhancer binding factor (TCF/LEF) transcription factors, leading to the transcription of *Wnt* target genes, such as cyclin D1, PPAR delta and engrailed [8].

Putative novel *Wnt* target genes (~540) were identified in the human genome (15,476 promoter

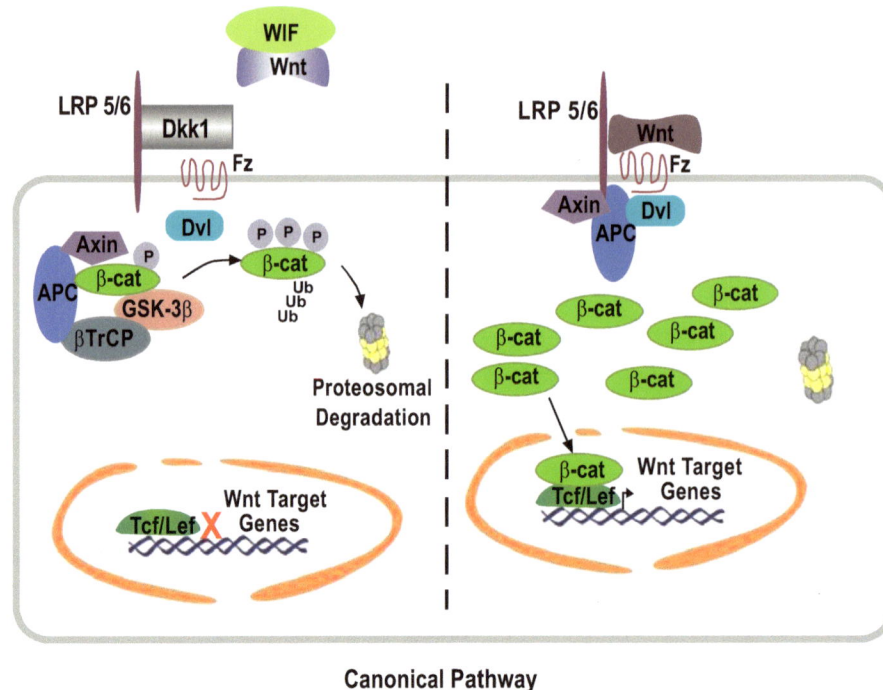

Canonical Pathway

Fig. (1). The Canonical *Wnt* signaling pathway. In the absence of a *Wnt* protein (Left Panel), GSK-3β phosphorylates β-catenin molecules and directs them to the ubiquitin mediated degradation pathway, preventing its binding to TCF/LEF transcription factors and the expression of *Wnt*-target genes. In the presence of a *Wnt* protein (Right Panel). Fzd receptor along with the LDL-related receptor protein LRP5/6 transduces its signal by activating Dvl protein, which in turn inactivates GSK-3β that resides in a protein complex together with APC, Axin and β-catenin. β–catenin molecules are stabilized and cytosolic levels rise, thus allowing β-catenin binding to TCF/LEF transcription factors and the subsequent expression of *Wnt*-target genes.

regions were studied), by using a representative matrix for TCF/LEF binding sequence present in the promoter regions of all known *Wnt* target genes. Based on this information, the CART method and additional 431 transcription factor binding sequences present in each promoter region, putative *Wnt* target genes were identified and classified according to their role in different cellular processes and their molecular function. Concerning *Wnt* neuroprotective effects, several interesting genes emerged including neuronal receptors, synaptic components, transcription factors and growth factors. Of all genes predicted as *Wnt* target genes, calcium/calmodulin dependent protein kinase IV (CaMKIV) showed the higher score, similar to those already known *Wnt* target genes [10]. CaMKIV is a very interesting candidate since it has been related to long-term memory [11]. *Wnt* signaling is also transduced independently of β-catenin. These pathways are referred to as non-canonical pathways, Fig. (**2**). These include the cell polarity pathway (PCP), which directs asymmetric cytoskeletal organization and Ca^{2+} pathway, via G-proteins and the *Wnt*/Ca^{2+} pathway which regulates cell movements during gastrulation and heart development. The PCP controls the orthogonal

polarity of cells in the epithelium and convergent extension movements during gastrulation [12, 13]. Signaling in this non-canonical pathway also involves *Dvl*, which can signal through small GTPase and Jun N-terminal Kinase (JNK) pathway. The *Wnt*/Ca^{2+} pathway regulate cell movements during gastrulation and heart development [14, 15]. This pathway signals through *Dvl* to induce calcium influx and the activation of protein kinase C (PKC) and calcium/calmodulin dependent protein kinase II (CaMKII) [15].

Historically, *Wnt* proteins were classified as either canonical, such as *Wnt-1* and *Wnt-3a*, or non-canonical, including *Wnt-4*, *Wnt-5* and *Wnt-11* [16-18]. The characterization of Fz and LRPs and other receptors had challenged this classification of individual *Wnts* proteins. Evidence suggests that *Wnt-5a*, for example, may activate the canonical pathway or inhibit it, depending on the receptor context [19]. Accordingly, the terms "canonical" and "non-canonical" are used to indicate molecular mechanisms, not specifically *Wnt* proteins. Current and update information about the *Wnt* signaling can be found at the *Wnt* Homepage (*http://www.stanford.edu/~rnusse/wntwindow.htm*).

The *Wnt* signaling has been characterized to modulate different biological systems. For the purpose of this chapter, we will focus on the link between central nervous system and *Wnt* signaling. While investigating the role of *Wnts* in the formation of the sensory-motor connections in mouse spinal cord, it was found that *Wnt-3* can guide and promote axonal branching and growth cone size from sensory axons from dorsal root ganglia neurons [20]. In motoneurons *Wnt-3* acts as a retrograde signal inhibiting axonal extension and promoting terminal arborization. However, this effect was only observed for neurotrophin-3 dependent sensory neurons. *Wnt-3* [20] and *Wnt-7a* ligands [21, 22], promote synaptogenesis inducing the clustering of synapsin I, a presynaptic protein involved in synapse formation and function [23, 24]. This effect is controlled by the canonical pathway and can be mimicked by the GSK-3β inhibition induced by lithium.

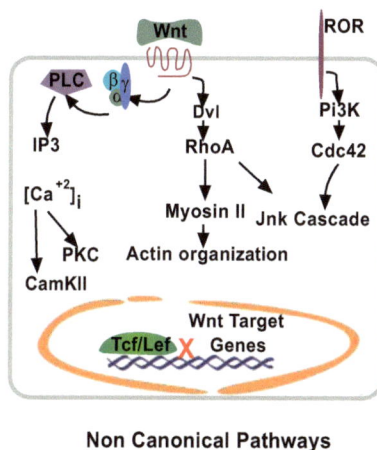

Non Canonical Pathways

Fig. (2). The No-Canonical *Wnt* signaling pathway. In the presence of *Wnt*, the Fzd receptor transduce it signal modulating cytoskeletal organization, which can signal through small GTPase and JNK pathway, after the activation of Dvl. In the *Wnt*/Ca²⁺ pathway signals Dvl induces calcium influx and activation of PKC and CaMKII. *Wnts* ligands can act through other types of receptors beside Fzds, both members of the tyrosine kinase family, Ryk and Ror. This activation is able to inhibit the canonical signaling through an unknown mechanism.

Wnt-7a and lithium induce axonal spreading and branching by the remodeling of axonal microtubules during postnatal cerebellar development [21, 22]. Moreover, the loss of function of *Wnt-7a* produces a failure in the distribution of presynaptic proteins and in the

morphology of the presynaptic axons [25]. The activation with *Wnt-7b*, apparently a ligand, previously shown to be specific for non-canonical *Wnt* signaling, induces synaptic vesicle clustering and enhances recycling of synaptic vesicles through Dvl-1. *Wnt-7a* has similar effects on synaptic vesicle clustering [26].

The role of *Wnt* ligands in synaptic plasticity in mouse hippocampal neurons has also been described. *Wnt-3a* was released in an activity dependent manner from glutamatergic synapses. Inhibition of *Wnt* signaling impairs long-term potentiation (LTP), while its activation facilitates LTP [27]. In addition, over-expression of GSK-3β in mice prevents the induction of LTP [28] and causes a decrease in spatial learning [29]. Inhibitors of GSK-3β have also been shown to block long-term depression (LTD) and GSK-3β activity is enhanced during LTD [30]. In immature hippocampal neurons, the activation of the *Wnt* signaling by *Wnt7b* signals through Dvl, Rac and JNK in a β-catenin independent manner induces an enhanced number and length of dendritic branching [31]. The lack of *Dvl*-1 resulted in the decay of dendritic morphogenesis, and the overexpression of *Dvl*-1 mimicked the effect of *Wnt-7b*.

Recently, we found that *Wnt-7a* modulates the synaptic vesicle cycle and synaptic transmission in rat hippocampal neurons [32]. In fact, when neurons where incubated with the *Wnt-7a* ligand an increase in the neurite clustering of presynaptic proteins was observed in comparison with control condition. *Wnt-5a* ligand did not show this effect. Also, when we used another canonical ligand like *Wnt-3a* the clustering of SV-2 was also increased. *Wnt-7a* induces recycling and exocytosis of synaptic vesicles as studied with the amphipathic fluorescence dye FM1-43. *Wnt-3a* has a moderate effect on recycling of synaptic vesicles, and no effect of *Wnt-1* and *Wnt-5a* was detected. Electrophysiological analysis on adult rat hippocampal slices (taken from P24-P30 rats) indicates that *Wnt-7a*, but not *Wnt-5a*, increases neurotransmitter release in CA3-CA1 synapses by decreasing paired pulse facilitation and increasing the miniature excitatory post-synaptic current frequency. These results indicate that *Wnt-7a*: (a) is a physiologically active *Wnt* ligand in postnatal hippocampal slices and (b) increases synaptic transmission by a presynaptic mechanism, probably involving an increase in neurotransmitter release. As a whole our results suggest a role of the *Wnt*/β-catenin signaling pathway in the organization of the pre-synaptic region.

All these evidences point toward a physiological role for the *Wnt* signaling in the development and function of the central nervous system.

2. β-AMYLOID PEPTIDE NEURO-TOXICITY AND *Wnt* SIGNALING

Alzheimer's disease (AD) is a neurodegenerative disorder associated with aging, characterized by fibrillar deposits of amyloid-β-peptide (Aβ) in subcortical brain regions. Typical features of AD are extracellular neuritic amyloid plaques (senile plaques) and intracellular neurofibrillary tangles. The main proteinaceous component of the amyloid deposited in AD is the Aβ peptide, a 40-to 42-

Fig. (3). Amyloid aggregates in a model of Alzheimer's disease. Brain sections of mice APPswe-PSEN1ΔE9 were stained against Aβ1-17 (A) and Thioflavin-S (B). Showing the amyloid aggregates presents in the brain. Silver Stain reveals an amyloid aggregate surrounded by neurites (C).

residue peptide that has been isolated from senile plaque cores, Fig. (3) [33]. The Aβ peptide is originated by proteolytic processing of the transmembrane protein amyloid precursor protein (APP). The generation of Aβ peptide from APP is the result of two enzymatic activities, designated as β and γ–secretase (reviewed at [34]). The γ-secretase activity resides in a complex of proteins, which is composed at least by presenilin (PS) with nicastrin, aph-1 and pen-2. Formation of neurofibrillary tangles results from a hyperphosphorylation of tau protein, which is in part driven by GSK-3β [35].

The accumulation of the Aβ peptide, initiate a series of pathological events that initiate with the impairment of synaptic plasticity, inflammation, astroglial hypertrophy and microglial activation, ionic homeostasis alteration and oxidative stress, events that are spatially correlated with Aβ plaques aggregates and cell death, Fig. (4) [36-39]. An increase in those pathological markers was found to be correlated with the cognitive decline observed in AD patients and in models of the disease.

At the beginning of this decade, we found a relationship between a loss of the *Wnt* signaling pathway activity and AD. Early studies in our laboratory suggested a relationship between Aβ-induced neurotoxicity and an impairment of this signaling pathway [40-43]. Several independent studies are consistent with the idea that *Wnt* signaling components are altered in AD [44-50]. As a consequence, we have studied whether or not the activation of the *Wnt* pathway may be used as a therapeutic strategy for the treatment of AD.

Active GSK-3β has been found in brains staged for AD neurofibrillary changes [51], a decrease in β-catenin levels and an increase in *tau* hyperphosphorylation. In addition, previous studies have shown that β-catenin levels are reduced in AD patients carrying presenilin-1 (PS-1)-inherited mutations [46]. In fact, several studies have shown that familial AD-linked PS proteins form multi-protein complexes with the cell adhesion/*Wnt* signaling β-catenin protein, α-catenin and GSK-3β. β-catenin and its homolog γ-catenin, commonly named plakoglobin; were initially described as intracellular proteins located near the cell surface and linked to cadherins.

A loss of *Wnt* signaling through the β-catenin-TCF pathway increases neuronal vulnerability to

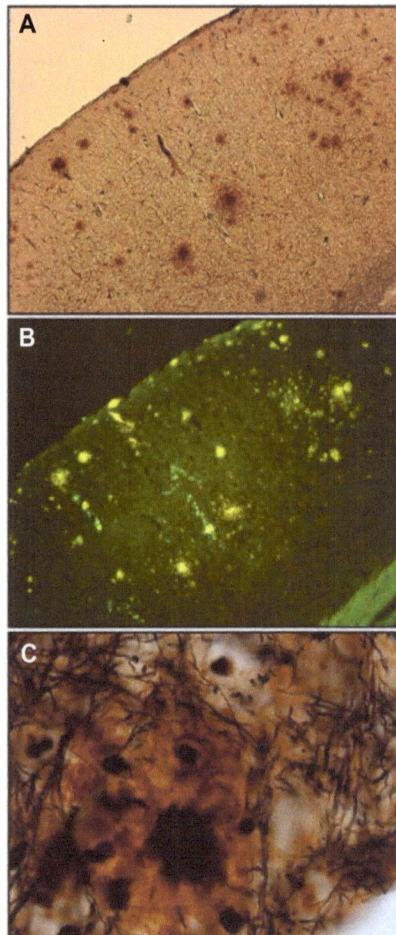

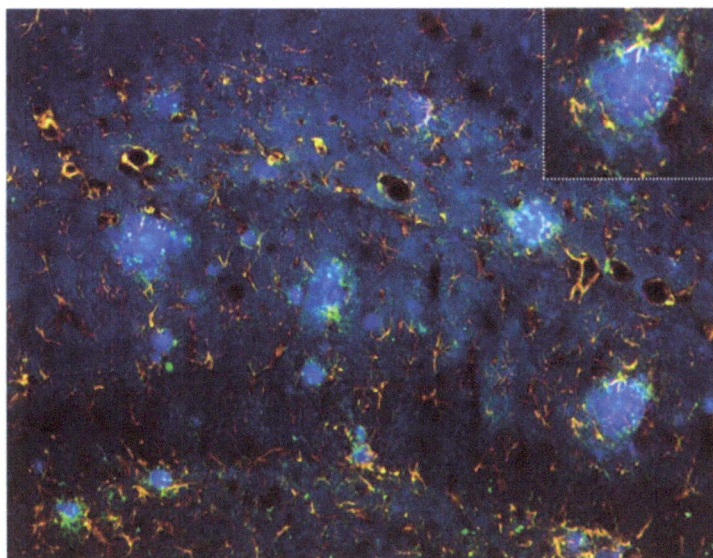

Fig. (4). Inflammatory Markers in a model of Alzheimer's disease. Brain sections of mice APPswe-PSEN1ΔE9 were co-stained against the inflammatory markers of astrocytes, microglia and amyloid. Plaques present in hippocampal section of the double transgenic were found surrounded with inflammatory markers. In blue X34 an amyloid stain, green CD11b a microglial marker, and red GFAP a astrocytes marker.

apoptosis induced by Aβ [46], and possible defects in *Wnt* signaling could contribute to the pathogenesis of AD [40, 52, 53]. Although the mechanism by which *Wnt* signaling plays a role in AD pathology remains unclear, there is evidence that shows that Aβ-dependent neurotoxicity induces a loss of function of *Wnt* signaling components [43, 54, 55]. Moreover, it was found that the up-regulation of β-catenin during tau hyperphosphorylation prevents the cell from going into apoptosis, and increasing levels of hyperphosphorylated tau was correlated with diminished levels of phospho-β-catenin and increased levels of nuclear β-catenin. Moreover, the knockdown of β-catenin produces an increase in the numbers of apoptotic cells; and also antagonizes the antiapoptotic effects of tau [56]. These results support the role of β-catenin as a survival element in AD.

Epidemiological data showed an increased risk for AD in populations with the allele 4 of apolipoprotein E (ApoE4) [57, 58] and recently, it was reported that ApoE4 causes the inhibition of the *Wnt* canonical signaling in PC12 cells upon stimulation with *Wnt-7a,* as determined by luciferase activities and nuclear β-catenin levels [59]. This antecedent also points toward a correlation between the loss of *Wnt* signaling and AD.

One negative modulator of the *Wnt* pathway is the extracellular protein Dickkopf-1 (*Dkk-1*), which

binds to LRPs, preventing their interaction with *Wnts* [60, 61]. In primary culture of cortical neurons *Dkk-1* is expressed when these cells were exposed to Aβ. Moreover, in brain tissue from AD patients a highly significant immunostaining for *Dkk-1* was found. On the other hand, no evidence of *Dkk-1* expression was found in control, non-demented age-matched brain tissue [47]. Interestingly, *Dkk-1* participates in ischemic damage, and treatment with *Dkk-1* antisense or lithium can protect against ischemic damage [62].

3. EFFECT OF β-AMYLOID FIBRILS

The last stage of aggregation of β-amyloid is the formation of fibrils (Aβ$_f$) with a predominant β-sheets organization of monomers, which have a different toxic target for smaller oligomeric species of β-amyloid [63-65]. Recently, was identified that dimmers of β-amyloid are the smallest toxic aggregates found in the brains of AD patients. It was shown that dimmers are able to cause impairment in synaptic plasticity, leaving the brain slices unable to respond to LTP or LTD [66].

Early studies in our laboratory, suggested a relationship between Aβ$_f$ - induced neurotoxicity and lower cytoplasmic levels of β-catenin, due to the increased activity of the enzyme GSK-3β. On the other hand, inhibition of GSK-3β by lithium protects rat neurons from Aβ-induced damage. This evidence led to the proposal that a sustained loss of *Wnt* signaling function may be involved in the Aβ dependent neurodegeneration observed in AD [40, 41].

In AD brain, active GSK-3β (also known as tau kinase I) is mainly found in neuronal cell bodies and neurites [67], where it is found co-localized with the neurofibrillary changes observed in AD brains. The activation of the enzyme GSK-3β, the hyperphosphorylation of tau protein, and the loss of the microtubular network have all been observed in primary cultures of rat hippocampal and human cortical neurons exposed to the Aβ peptide [68, 69]. Interestingly, it has been observed that blocking GSK-3β activity prevents tau hyper-phosphorylation and promotes its binding to the microtubular network [70]. Lithium, which has long been used to treat bipolar disorders [71], has been shown to be a competitive inhibitor of GSK-3 with respect to magnesium, a property not found in other group I metal ions [72]. This may account for its ability to act as a mood-stabilizing drug [73], though other actions of lithium, such as its well-known ability to inhibit inositol-1,4 bis-phosphate 1-phosphatase and inositol-1(or 4)-mono-phosphatase, could also explain or contribute to its therapeutic effects [74]. Recent evidence suggests that lithium, through the inhibition of GSK-3β, is neuroprotective against a variety of neurodegenerative conditions [71, 75], and it is noteworthy that lithium reduces the prevalence of AD in elderly patients with bipolar disorder [76].

The direct activation of *Wnt* signaling with the ligand *Wnt-3a* has been demonstrated to prevent neuronal cell death in Aβ treated rat hippocampal cultures [54]. Frzb-1, a secreted *Wnt* antagonist protein was able to reverse the *Wnt-3a* neuroprotective effect on cell survival against $A\beta_f$ toxicity. Furthermore, when hippocampal neurons were exposed to $A\beta_f$ a decrease in their cytosolic β-catenin level was observed. This effect was also reversed when the *Wnt*-3a ligand was co-incubated with Frzb-1. These results suggest that *Wnt-3a* is able to enhance the *Wnt*/β-catenin signaling, playing an important role in neuroprotection against Aβ toxicity and its loss of function may play a role in triggering the neurodegeneration observed in AD.

4. EFFECT OF β-AMYLOID OLIGO-MERS ON POST-SYNAPTIC REGION

The toxics effects of β-amyloid over the neurons are not limited to impairment in cell homeostasis. When transgenic animals models of AD were analyzed one of the earliest changes caused by the production of β-amyloid was impairment in the synaptic transmission [36]. Further analysis has shown that Aβ oligomers are able to induce changes in the synapse composition and function, *in vitro* [77, 78] and *in vivo* [79].

Some evidence obtained in hippocampal culture neurons indicated that Aβ oligomers are associated with the post-synaptic density protein 95 (PSD-95) at synaptic terminals [77]. Indeed, Aβ oligomers decrease the levels of this protein in the neurons. Similar results were found in APP (Tg2576) transgenic mice [80].

We have confirmed the reduction of PSD-95 by treatment with Aβ oligomers. [81]. The decrease in PSD-95 levels by Aβ oligomers has been related to a reduction in the GluR1 subunit of the AMPA glutamate receptor levels in primary cultures of APP mutant neurons, compared with neurons of wild-type mice [80]. Other authors suggested that the main targets of Aβ peptide are the NMDA glutamate receptors. Aβ promotes the endocytosis of NMDA channels in cortical neurons and the subsequent NMDA-dependent current decrease [82]. Since PSD-95 recruits glutamate receptor subunits to the postsynaptic density, our results suggest that Aβ oligomers decrease the glutamatergic transmission by interfering with the stabilization of glutamate receptors at the synapse [65].

We found that *Wnt-5a*, a *Wnt* ligand highly concentrated at the hippocampus, Fig. (**5**) [83], was able to overcome the neurotoxic effects of Aβ oligomers [81]. Mature hippocampal neurons were exposed to Aβ oligomers in the absence or presence of conditioned media of *Wnt-5a*. The exposure of neurons to Aβ oligomers decreases the level of the postsynaptic proteins PSD-95 and NMDA glutamate receptor subunit NR2 [65]. The co-exposure of oligomers of Aβ with *Wnt-5a* ligand was able to maintain the levels of PSD-95, protecting the postsynaptic structure upon Aβ exposure [65, 81]. As a whole, these results indicated that *Wnt-5a* modulates the postsynaptic region of central mammalian synapses and indicate that the activation of the *Wnt* pathway by *Wnt*-5a protects neurons from Aβ-oligomers, suggesting a therapeutic potential for this signaling pathway in the treatment of AD.

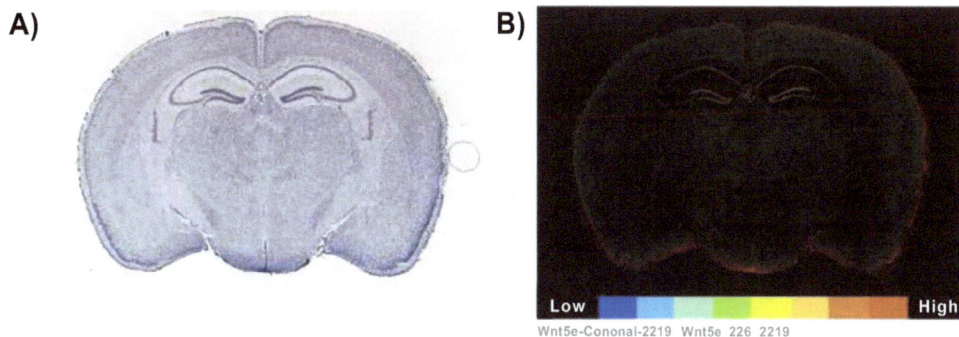

Fig. (5). **Expression of *Wnt*-5A in adult brain mouse**. Coronal View of ISH (Series Id=2733 - position 5650) with a probe antisense of *Wnt*-5a. (A) Shows the distribution of the mRNA of *Wnt*-5A in adult mouse brain. (B) Presents the quantification of the hybridization showing higher amount of signals in the cortex and hippocampus. Images obtained from the Allen Brain Atlas [Internet]. Seattle (WA): Allen Institute for Brain Science. © 2007. Available from: http://www.brain-map.org

In addition, we recently showed that *Wnt-3a* protects hippocampal neurons against the toxicity of Aβ oligomers. This effect was modulated by Fz1 which we found to mediate the activation of the canonical *Wnt*/β-catenin pathway by *Wnt-3a*. Over-expression of Fz1 significantly increased cell survival induced by *Wnt-3a* and diminished caspase-3 activation and β-catenin degradation, while knocking-down Fz1 expression by antisense oligonucleotides decreased the *Wnt-3a* protection [84]. Co-transfecting Fz1 and a transcriptionally inactive mutated version of β-catenin decreased the protection against Aβ oligomers, suggesting that the transcription of *Wnt* target genes may be involved in the protective effect of *Wnt-3a*/Fz1 signaling. Fz1 is expressed in the adult rat hippocampus and cortex, and in cultured hippocampal neurons [84], and interestingly, we have determined that some Fz receptors are distributed synaptically (Varela-Nallar, Grabowsky & Inestrosa, submitted for publication), as is the case of Fz3, Fig. (**6**). So, it is possible that the *Wnt* signaling could be locally activated at the synapse, where it could have a neuroprotective role against

Aβ oligomers synaptotoxicity. The involvement of *Wnt*/Fz signaling in Aβ toxicity was also suggested by a recent publication. Using phage display of peptide libraries it was identified a cysteine-linked cyclic heptapeptide (cSP5) that binds Aβ with high affinity and is homologous to the extracellular cysteine-rich domain of several Fz receptors [50]. Furthermore, it was determined that Aβ directly binds to Fz5 cysteine-rich domain at or in close proximity to the *Wnt*-binding site, and inhibits the canonical *Wnt* signaling pathway, suggesting that Aβ binding to Fz could mediate the loss of *Wnt* signaling function observed by Aβ treatments and that interfering with this interaction could be a therapeutic target for AD. So in this scenario, the binding of the *Wnt* ligand to the Fz receptor is obstructed by Aβ, therefore, the *Wnt* signaling is inhibited and β-catenin is phosphorylated and degraded by the proteasome. We have shown in PC12 cells that overexpression of Fz1 potentiates the activation of the canonical *Wnt*/β-catenin pathway by *Wnt*-3a ligand, and the neuroprotective role of this ligand against the toxicity of Aβ oligomers [84]. This data suggests that in a

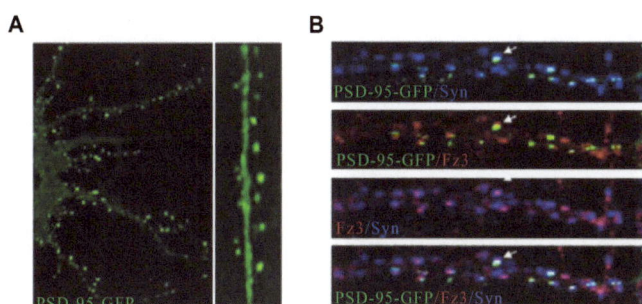

Fig. (6). Fz3 is located at synaptic sites. (A) Hippocampal neurons were transfected with GFP-tagged PSD-95 plasmid (kindly donated by Dr Roger Nicoll) before plating. After 14 days in vitro, PSD-95-GFP is located in dendritic spines, allowing the clear identification of the postsynaptic region. (B) Immunodetection of Fz3 and synapsin I (Syn) in hippocampal neurons transfected with PSD-95-GFP. Co-localization analysis reveals that Fz3 clusters co-localize with Syn in close apposition to PSD-95-GFP puncta (arrow).

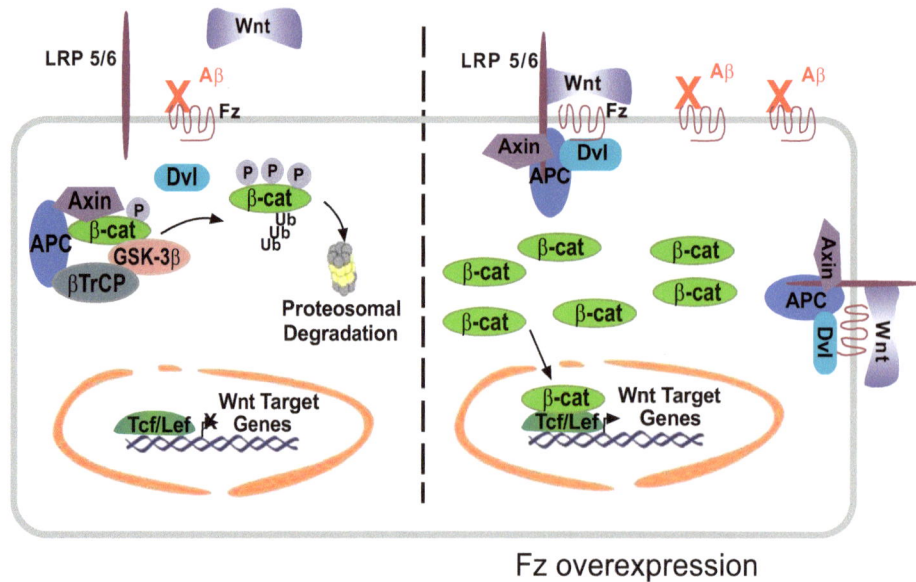

Fz overexpression

Fig (7). Schematic model for the potential mechanism of Aβ-mediated inhibition of the *Wnt* pathway. Aβ interacts with Fz receptor interfering with the binding of the *Wnt* ligand, thus the *Wnt* signaling is inhibited and β-catenin is phosphorylated and degraded by the proteasome. In a condition of Fz overexpression, elevated levels of the receptor allow the activation of the *Wnt* pathway even in the presence of Aβ.

condition of Fz overexpression, the *Wnt* pathway could be activated even in the presence of Aβ, allowing the expression of neuroprotective genes, Fig. (7).

5. CONCLUSION

In this review we discussed recent evidence indicating that deregulation of the *Wnt* signaling may play a role in the pathogenesis of AD. So far, the mechanisms by which extracellular Aβ causes its different intraneuronal effects have not been clarified. *Wnt-7a* signaling stimulates clustering of presynaptic proteins and modulates the synaptic vesicle cycle by inducing recycling and exocytosis of synaptic vesicles. Aβ oligomers bind to the central synapse at the postsynaptic region, and we have found that *Wnt-5a* and *Wnt-3a* play an attenuating role in Aβ neurotoxicity. All of these data opens a novel therapeutic window in AD treatment.

6. ACKNOWLEDGEMENTS

This work was supported by grants from Conicyt, FONDAP-Biomedicine N° 13980001, the Millennium Institute for Fundamental and Applied Biology (MIFAB), Bicentennial Project R-18, a FONDECYT Postdoctoral Fellowship to LV-N (N° 3070017).

6. REFERENCE

1.   Mason, J.O.; J. Kitajewski and H.E. Varmus. Mutational analysis of mouse Wnt-1 identifies two temperature-sensitive alleles and attributes of Wnt-1 protein essential for transformation of a mammary cell line. Mol Biol Cell, **1992**. 3(5): p. 521-33.
2.   Willert, K.; J.D. Brown; E. Danenberg; A.W. Duncan; I.L. Weissman; T. Reya; J.R. Yates, 3rd and R. Nusse. *Wnt proteins are lipid-modified and can act as stem cell growth factors.* Nature, **2003**. 423(6938): p. 448-52.
3.   Kurayoshi, M.; H. Yamamoto; S. Izumi and A. Kikuchi. *Post-translational palmitoylation and glycosylation of Wnt-5a are necessary for its signalling.* Biochem J, **2007**. 402(3): p. 515-23.
4.   Tamai, K.; M. Semenov; Y. Kato; R. Spokony; C. Liu; Y. Katsuyama; F. Hess; J.P. Saint-Jeannet and X. He. *LDL-receptor-related proteins in Wnt signal transduction.* Nature, **2000**. 407(6803): p. 530-5.
5.   Davidson, G.; W. Wu; J. Shen; J. Bilic; U. Fenger; P. Stannek; A. Glinka and C. Niehrs. *Casein kinase 1 gamma couples Wnt receptor activation to cytoplasmic signal transduction.* Nature, **2005**. 438(7069): p. 867-72.
6.   Zeng, X.; K. Tamai; B. Doble; S. Li; H. Huang; R. Habas; H. Okamura; J. Woodgett and X. He. *A dual-kinase mechanism for Wnt co-receptor phosphorylation and activation.* Nature, **2005**. 438(7069): p. 873-7.
7.   Dale, T.C., *Signal transduction by the Wnt family of ligands.* Biochem J, **1998**. 329 (Pt 2): p. 209-23.
8.   Logan, C.Y. and R. Nusse. *The Wnt signaling pathway in development and disease.* Annu Rev Cell Dev Biol, **2004**. 20: p. 781-810.
9.   Chen, R.H.; W.V. Ding and F. McCormick. *Wnt signaling to beta-catenin involves two interactive components. Glycogen synthase kinase-3beta inhibition and activation of protein kinase C.* J Biol Chem, **2000**. 275(23): p. 17894-9.
10. Arrazola, M., Varela-Nallar, L., Colombres, M., Assar, R., Aravena, A., Maass, A., Martínez S. and Inestrosa

N.C. . *Calcium/calmodulin-dependent protein kinase type IV (CaMKIV) is a target gene of the Wnt/beta-catenin signaling pathway.* J Cell Physiol, **2008**. (Submitted for publication).

11. Fukushima, H.; R. Maeda; R. Suzuki; A. Suzuki; M. Nomoto; H. Toyoda; L.J. Wu; H. Xu; M.G. Zhao; K. Ueda; A. Kitamoto; N. Mamiya; T. Yoshida; S. Homma; S. Masushige; M. Zhuo and S. Kida. *Upregulation of calcium/calmodulin-dependent protein kinase IV improves memory formation and rescues memory loss with aging.* J Neurosci, **2008**. 28(40): p. 9910-9.

12. Shulman, J.M.; N. Perrimon and J.D. Axelrod. *Frizzled signaling and the developmental control of cell polarity.* Trends Genet, **1998**. 14(11): p. 452-8.

13. Yamanaka, H.; T. Moriguchi; N. Masuyama; M. Kusakabe; H. Hanafusa; R. Takada; S. Takada and E. Nishida. *JNK functions in the non-canonical Wnt pathway to regulate convergent extension movements in vertebrates.* EMBO Rep, **2002**. 3(1): p. 69-75.

14. Saneyoshi, T.; S. Kume; Y. Amasaki and K. Mikoshiba. *The Wnt/calcium pathway activates NF-AT and promotes ventral cell fate in Xenopus embryos.* Nature, **2002**. 417(6886): p. 295-9.

15. Sheldahl, L.C.; D.C. Slusarski; P. Pandur; J.R. Miller; M. Kuhl and R.T. Moon. *Dishevelled activates Ca2+ flux, PKC, and CamKII in vertebrate embryos.* J Cell Biol, **2003**. 161(4): p. 769-77.

16. Moon, R.T.; A. DeMarais and D.J. Olson. *Responses to Wnt signals in vertebrate embryos may involve changes in cell adhesion and cell movement.* J Cell Sci Suppl, **1993**. 17: p. 183-8.

17. Du, S.J.; S.M. Purcell; J.L. Christian; L.L. McGrew and R.T. Moon. *Identification of distinct classes and functional domains of Wnts through expression of wild-type and chimeric proteins in Xenopus embryos.* Mol Cell Biol, **1995**. 15(5): p. 2625-34.

18. Gordon, M.D. and R. Nusse. *Wnt signaling: multiple pathways, multiple receptors, and multiple transcription factors.* J Biol Chem, **2006**. 281(32): p. 22429-33.

19. Mikels, A.J. and R. Nusse. *Purified Wnt5a protein activates or inhibits beta-catenin-TCF signaling depending on receptor context.* PLoS Biol, **2006**. 4(4): p. e115.

20. Krylova, O.; J. Herreros; K.E. Cleverley; E. Ehler; J.P. Henriquez; S.M. Hughes and P.C. Salinas. *WNT-3, expressed by motoneurons, regulates terminal arborization of neurotrophin-3-responsive spinal sensory neurons.* Neuron, **2002**. 35(6): p. 1043-56.

21. Hall, A.C.; F.R. Lucas and P.C. Salinas. *Axonal remodeling and synaptic differentiation in the cerebellum is regulated by WNT-7a signaling.* Cell, **2000**. 100(5): p. 525-35.

22. Lucas, F.R. and P.C. Salinas. *WNT-7a induces axonal remodeling and increases synapsin I levels in cerebellar neurons.* Dev Biol, **1997**. 192(1): p. 31-44.

23. Chin, L.S.; L. Li; A. Ferreira; K.S. Kosik and P. Greengard. *Impairment of axonal development and of synaptogenesis in hippocampal neurons of synapsin I-deficient mice.* Proc Natl Acad Sci U S A, **1995**. 92(20): p. 9230-4.

24. Greengard, P.; F. Valtorta; A.J. Czernik and F. Benfenati. *Synaptic vesicle phosphoproteins and regulation of synaptic function.* Science, **1993**. 259(5096): p. 780-5.

25. Ahmad-Annuar, A.; L. Ciani; I. Simeonidis; J. Herreros; N.B. Fredj; S.B. Rosso; A. Hall; S. Brickley and P.C. Salinas. *Signaling across the synapse: a role for Wnt and Dishevelled in presynaptic assembly and*

neurotransmitter release. J. Cell Biol., **2006**. 174(1): p. 127-139.

26. Farias, G.G.; A.S. Valles; M. Colombres; J.A. Godoy; E.M. Toledo; R.J. Lukas; F.J. Barrantes and N.C. Inestrosa. *Wnt-7a induces presynaptic colocalization of alpha 7-nicotinic acetylcholine receptors and adenomatous polyposis coli in hippocampal neurons.* J Neurosci, **2007**. 27(20): p. 5313-25.

27. Chen, J.; C.S. Park and S.-J. Tang. *Activity-dependent Synaptic Wnt Release Regulates Hippocampal Long Term Potentiation.* J. Biol. Chem., **2006**. 281(17): p. 11910-11916.

28. Hooper, C.; V. Markevich; F. Plattner; R. Killick; E. Schofield; T. Engel; F. Hernandez; B. Anderton; K. Rosenblum; T. Bliss; S.F. Cooke; J. Avila; J.J. Lucas; K.P. Giese; J. Stephenson and S. Lovestone. *Glycogen synthase kinase-3 inhibition is integral to long-term potentiation.* Eur J Neurosci, **2007**. 25(1): p. 81-6.

29. Hernandez, F.; J. Borrell; C. Guaza; J. Avila and J.J. Lucas. *Spatial learning deficit in transgenic mice that conditionally over-express GSK-3beta in the brain but do not form tau filaments.* J Neurochem, **2002**. 83(6): p. 1529-33.

30. Peineau, S.; C. Taghibiglou; C. Bradley; T.P. Wong; L. Liu; J. Lu; E. Lo; D. Wu; E. Saule; T. Bouschet; P. Matthews; J.T. Isaac; Z.A. Bortolotto; Y.T. Wang and G.L. Collingridge. *LTP inhibits LTD in the hippocampus via regulation of GSK3beta.* Neuron, **2007**. 53(5): p. 703-17.

31. Rosso, S.B.; D. Sussman; A. Wynshaw-Boris and P.C. Salinas. *Wnt signaling through Dishevelled, Rac and JNK regulates dendritic development.* Nat Neurosci, **2005**. 8(1): p. 34-42.

32. Cerpa, W.; J.A. Godoy; I. Alafaro; G.G. Farias; M.J. Metcalfe; R. Fuentealba; C. Bonansco and N.C. Inestrosa. *WNT-7a modulates the synaptic vesicle cycle and synaptic transmission in hippocampal neurons.* J Biol Chem, **2008**. 283: p. 5918-5927.

33. Selkoe, D.J., *Alzheimer's disease: genes, proteins, and therapy.* Physiol Rev, **2001**. 81(2): p. 741-66.

34. Wilquet, V. and B. De Strooper. *Amyloid-beta precursor protein processing in neurodegeneration.* Curr Opin Neurobiol, **2004**. 14(5): p. 582-8.

35. Takashima, A.; T. Honda; K. Yasutake; G. Michel; O. Murayama; M. Murayama; K. Ishiguro and H. Yamaguchi. *Activation of tau protein kinase I/glycogen synthase kinase-3beta by amyloid beta peptide (25-35) enhances phosphorylation of tau in hippocampal neurons.* Neurosci Res, **1998**. 31(4): p. 317-23.

36. Selkoe, D.J., *Alzheimer's disease is a synaptic failure.* Science, **2002**. 298(5594): p. 789-91.

37. Ferreira, S.T.; M.N. Vieira and F.G. De Felice. *Soluble protein oligomers as emerging toxins in Alzheimer's and other amyloid diseases.* IUBMB Life, **2007**. 59(4-5): p. 332-45.

38. Green, K.N. and F.M. LaFerla. *Linking Calcium to A[beta] and Alzheimer's Disease.* Neuron, **2008**. 59(2): p. 190-194.

39. Busche, M.A.; G. Eichhoff; H. Adelsberger; D. Abramowski; K.-H. Wiederhold; C. Haass; M. Staufenbiel; A. Konnerth and O. Garaschuk. *Clusters of Hyperactive Neurons Near Amyloid Plaques in a Mouse Model of Alzheimer's Disease.* Science, **2008**. 321(5896): p. 1686-1689.

40. De Ferrari, G.V. and N.C. Inestrosa. *Wnt signaling function in Alzheimer's disease.* Brain Res Brain Res Rev, **2000**. 33(1): p. 1-12.

41. Inestrosa, N.; G.V. De Ferrari; J.L. Garrido; A. Alvarez; G.H. Olivares; M.I. Barria; M. Bronfman and M.A. Chacon. *Wnt signaling involvement in beta-*

amyloid-dependent neurodegeneration. Neurochem Int, **2002**. 41(5): p. 341-4.

42. Garrido, J.L.; J.A. Godoy; A. Alvarez; M. Bronfman and N.C. Inestrosa. *Protein kinase C inhibits amyloid beta peptide neurotoxicity by acting on members of the Wnt pathway.* FASEB J, **2002**. 16(14): p. 1982-4.

43. De Ferrari, G.V.; M.A. Chacon; M.I. Barria; J.L. Garrido; J.A. Godoy; G. Olivares; A.E. Reyes; A. Alvarez; M. Bronfman and N.C. Inestrosa. *Activation of Wnt signaling rescues neurodegeneration and behavioral impairments induced by beta-amyloid fibrils.* Mol Psychiatry, **2003**. 8(2): p. 195-208.

44. Alvarez, G.; J.R. Munoz-Montano; J. Satrustegui; J. Avila; E. Bogonez and J. Diaz-Nido. *Regulation of tau phosphorylation and protection against beta-amyloid-induced neurodegeneration by lithium. Possible implications for Alzheimer's disease.* Bipolar Disord, **2002**. 4(3): p. 153-65.

45. Takashima, A.; M. Murayama; O. Murayama; T. Kohno; T. Honda; K. Yasutake; N. Nihonmatsu; M. Mercken; H. Yamaguchi; S. Sugihara and B. Wolozin. *Presenilin 1 associates with glycogen synthase kinase-3beta and its substrate tau.* Proc Natl Acad Sci U S A, **1998**. 95(16): p. 9637-41.

46. Zhang, Z.; H. Hartmann; V.M. Do; D. Abramowski; C. Sturchler-Pierrat; M. Staufenbiel; B. Sommer; M. van de Wetering; H. Clevers; P. Saftig; B. De Strooper; X. He and B.A. Yankner. *Destabilization of beta-catenin by mutations in presenilin-1 potentiates neuronal apoptosis.* Nature, **1998**. 395(6703): p. 698-702.

47. Caricasole, A.; A. Copani; F. Caraci; E. Aronica; A.J. Rozemuller; A. Caruso; M. Storto; G. Gaviraghi; G.C. Terstappen and F. Nicoletti. *Induction of Dickkopf-1, a negative modulator of the Wnt pathway, is associated with neuronal degeneration in Alzheimer's brain.* J Neurosci, **2004**. 24(26): p. 6021-7.

48. Ghanevati, M. and C.A. Miller. *Phospho-beta-Catenin Accumulation in Alzheimer's Disease and in Aggresomes Attributable to Proteasome Dysfunction.* J Mol Neurosci, **2005**. 25(1): p. 79-94.

49. De Ferrari, G.V.; A. Papassotiropoulos; T. Biechele; F. Wavrant De-Vrieze; M.E. Avila; M.B. Major; A. Myers; K. Saez; J.P. Henriquez; A. Zhao; M.A. Wollmer; R.M. Nitsch; C. Hock; C.M. Morris; J. Hardy and R.T. Moon. *Common genetic variation within the low-density lipoprotein receptor-related protein 6 and late-onset Alzheimer's disease.* Proc Natl Acad Sci U S A, **2007**. 104(22): p. 9434-9.

50. Magdesian, M.H.; M.M. Carvalho; F.A. Mendes; L.M. Saraiva; M.A. Juliano; L. Juliano; J. Garcia-Abreu and S.T. Ferreira. *Amyloid-beta binds to the extracellular cysteine-rich domain of Frizzled and inhibits Wnt/beta-catenin signaling.* J Biol Chem, **2008**. 283(14): p. 9359-68.

51. Pei, J.J.; E. Braak; H. Braak; I. Grundke-Iqbal; K. Iqbal; B. Winblad and R.F. Cowburn. *Distribution of active glycogen synthase kinase 3beta (GSK-3beta) in brains staged for Alzheimer disease neurofibrillary changes.* J Neuropathol Exp Neurol, **1999**. 58(9): p. 1010-9.

52. Mudher, A. and S. Lovestone. *Alzheimer's disease-do tauists and baptists finally shake hands?* Trends Neurosci, **2002**. 25(1): p. 22-6.

53. Caricasole, A.; A. Copani; A. Caruso; F. Caraci; L. Iacovelli; M.A. Sortino; G.C. Terstappen and F. Nicoletti. *The Wnt pathway, cell-cycle activation and beta-amyloid: novel therapeutic strategies in Alzheimer's disease?* Trends Pharmacol Sci, **2003**. 24(5): p. 233-8.

54. Alvarez, A.R.; J.A. Godoy; K. Mullendorff; G.H.

55. Olivares; M. Bronfman and N.C. Inestrosa. *Wnt-3a overcomes beta-amyloid toxicity in rat hippocampal neurons.* Exp Cell Res, **2004**. 297(1): p. 186-96.

55. Fuentealba, R.A.; G. Farias; J. Scheu; M. Bronfman; M.P. Marzolo and N.C. Inestrosa. *Signal transduction during amyloid-beta-peptide neurotoxicity: role in Alzheimer disease.* Brain Res Brain Res Rev, **2004**. 47(1-3): p. 275-89.

56. Li, H.-L.; H.-H. Wang; S.-J. Liu; Y.-Q. Deng; Y.-J. Zhang; Q. Tian; X.-C. Wang; X.-Q. Chen; Y. Yang; J.-Y. Zhang; Q. Wang; H. Xu; F.-F. Liao and J.-Z. Wang. *Phosphorylation of tau antagonizes apoptosis by stabilizing beta-catenin, a mechanism involved in Alzheimer's neurodegeneration.* PNAS, **2007**. 104(9): p. 3591-3596.

57. Raber, J.; Y. Huang and J.W. Ashford. *ApoE genotype accounts for the vast majority of AD risk and AD pathology.* Neurobiol Aging, **2004**. 25(5): p. 641-50.

58. Strittmatter, W.J. and A.D. Roses. *Apolipoprotein E and Alzheimer disease.* Proc Natl Acad Sci U S A, **1995**. 92(11): p. 4725-7.

59. Caruso, A.; M. Motolese; L. Iacovelli; F. Caraci; A. Copani; F. Nicoletti; G.C. Terstappen; G. Gaviraghi and A. Caricasole. *Inhibition of the canonical Wnt signaling pathway by apolipoprotein E4 in PC12 cells.* J Neurochem, **2006**. 98(2): p. 364-371.

60. Mao, B.; W. Wu; Y. Li; D. Hoppe; P. Stannek; A. Glinka and C. Niehrs. *LDL-receptor-related protein 6 is a receptor for Dickkopf proteins.* Nature, **2001**. 411(6835): p. 321-5.

61. Zorn, A.M., *Wnt signalling: antagonistic Dickkopfs.* Curr Biol, **2001**. 11(15): p. R592-5.

62. Cappuccio, I.; A. Calderone; C.L. Busceti; F. Biagioni; F. Pontarelli; V. Bruno; M. Storto; G.T. Terstappen; G. Gaviraghi; F. Fornai; G. Battaglia; D. Melchiorri; S. Zukin; F. Nicoletti and A. Caricasole. *Induction of Dickkopf-1, a negative modulator of the Wnt pathway, is required for the development of ischemic neuronal death.* J Neurosci, **2005**. 25(10): p. 2647-57.

63. Inestrosa, N.C.; A. Alvarez; M.C. Dinamarca; T. Perez-Acle and M. Colombres. *Acetylcholinesterase-amyloid-beta-peptide interaction: effect of Congo Red and the role of the Wnt pathway.* Curr Alzheimer Res, **2005**. 2(3): p. 301-6.

64. Cerpa, W.; M.C. Dinamarca and N. Inestrosa. *Structure-Function Implications in Alzheimer's Disease: Effect of Abeta Oligomers at Central Synapses.* Current Alzheimers Research, **2008**. 5: p. 233-243.

65. Dinamarca, M.C.; M. Colombres; W. Cerpa; C. Bonansco and N.C. Inestrosa. *Beta-amyloid oligomers affect the structure and function of the postsynaptic region: role of the Wnt signaling pathway.* Neurodegener Dis, **2008**. 5(3-4): p. 149-52.

66. Shankar, G.M.; S. Li; T.H. Mehta; A. Garcia-Munoz; N.E. Shepardson; I. Smith; F.M. Brett; M.A. Farrell; M.J. Rowan; C.A. Lemere; C.M. Regan; D.M. Walsh; B.L. Sabatini and D.J. Selkoe. *Amyloid-[beta] protein dimers isolated directly from Alzheimer's brains impair synaptic plasticity and memory.* Nat Med, **2008**. 14(8): p. 837-842.

67. Takahashi, M.; K. Tomizawa; R. Kato; K. Sato; T. Uchida; S.C. Fujita and K. Imahori. *Localization and developmental changes of tau protein kinase I/glycogen synthase kinase-3 beta in rat brain.* J Neurochem, **1994**. 63(1): p. 245-55.

68. Bhat, R.V.; S.L. Budd Haeberlein and J. Avila. *Glycogen synthase kinase 3: a drug target for CNS therapies.* J Neurochem, **2004**. 89(6): p. 1313-7.

69. Plattner, F.; M. Angelo and K.P. Giese. *The roles of*

cyclin-dependent kinase 5 and glycogen synthase kinase 3 in tau hyperphosphorylation. J Biol Chem, **2006**. 281(35): p. 25457-65.

70.   Avila, J.; J.J. Lucas; M. Perez and F. Hernandez. *Role of tau protein in both physiological and pathological conditions.* Physiol Rev, **2004**. 84(2): p. 361-84.

71.   Gould, T.D. and H.K. Manji. *Glycogen synthase kinase-3: a putative molecular target for lithium mimetic drugs.* Neuropsychopharmacology, **2005**. 30(7): p. 1223-37.

72.   Ryves, W.J. and A.J. Harwood. *Lithium inhibits glycogen synthase kinase-3 by competition for magnesium.* Biochem Biophys Res Commun, **2001**. 280(3): p. 720-5.

73.   Grimes, C.A. and R.S. Jope. *The multifaceted roles of glycogen synthase kinase 3beta in cellular signaling.* Prog Neurobiol, **2001**. 65(4): p. 391-426.

74.   Harwood, A.J., *Lithium and bipolar mood disorder: the inositol-depletion hypothesis revisited.* Mol Psychiatry, **2005**. 10(1): p. 117-26.

75.   Wada, A.; H. Yokoo; T. Yanagita and H. Kobayashi. *Lithium: potential therapeutics against acute brain injuries and chronic neurodegenerative diseases.* J Pharmacol Sci, **2005**. 99(4): p. 307-21.

76.   Nunes, P.V.; O.V. Forlenza and W.F. Gattaz. *Lithium and risk for Alzheimer's disease in elderly patients with bipolar disorder.* Br J Psychiatry, **2007**. 190: p. 359-60.

77.   Lacor, P.N.; M.C. Buniel; P.W. Furlow; A.S. Clemente; P.T. Velasco; M. Wood; K.L. Viola and W.L. Klein. *Abeta oligomer-induced aberrations in synapse composition, shape, and density provide a molecular basis for loss of connectivity in Alzheimer's disease.* J Neurosci, **2007**. 27(4): p. 796-807.

78.   Shankar, G.M.; B.L. Bloodgood; M. Townsend; D.M. Walsh; D.J. Selkoe and B.L. Sabatini. *Natural oligomers of the Alzheimer amyloid-beta protein induce reversible synapse loss by modulating an NMDA-type glutamate receptor-dependent signaling pathway.* J Neurosci, **2007**. 27(11): p. 2866-75.

79.   Walsh, D.M.; I. Klyubin; J.V. Fadeeva; W.K. Cullen; R. Anwyl; M.S. Wolfe; M.J. Rowan and D.J. Selkoe. *Naturally secreted oligomers of amyloid [beta] protein potently inhibit hippocampal long-term potentiation in vivo.* Nature, **2002**. 416(6880): p. 535-539.

80.   Almeida, C.G.; D. Tampellini; R.H. Takahashi; P. Greengard; M.T. Lin; E.M. Snyder and G.K. Gouras. *Beta-amyloid accumulation in APP mutant neurons reduces PSD-95 and GluR1 in synapses.* Neurobiol Dis, **2005**. 20(2): p. 187-98.

81.   Inestrosa, N.C.; L. Varela-Nallar; C.P. Grabowski and M. Colombres. *Synaptotoxicity in Alzheimer's disease: the Wnt signaling pathway as a molecular target.* IUBMB Life, **2007**. 59(4-5): p. 316-21.

82.   Snyder, E.M.; Y. Nong; C.G. Almeida; S. Paul; T. Moran; E.Y. Choi; A.C. Nairn; M.W. Salter; P.J. Lombroso; G.K. Gouras and P. Greengard. *Regulation of NMDA receptor trafficking by amyloid-beta.* Nat Neurosci, **2005**. 8(8): p. 1051-8.

83.   Lein, E.S.; M.J. Hawrylycz; N. Ao; M. Ayres; A. Bensinger; A. Bernard; A.F. Boe; M.S. Boguski; K.S. Brockway; E.J. Byrnes; L. Chen; L. Chen; T.M. Chen; M.C. Chin; J. Chong; B.E. Crook; A. Czaplinska; C.N. Dang; S. Datta; N.R. Dee; A.L. Desaki; T. Desta; E. Diep; T.A. Dolbeare; M.J. Donelan; H.W. Dong; J.G. Dougherty; B.J. Duncan; A.J. Ebbert; G. Eichele; L.K. Estin; C. Faber; B.A. Facer; R. Fields; S.R. Fischer; T.P. Fliss; C. Frensley; S.N. Gates; K.J. Glattfelder; K.R. Halverson; M.R. Hart; J.G. Hohmann; M.P. Howell; D.P. Jeung; R.A. Johnson; P.T. Karr; R. Kawal; J.M. Kidney; R.H. Knapik; C.L. Kuan; J.H. Lake; A.R. Laramee; K.D. Larsen; C. Lau; T.A. Lemon; A.J. Liang; Y. Liu; L.T. Luong; J. Michaels; J.J. Morgan; R.J. Morgan; M.T. Mortrud; N.F. Mosqueda; L.L. Ng; R. Ng; G.J. Orta; C.C. Overly; T.H. Pak; S.E. Parry; S.D. Pathak; O.C. Pearson; R.B. Puchalski; Z.L. Riley; H.R. Rockett; S.A. Rowland; J.J. Royall; M.J. Ruiz; N.R. Sarno; K. Schaffnit; N.V. Shapovalova; T. Sivisay; C.R. Slaughterbeck; S.C. Smith; K.A. Smith; B.I. Smith; A.J. Sodt; N.N. Stewart; K.R. Stumpf; S.M. Sunkin; M. Sutram; A. Tam; C.D. Teemer; C. Thaller; C.L. Thompson; L.R. Varnam; A. Visel; R.M. Whitlock; P.E. Wohnoutka; C.K. Wolkey; V.Y. Wong; M. Wood; M.B. Yaylaoglu; R.C. Young; B.L. Youngstrom; X.F. Yuan; B. Zhang; T.A. Zwingman and A.R. Jones. *Genome-wide atlas of gene expression in the adult mouse brain.* Nature, **2007**. 445(7124): p. 168-76.

84.   Chacon, M.A.; L. Varela-Nallar and N.C. Inestrosa. *Frizzled-1 is involved in the neuroprotective effect of Wnt3a against Abeta oligomers.* J Cell Physiol, **2008**.

β-Amyloid Peptide, Endoplasmic Reticulum Stress, and Alzheimer's Disease

Othman Ghribi

Department of Pharmacology, Physiology and Therapeutics, University of North Dakota School of Medicine, Grand Forks, ND, 58202, USA

Abstract: Accumulation of β-amyloid (Aβ) peptide in the brain is suggested to play a key role in the pathogenesis of Alzheimer's disease (AD). Both the inherited familial and the sporadic forms of AD are characterized by increased levels of $A\beta_{42}$. Incubation of cells with synthetic Aβ or administration of this peptide to animals is also associated with cellular degeneration. Currently, the mechanisms by which Aβ accumulates as well as the mechanisms that underlie Aβ-induced neurodegeneration in AD are not fully understood. Aβ is generated in part in the endoplasmic reticulum of neurons, degraded chiefly by the insulin degrading enzyme, and cleared out of the brain primarily by the low-density lipoprotein receptor-related protein. Stress in the endoplasmic reticulum can affect the processes involved in Aβ generation, degradation, and clearance, thus resulting in increased levels of this peptide in the brain. In this chapter, *first*, supportive data of role of disturbances in the endoplasmic reticulum homeostasis as an underlying mechanism of Aβ accumulation will be provided. *Second*, evidence from in *vitro* and in *vivo* studies showing that the endoplasmic reticulum is a target organelle for exogenous Aβ will be demonstrated. When applied to cells or administered to animals Aβ triggers endoplasmic reticulum stress that is ultimately deleterious to cells. Collectively, data from AD brains, animal models for AD, and in *vitro* studies converge to present compelling evidence that the endoplasmic reticulum stress is relevant to the pathogenesis of AD.

INTRODUCTION

Bronchial Alzheimer's disease (AD), a devastating neurodegenerative disorder, has a complex and not well-defined etiology. Histopathologically, AD is characterized by the presence of neurofibrillary tangles and senile plaques. Neurofibrillary tangles are formed of tau protein that deposits in a hyperphoshorylated and aggregated form. Plaques are primarily constituted by the accumulation of β-amyloid$_{42}$ ($A\beta_{42}$) peptide in the form of pleated sheet fibrils [1, 2]. In addition to plaques and tangles, oxidative stress, inflammation, and axonal transport inhibition are also pathological hallmarks of AD. $A\beta_{42}$ is generated from β-amyloid precursor protein (β-APP) through sequential cleavage by membrane proteases referred to as β and γ-secretases. The β-secretase, BACE1, first cleaves β-APP to generate a C-terminus fragment (β-CTF), the immediate substrate for γ-secretase [3, 4]. Because mutations in β-amyloid precursor protein (β-APP) gene (located on chromosome 21) cause the accumulation of $A\beta_{42}$ and lead to some forms of familial AD, $A\beta_{42}$ has been suggested to be the key factor in the etiology of AD [5-7]. In support of this hypothesis, mutations in presenilin 1 (on chromosome 14) and presenilin 2 (chromosome 1) that also cause familial AD are associated with increased Aβ plaques [8]. Mutations in these three

genes account for about 5% of all cases of AD. The fact that mutation in tau does not cause AD has suggested that aberrant Aβ metabolism is the trigger of the neuronal death in AD. However, presenilin 1 and 2 have been shown to regulate tau phosphorylation and cell survival without affecting Aβ [9], and suppression of transgenic tau in mice restores memory function and prevents neuronal death [10], suggesting that tau accumulation may also play a role in neuronal impairment in AD. Polymorphisms in four genes, apolipoprotein E (apo E) [11, 12], α-2 macroglobulin [13, 14] very low density lipoprotein receptor [15], and the low-density lipoprotein receptor -related protein, LRP [16, 17], are considered as risk factors for AD pathogenesis. Over the past two decades, the identification of genetic defects in presenilins and β-APP has led to the development of cellular and animal models that have helped in understanding aspects of the pathophysiology of the inherited forms of AD. While genetic mutations in β-APP and presenilins are responsible for the accumulation of Aβ in familial AD, the causative factors for accumulation of Aβ in sporadic AD, which represents the majority of AD cases, are not known. This raises the possibility that, in the absence of genetic mutations in APP and presenilins, factors that affect pathways of generation or clearance of Aβ may alter the level of this peptide, causing sporadic forms of AD.

Despite the accumulation of Aβ peptide in both familial and sporadic AD forms, the mechanisms by which Aβ accumulates or the mechanisms by which Aβ kills neurons are not well known. In this chapter, *first*, data suggesting a potential role of dysfunction of the endoplasmic reticulum (ER) in the aberrant accumulation of Aβ in cellular, animal, and human tissue for familial and sporadic AD forms will be summarized. *Second*, potential mechanisms by which ER stress induces Aβ accumulation will be demonstrated. *Third*, evidence from the literature pointing to the dysregulation of ER function by Aβ as a mechanism by which this peptide may exert neurotoxic effects will be presented.

ER STRESS AND FAMILIAL AD

Presenilin-1 and 2 are critical components of the γ-secretase complex which with β-secretase cleaves the β-APP, producing the Aβ peptide. β-APP is formed in the ER and cleavage of β-APP by β and γ secretases to yield Aβ occurs at least in part in the ER [18-21]. Presenilin-1 and 2 are located primarily in the ER and their mutations, which also occur in the ER, increase the generation of Aβ and calcium dyshomeostasis [22-25]. Familial AD forms are associated with mutations in the genes encoding β-APP and more than 100 mutations, the vast majority of which occurs with presenilin-1, have also been reported to be associated with early onset AD. Thus, the ER appears to be central to the pathogenesis of the inherited forms of AD. Because the ER is the major calcium store in cells, in addition to its role in protein folding, mutation in β-APP and presenilns as well as the subsequent Aβ accumulation would have significant effects on ER homeostasis. In the following paragraphs, data related to the functional link between ER and presenilins as well as β-APP mutations will be presented.

The ER Calcium Dyshomeostasis Hypothesis

The ER serves as a dynamic store for calcium, with a high free calcium concentration being maintained within its lumen. Inside the lumen of the ER, most of the calcium is buffered and bound to ER resident chaperones, however a significant portion of it is free [26, 27]. Calcium concentrations can reach 5 mM in the ER lumen, whereas in the cytosol, calcium concentrations are only at the nanomolar levels [28]. Maintenance of the steep concentration gradient between the ER lumen and cytoplasm is regulated by calcium uptake through the sarcoplasmic/endoplasmic calcium-ATPase (SERCA) pathway and is released via ryanodine receptors (RyRs) and the inositol-1,4,5-triphosphate receptors (IP$_3$Rs). Calreticulin, a protein that is localized in the lumen of the ER, controls SERCA, binds calcium with high capacity, and is involved in the folding of newly synthesized proteins [26]. Maintenance of the equilibrium between calcium influx into the ER and calcium efflux from the ER to the cytoplasm is critical for cell functioning.

The calcium hypothesis in the pathogenesis of Alzheimer's disease was first proposed by Khachaturian [29] and implicates calcium dysregulation as a cause of the synaptic dysfunction and neurodegeneration that are manifestations of the disease (see for review [30, 31]). Presenilin 1 and 2 are integral membrane proteins that localize primarily in the ER. Mutations in the genes encoding for presenilin 1 and 2 cause disturbances in calcium homeostasis in diverse cell lines, increase Aβ$_{42}$ accumulation [8] and lead to early onset familial AD [32, 33]. The development of mutant presenilin1 mouse models [34] provides an *in vivo* tool to study the effect of mutant presenilin 1 on calcium and on downstream signaling pathways. Cortical neurons from transgenic presenilin 1 mice have demonstrated an increased release of calcium [35, 36]. Mutant presenilin 1 dysregulates neuronal calcium homeostasis, either directly or indirectly, via processing of APP and generation of Aβ peptide in hippocampal neurons from mice [37]. Triple transgenic mice (APP swe and tau $_{p301L}$ in the presenilin 1 mutant knock-in mouse) model for AD have shown altered ER calcium levels [38]. In cell lines and in the presenilin 1 knock-in mice and triple transgenic mice, ER-ryanodine receptors overexpression mediates increased calcium release from the ER [35, 38]. Caffeine, an agonist of the ryanodine receptors, exacerbates the increased release of calcium from the ER [35, 38]. The caffeine effect on calcium release from the ER may link this commonly ingested psychoactive drug to the pathogenesis of AD. Indeed, caffeine has been shown to increase levels of Aβ peptide and to enhance neurodegenerative processes in cellular and animal models of familial AD [35, 38-41]. Caffeine-induced overproduction of Aβ has been attributed to its facilitatory effect on calcium release through ryanodine receptors, and these results suggest that activation of the ryanodine receptors may be linked to familial AD. However, currently the mechanisms by which dysregulation of calcium increases ryanodine receptors levels or the mechanisms by which caffeine increases the levels of Aβ are still to be determined. Syntaxin 5, a member of the mammalian syntaxin family, is an ER—Golgi-resident protein that has been shown to bind to presenilins, affecting β-APP processing and altering the production of Aβ peptides in neuronal cells [42, 43]. On the other hand, the ER stress-inducible protein, Herp, an ER-localized membrane protein, increases Aβ generation through its binding to presenilins; in presenilin-deficient cells, overexpression of Herp does not affect Aβ levels [44].

The Unfolded Protein Response (UPR) is Involved in the Pathology of AD

In eukaryotic cells, the ER plays a key role in the secretory pathway, which in addition to the ER, comprises the Golgi apparatus and plasma membrane. The ER is the subcellular site where surface and secreted proteins are synthesized and folded (see for review, [45]). The folding of proteins in the ER is facilitated by an oxidizing environment; folding enzymes, such as the protein disulfide isomerase (PDI); and chaperones residing in the lumen of the ER, such as glucose-regulated protein (grp)78 and 94. Other ER-resident chaperones, such as calreticulin and calnexin, facilitate release of the correct folded protein to their target sites through the secretory pathway and the extracellular space. Protein synthesis, folding, assembly and transport are all calcium-dependent processes. Perturbation of the ER calcium pool may therefore affect the ER-resident chaperone activity and correct folding of proteins. A variety of conditions can cause incorrect folding of proteins. In response, the ER triggers a signaling response by two distinct pathways, the unfolded protein response (UPR) and the ER overload response (EOR) (for review see [46, 47]).

The UPR is a signaling cascade that senses misfolded proteins in the ER-lumen and signals an accumulation of abnormal proteins to the cell nucleus. The primary pro-survival mechanism triggered by the UPR involves the activation of the ER-resident transmembrane proteins, the double-stranded RNA-activated protein kinase (PKR)-like ER kinase (PERK), the eukaryotic translation initiation factor 2-α (eIF2-α), and the basic leucine-zipper transcription factor activating transcription factor (ATF6), all acting as transducers of ER stress signaling [48]. In a non-stress condition, the ER-resident glucose-regulated protein chaperone, grp78 (also called BIP), binds to the N-terminus of PERK, ATF6, and eIF2-α, thus preventing their activation. Stress in the ER causes down-

regulation or translocation from the ER to the cytoplasm and nuclei of grp78, resulting in the release of PERK, ATF6 and/or eIF2-α and their oligomerization in ER membranes. Oligomerized Ire1-α binds TRAF2 and produces XBP-1, PERK causes the phosphorylation of the α subunit of the eukaryotic initiation factor 2 (eIF2α), and ATF6 translocates to the Golgi apparatus for proteolytic processing to release active ATF6 (see for review,[45, 49]). This signaling is intended to protect cells from the consequences of changes in calreticulin levels and the buildup of misfolded proteins.

In contrast to this adaptive ER signaling, sustained or intense ER stress causes cell death. ER stress involves grp78 and other ER-resident chaperones, like grp94 and calreticulin, and the activation of the growth arrest-and DNA damage-inducible gene 153 (gadd153). Gadd153 (also called CHOP) triggers cell death by mechanisms that may include depletion of glutathione, generation of ROS, downregulation of Bcl-2, and upregulation of Bax [50, 51]. NF-κB is activated by the EOR or by binding to the adapter protein, TRAF2, via Ire-1α. TRAF2 activates kinases linked to NF-κB activation. Activated NF-κB translocates to the nucleus, where it regulates cell survival and death. Gadd153 can also induce cell death by activating Gadd34, a regulatory subunit in a protein phosphatase-containing complex that dephosphorylates eIF2α and promotes protein synthesis; gadd153 deletion and gadd34 mutation protect cells against deleterious consequences of these two factors [52].

β-APP plays an important physiological role in protecting neurons from the consequences of prolonged ER stress and UPR. PC12 cells over-expressing human wild-type APP (APPwt) show increased resistance to tunicamycin- or brefeldin A, two agents that induce the unfolded protein response and apoptosis [53]. Conversely, cells expressing the Swedish mutation of APP (KM670/671NL) demonstrate a diminished neuroprotective effect following tunicamycin and berfeldin A [53]. Mutant versions of presenilin-1 also interfere with the UPR [54]. Spontaneous apoptosis or apoptosis induced by brefeldin A, which is known to induce the UPR, is enhanced in primary cultured neurons from transgenic mice which overexpress mutated presenilin 1 [55]. Presenilin-1 mutations increase gadd153 protein levels and apoptosis in presenilin-1 mutant cells challenged with ER stress inducers, effects that are attenuated by the anti-sense-mediated suppression of gadd153 production [56]. Presenilin-1 affects the substrates and effector proteins of the UPR pathway, Ire1α, PERK, or the phosphorylation of eIF2-α [57], and directly cleaves Ire1α, releasing the cytosolic domain to translocate to the nucleus [58]. In postmortem tissue from AD patients, protein levels of grp78 and p-PERK are also found to be increased in the temporal cortex and hippocampus [59]. Although consistent data clearly demonstrate the involvement of presenilins and β-APP and the mutations of genes coding for these two proteins in calcium dyshomeostasis and ER stress response, the mechanisms by which Aβ accumulates in such an environment are not well known. Because ER-resident chaperones are involved in maintaining calcium homeostasis and in the normal folding and degradation of proteins, depletion of ER calcium stores and disturbances in the levels, expression and activity of these chaperones may directly or indirectly affect β-APP processing, thus increasing Aβ generation or decreasing its clearance.

ER STRESS AND SPORADIC AD

While hereditary familial forms of AD are caused by genetic mutations in β-APP and presenilins, the causes of sporadic cases of AD are not known. Environmental factors, in addition to a possible genetic predisposition, can lead to increased accumulation of Aβ in sporadic AD cases. Reduced catabolism or clearance of Aβ peptide could be due to various factors that may include alteration in the expression of the enzymes that degrade Aβ in the brain or transport this peptide out of the brain. Diet, oxidative stress induced by environmental agents, and disturbances in the insulin pathway may all contribute to the development of sporadic AD forms. In the following paragraphs, the existence of a link between potential causative factors of sporadic AD and disturbances in ER functions will be discussed.

Hypercholesterolemia

Abnormalities in cholesterol metabolism are emerging as possible contributors in the etiology of AD by increasing Aβ accumulation. However, in spite of abundant reports, a clear association between cholesterol and AD has not yet been established. Although some of the cholesterol-lowering drugs (the statins) have been reported to decrease Aβ levels and to lower the risk of AD [60, 61], the neuroprotective effect of the statins might be cholesterol-independent. Nevertheless, it may be possible that abnormalities in cholesterol metabolism at mid-age may take part in initiating AD. At late-age when AD progresses the correlation between AD and cholesterol levels is no longer consistent. The first indication of a

connection between cholesterol and Aβ was reported in rabbits [62]. The rabbit demonstrates a marked response to a high cholesterol diet by exhibiting Aβ deposition [63, 64]. High cholesterol levels have also been shown to increase Aβ production in the mouse [65, 66] and in cultured cells [67-71]. Despite abundant studies showing cholesterol-induced Aβ accumulation, the molecular mechanisms by which cholesterol promotes Aβ accumulation are still to be determined.

Cholesterol homeostasis in the brain is regulated through *de novo* synthesis, with no or very poor transfer from the peripheral circulation due to the impermeability of the blood brain barrier (BBB) to plasma lipoproteins [72]. The poor passage of cholesterol from the circulation to the brain however implies that dietary cholesterol does not affect the outcome of Aβ production or accumulation in the brain. Understanding cellular distribution of cholesterol in the brain and its consequences may represent the cornerstone to identifying mechanisms and signaling pathways associated with the cholesterol-Aβ association. In the brain, cells either produce their own cholesterol or import the cholesterol they require from neighboring cells. Oligodendrocytes use large amounts of brain-made cholesterol for the synthesis of myelin [73], and are capable of independently producing cholesterol [74]. Neurons are suggested to depend, at least in part, on cholesterol derived from neighboring cells (for review, see reference [75]). We have found that the cholesterol-enriched diet, while decreasing cholesterol content in oligodendrocytes, causes an increase in cholesterol content in neurons from rabbit hippocampus.

Whether increased neuronal cholesterol derives from oligodendrocytes or is due to an increased production and/or decreased clearance of cholesterol from neurons remains to be determined. The rate-limiting enzyme of cholesterol synthesis, HMG-CoA reductase, and acyl-coenzyme A: cholesterol acyltransferase (ACAT), the enzyme that catabolizes cholesterol, are both ER-resident enzymes. Because ER cholesterol levels are normally low [76], ER homeostasis may be compromised by an abnormal increase in cholesterol levels in the cell. Excess cholesterol has indeed been shown to induce disturbances in ER homeostasis in macrophages [77], and inhibition of ACAT has been shown to reduce amyloid pathology in transgenic mice of AD-expressing human APP751 containing London and Swedish mutations [78]. There is also evidence of a spatial and functional relationship between cholesterol and BACE1, the enzyme that initially cleaves β-APP to generate Aβ. BACE1, like cholesterol, is initially synthesized in the ER and also can process β-APP in the ER compartment [79]. Furthermore, processing of β-APP to the Aβ peptide by BACE1 occurs predominantly in cholesterol-rich lipid domains [80]. Accumulation of cholesterol in neurons would be expected to foster the generation and/or activation of BACE 1, potentially leading to Aβ overproduction. However, the extent to which this mechanism might explain the accumulation of Aβ in cholesterol-fed animals has not been examined. We have found that in neurons, the cholesterol content in the ER markedly increases, and that gadd153 is activated [81]. Factors such as the alteration in cholesterol distribution, the dysregulation in levels of ER chaperones grp78 and grp94, and the activation of the transcription factor, gadd153, may all participate in the intracellular events underlying the accumulation of Aβ peptide in cholesterol-fed rabbits.

Cholesterol may have multifaceted actions in that, in addition to increasing BACE1, high cholesterol-induced ER stress-evoked ROS generation can modify cholesterol itself to generate derivatives containing aldehyde groups. An aldehyde is a functional group or a compound containing a terminal carbonyl group one which, when reacted with Aβ, makes this peptide more hydrophobic and thus more prone to aggregate formation. Although levels of the cholesterol aldehydes in AD patients appear not to be potentially elevated, only small amounts of these metabolites are required to trigger Aβ aggregation. Zhang and colleagues recently have demonstrated that cholesterol aldehydic derivatives accelerate the aggregation of Aβ *in vitro*, and are present in brains from AD patients [82]. These finding confirm earlier work showing that aldehydes from lipid peroxidation are associated with Aβ plaques [83-87]. Despite the above mentioned findings, however, a clear association between the high cholesterol environment-induced ROS generation, an increase in BACE1 levels, generation of cholesterol aldehydic derivatives, and Aβ accumulation remains to be determined. Currently, there are only a few models of sporadic AD that exhibit Aβ accumulation without genetic manipulations, and the rabbit model has advantages over others because rabbit Aβ sequence is similar to that of humans [88]. Additionally, the rabbit phylogeny is close to that of the human [89]. The cholesterol-fed rabbit model may thus provide a model complementary to current mouse models for autosomal dominant forms of AD.

Oxidative Stress and Trace Metals

Oxidative stress is a major risk factor for AD that has been suggested to be the trigger of AD pathology. However, whether oxidative damage precedes and contributes directly to the accumulation of Aβ peptide is still a matter of debate (see for review [90]). Nevertheless, it has been recently shown that free radicals causes exacerbation of the amyloid pathology in Aβ in mice crossed with a knockout of one allele of manganese superoxide dismutase (MnSOD), a critical antioxidant enzyme, with Tg19959 mice, which overexpress a doubly mutated human beta-amyloid precursor protein (APP) [91]. Although the mitochondrial pathway is the main generator of oxidative damage, stress in the ER can also mediate or be targeted by oxidative stress. Primary neuronal cell cultures exposed to H_2O_2 lead to a decrease in the mRNA levels of the ER-resident chaperones, grp78 and grp94 [92]. Also, bombesin-releasable calcium stores (BRCS), an endoplasmic reticulum calcium store has also been demonstrated to be a target for oxidative stress [93, 94].

The trace metals copper, zinc and iron, have been strongly suggested as a potential trigger of AD by generating oxidative stress. Of the trace metal elements, excess iron accumulation in the brain has been a consistent observation in AD, and iron reaction product is found in the proximity of plaques and in cells associated with the plaques [95-97]. Iron promotes aggregation of Aβ in vitro [98], and incubation of Aβ with excess free iron induces oxidative stress [99]. Of relevance, increased iron deposition has been recently demonstrated in the cerebral cortex of cholesterol-fed rabbits [100]. Although Aβ production may be central to AD, its production, and eventually its effects, can be enhanced by other agents. The metals, copper and aluminum, can enhance Aβ deposition *in vivo*. We have previously shown that aluminum causes ER stress involving the activation of gadd153 and the ER-specific caspase, caspase-12 [101, 102]. Trace amounts of copper in water foster Aβ plaque formation and induce learning deficits in rabbit [63], and dietary aluminum increases brain amyloidosis in APP transgenic mice [103]. It appears therefore that metals enhance the deposition of Aβ. Chronic exposure to aluminium sulphate in drinking water resulted in deposition of Abeta and reduction in neuronal expression of GRP78 similar to what has previously been observed in Alzheimer's disease [104].

A recent population-based cohort study, demonstrating that the risk of developing AD is much greater in patients with elevated cholesterol and iron than in patients having either high cholesterol or elevated iron concentrations [105], further suggests a potential link between cholesterol, iron, Aβ and AD. The mechanisms that underlie iron toxicity are poorly understood. It has been shown that iron is a modulator of the ryanodine receptors, which play an important role in maintaining calcium homeostasis in the ER. Also iron has been shown to modulate calreticulin, a major calcium binding protein and a chaperone involved in the correct folding of proteins in the ER, leading to oxidative stress. Disturbances of calcium and ER homeostasis may explain at least in part the oxidative stress and potential Aβ aggregation mediated by iron.

Insulin Metabolism

Mounting evidence suggests that insulin deregulation in the brain is involved in the pathophysiologic events of AD [106]. The insulin receptor density has been shown to be up-regulated in sporadic AD [107] in a manner similar to that occurring in non-insulin dependent-type II diabetes mellitus, suggesting an impairment in the insulin transduction pathway rather than alterations in concentration or activity of insulin (reviewed in [108]). In regard to its action on Aβ, insulin significantly reduces the intracellular accumulation of Aβ and increases its extracellular level in neuronal cultures, both by promoting its secretion and by inhibiting its degradation, via an insulin-degrading enzyme (IDE) [109]. Impairment of ER functioning may be linked to insulin deregulation. Several studies have indeed shown that pancreatic β-cells have highly developed ER machinery and abundantly express ER stress-proteins (see for review, [110, 111], characteristics that may render these cells particularly vulnerable to disturbances in ER functions . More recently, insulin knockout mice have been shown to demonstrate swollen ER and hyperphosphorylation of JNK in the brain [112]. Treatment of macrophages with insulin also causes ER stress, indicating that both increased or decreased insulin levels alter ER homeostasis [113]. Furthermore, in a model for streptozotocin-induced diabetes, calcium release from the ryanodine receptors, which control the efflux of calcium from the ER into the cytoplasm, were down-regulated in rat neurons [114]. Recent findings also demonstrate that ER stress is a central feature of insulin resistance and type II diabetes in cell culture and mouse models. High lipid levels, which contribute to type II diabetes, have been shown to cause ER stress and to suppress insulin receptor signaling [115]. Mice

deficient in X-box–binding protein–1 (XBP-1), a transcription factor that modulates the ER stress response, develop insulin resistance [115]. Additionally, treatment of mouse insulinoma with insulin-like growth factor (IGF-1) inhibits apoptosis initiated by ER stress inducers [116]. Further studies are still needed to demonstrate a link between disturbances in insulin metabolism and the metabolism of Aβ peptide. In summary, alterations in insulin receptors, levels or signaling transduction pathways may reduce the availability of ATP, disturb calcium homeostasis and affect the correct functioning of the ER, thus leading to the generation of misfolded proteins and the accumulation of Aβ.

MECHANISMS INVOLVED IN ER STRESS-INDUCED Aβ ACCUMULATION IN AD BRAINS AND IN MODELS FOR AD.

Dysregulation in Calreticulin Expression

Disturbances in levels of the ER chaperone calreticulin may have devastating effects on calcium homeostasis and on the correct folding of proteins in the ER. The role of calreticulin in the pathophysiology of AD is not well known. Nevertheless, evidence indicates that calreticulin functions as a molecular chaperone for the β-amyloid precursor protein [117]. A decrease in levels and expression of calreticulin is indeed found in neurons from AD brains [118], and an NH$_2$-terminally truncated form of Aβ has been shown in ER of aged cell cultures [119]. In human cerebrospinal fluid, Aβ peptides bind to the ER chaperones, calreticulin and ERp57, suggesting that these proteins may be carrier proteins which prevent aggregation of Aβ; failure in the association of Aβ to these carriers may explain the aggregation of Aβ in plaques [120].

Alterations in glucose-related proteins (grps) expression

Activation of grp94 and grp78 is considered to be a mechanism for cells to cope with the toxic buildup of misfolded proteins and with changes in Ca^{2+} levels. However, sustained or intense ER stress leads to activation of the transcription factor gadd 153, a mediator of apoptosis. Expressional patterns of ER chaperones in the brain of AD subjects has shown that grp78 is increased only in surviving neurons, especially in the CA3 subfield of the hippocampus and in the deep layers of the entorhinal cortex, suggesting that this protein may protect such cells from AD-specific damage [121].

Other studies have demonstrated that grp78 immunostaining is diminished in AD choroid plexus [122]. It has also been found that administration of 2-deoxy-d-glucose to adult rats procures the resistance of synaptic terminals to the dysfunction and degeneration induced by Aβ peptide, effects that correlate with increased levels of grp78 in synaptosomes [123]. In human embryonic kidney 293 cells, grp78 has been found to bind to β-APP in the ER and to decrease the levels of $A\beta_{40}$ and $A\beta_{42}$ secretion, suggesting that grp78 facilitates the correct folding of β-APP in the ER [124]. The addition of exogenous grp78 has been demonstrated in rat mixed glial cell cultures to stimulate $A\beta_{42}$ clearance by increasing phagocytosis by microglia, suggesting that ER stress-induced alterations in grp78 levels may cause the accumulation of extracellular $A\beta_{42}$ [125]. Overexpression of grp78 or inhibition of its basal expression decreased and increased respectively the level of Aβ40 and Aβ42 in cultured cells which produce a mutant type of APP [126]. While changes in grp78 expression are relevant to the pathology of AD, little is known about grp94 expression. Yoo and co-workers [127] have found that the expression of grp94, but not grp78, is increased in the parietal cortex of AD patients, and have suggested that this increase may account for abnormalities in the intracellular translocation of protein kinases and the intracellular signal transduction in AD brain.

Activation of Gadd153

Intense or sustained stress in the ER activates the transcription factor gadd153 which in turn can trigger the generation of reactive oxygen species (ROS). It has been demonstrated that gadd153 sensitizes cells to ER stress by perturbing the cellular redox state in a cell model system in which gadd153 is constitutively over-expressed [128]. Gadd153-induced ROS can foster the production of BACE1, the rate limiting enzyme in β-APP processing to yield Aβ, thus leading to increased Aβ levels. Incubation of NT2 neurons with the pro-oxidant ascorbate/ $FeSO_4$ or $H_2O_2/FeSO_4$ has indeed resulted in increased BACE1 protein level [129, 130]. These results strongly suggest that ER stress-induced gadd153 activation can trigger oxidative stress, increasing BACE1 generation and potentially resulting in Aβ overproduction.

Impairment of the ERAD and UPS

The essential role of the endoplasmic reticulum associated protein degradation (ERAD) and the ubiquitin proteasome system (UPS) is the removal and degradation of misfolded, unfolded or damaged proteins. Therefore, one possible cause of the accumulation of Aβ in AD is the malfunction of these systems [131, 132]. The UPS has a central role in degradation of intracellular proteins (see for review, [133]). Both normal and misfolded proteins can be destroyed by the UPS [134, 135]. UPS is a multi-step process that requires the activation of three proteins, ubiquitin-activating enzyme (E1), ubiquitin-conjugating enzyme (E2), and ubiquitin ligase complex (E3). Disturbances in the UPS have been suggested to result in a variety of human diseases, including Alzheimer's, Parkinson's, Huntington's, prion and Pick's diseases, as well as amyotrophic lateral sclerosis (see for review, [136]). Previous studies have indicated that the UPS could also be functionally impaired under conditions of increased endogenous oxidative stress [137-139].

Mounting evidence suggests that the activities of the proteasome and ubiquitination are reduced in patients with AD [140-143]. The degradation of BACE 1, the enzyme that intiates cleavage of β-APP to yield Aβ, is regulated by the UPS [144]. Malfunction of the UPS may thus prevent BACE 1 degeradation, leading to excessive β-APP cleavage and Aβ production. In ER-derived brain microsomes, Aβ42 generated in the ER has been shown to be exported distinctly from that of other ERAD substrates in that it is degraded by proteasome-dependent and proteasome-independent pathways; the latter pathway has been identified as involving the IDE. The IDE-mediated clearance mechanism for ER-localized Aβ thus represents a distinct proteasome- independent ERAD [145]. Although only small amounts of $A\beta_{42}$ are normally found in the ER, because of the progressive nature of the AD pathology, alterations in levels or expression of IDE may over the long-term cause significant accumulation of $A\beta_{42}$.

LRP is a large endocytic receptor that carries Aβ out of brain and into the periphery [146]. As a first step in the LRP-mediated clearance of Aβ peptide, Aβ forms a complex with α-2-macroglobulin (α-2M) or apolipoprotein E (apoE), two ligands of LRP (reviewed in [147]). Polymorphism in α-2M has been linked to the pathogenesis of AD [148]. Interestingly, suppressing the expression of the ER-resident chaperone grp78, which plays an important role in calcium homeostasis, protein folding and misfolded protein degradation, leads to the loss of the α-2M signalling receptor [149]. This same group has also previously demonstrated that, beside being essential for activated α-2M - induced signal transduction, grp78 is also associated with LRP [150].

Another specialized chaperone that is present in the ER, receptor-associated protein (RAP), also interacts with LRP, binds to LRP immediately following its biosynthesis and assists in its exocytic transport [151]. RAP -/- mice show reduced LRP expression in certain cell types [151]. In another study in RAP-deficient mice, RAP was found to be required for the proper folding and export of LRP from the ER by preventing the premature binding of co-expressed ligands [152]. In these same studies, overexpression of apoE, a high affinity ligand for LRP, resulted in reduced cellular LRP expression, an effect that is prevented by co-expression of RAP. RAP down-regulation may thus cause the aggregation in the ER of newly synthesized proteins. Potential interaction of other ER-resident chaperones, such as grp94, also needs to be tested. In addition to grp78, the three ER chaperones, calnexin, calreticulin, and PDI, also have the ability to associate with LRP [151]. Alterations in ER chaperone expression following ER stress may affect LRP capacity in clearing Aβ from the secretory pathway. Further studies are needed to determine a functional link between the ER-resident chaperones, α-2M, LRP and Aβ accumulation in AD.

Apoptosis

A number of reports have demonstrated in cultured cells that β-APP can also be cleaved by the executioner caspase, caspase-3, thus contributing to increased Aβ production [153, 154]. Stress in the ER has been shown to cause apoptosis, either in concert with mitochondria or independent of the mitochondrial pathway, involving the activation of caspases. Indeed a "cross-talk" between stressed ER and mitochondria exists, and both organelles can work in concert [102]. ER dyshomeostasis can increase calcium levels in mitochondria, resulting in the release of cytochrome *c* and the induction of apoptosis [155]. Cytochrome *c* released from stressed mitochondria can also translocate into the ER and triggers ER stress [156, 157]. Three major caspase recognition sites have been identified in the β-APP; Asp^{720} at the C terminus, and Asp^{197} and Asp^{219} at the N terminus. Cleavage at Asp^{720} has been suggested as the site leading to Aβ overproduction.

Cleavage of β-APP by caspases suggests that apoptosis may be an early event activated in the early stages of AD [158]. However, whether the proteolysis of β-APP by caspases precedes, is concomitant or exacerbates BACE 1 and γ-secretase-mediated Aβ production is not known. The role of cleavage of β-APP by caspases in the accumulation of Aβ has been questioned by Soriano and colleagues [159], demonstrating that

caspase cleavage of β-APP resulted in reduced secretion of Aβ in B103 cells. However, more recently, it has been shown that staurosporine and etoposide-induced caspase activation increases Aβ production in CHO cell lines overexpressing β-APP [160]. Furthermore, this increased Aβ production has been shown to be independent of caspase cleavage of the β-APP at its Asp$^{197, 219}$ or ^{720} sites, suggesting that caspase-dependant cleavage at sites of β-APP other than Asp$^{197, 219,720}$ may increase Aβ levels. Caspase-6, -8, and -9 have been reported to cleave β-APP between Asp^{664} and Ala^{665} [153, 161-163]. Alternatively, caspases can increase Aβ generation independently of caspase-dependent cleavage of β-APP [160, 161]. Stress in the ER, induced by environmental or biochemical factors, may therefore activate caspases leading to Aβ accumulation.

ER STRESS AS A MECHANISM UNDERLYING EXOGENOUS Aβ-INDUCED NEUROTOXICITY

Aβ induces an ER-specific Apoptosis

Caspase-12 has been implicated in ER stress-induced specific apoptosis and Aβ-induced apoptosis in cells and rodents [164]. Caspase-12 exists as a pro–caspase, predominantly localized to the ER, and is specifically cleaved by ER stress. However, it was reported that caspase-12 has acquired deleterious mutations in human [165]. Caspase-4 has also been shown to be activated by administration of Aβ, and small interference RNAs to caspase-4 attenuated Aβ-induced apoptosis, suggesting that caspase-4 may function as an ER stress-specific caspase in the human [165]. It has been demonstrated that although ER stress-induced apoptosis is caspase-dependent, this process does not require the expression of caspase-12 or caspase-4 but can be inhibited by overexpression of Bcl-xL or a dominant negative caspase-9 [165]. We have shown that the injection of Aβ into New Zealand white rabbit brain activates caspase-12, grp78 and grp94, and the transcription factor, gadd 153. These effects correlate with the activation of JNK and ERK as well as of microglia, and with the phosphorylation of tau protein. Treatment with lithium or with glial cell line-derived neurotrophic factor (GDNF) inhibits apoptosis, modulates JNK and ERK and does not affect the phosphorylation of tau [101, 166-168].

Aβ Affects ER Calcium Homeostasis

Synthetic Aβ, when applied *in vitro*, destabilizes neuronal calcium homeostasis and renders neurons more vulnerable to neuronal death [169, 170].

Incubation of cortical cultures with Aβ peptides induces a significant increase in intracellular calcium concentrations, an effect that is inhibited by dantrolene and xestospongin C, inhibitors of ER-Ca^{2+} release through ryanodine and IP_3 receptors [171]. However in a different study, reduction of ER calcium release only partially attenuates Aβ peptide neurotoxicity, suggesting that Aβ-induced ER stress is not the unique pathway that mediates Aβ toxicity [172]. In addition to an action on ryanodine and IP_3 receptors, proposed mechanisms for the Aβ-induced Ca^{2+} dysregulation include disruption of membrane integrity or fluidity [173-175], and formation of ion channels by Aβ peptide itself [176-181]. Oligomeric Aβ42 depletes ER Ca^{2+} levels leading to intracellular Ca^{2+} dyshomeostasis involving phospholipase C activation in primary rat embryo cortical neuronal cultures [182]. Moreover, in the presence of dantrolene, an inhibitor of ER Ca^{2+} release through ryanodine receptors, the oligomer-induced apoptosis was prevented demonstrating the involvement of ER Ca^{2+} release[182].

Exposure of neurons containing AD-linked mutant presenilins (mPS1) to Aβ induced IP3-mediated calcium release from ER as well as increased gadd153 [183]. Gadd153 is a death effector of ER stress, which acts to transcriptionally inhibit protective cellular molecules such as Bcl-2 and glutathione

Aβ Inhibits the Ubiquitin-proteasome System

Previous studies have indicated that the UPS could be functionally impaired under conditions of increased endogenous oxidative stress associated with coronary occlusion/ reperfusion in the rat [137] or with Parkinson's disease [138, 139]. In regard to the Aβ/AD hypothesis, Aβ *per se* has been shown to inhibit the UPS and to induce neuronal death when applied to primary cultures of neurons [184]. These Aβ effects correlate with an over- expression of E2-25K/Hip-2, a component of the gene encoding UPS that functions as an E2-ubiquitin conjugating enzyme. Thus, a reduction of E2-25K/Hip-2 has been shown to block the proteasome inhibition and neurotoxicty induced by Aβ. On the other hand, a mutant form of ubiquitin, called Ub+1, has been observed in the brains of AD patients [185]. Ub+1 has been shown to occur in a variety of neurodegenerative diseases including AD, suggesting that expression of Ub+1 may inhibit the ubiquitn-proteasome system [186, 187]. E2-25K/Hip-2, an E2 ubiquitin-conjugating enzyme, regulates the activation of caspase-12 and ER stress responses during Aβ neurotoxicity, and

that E2-25K/Hip-2–deficient cortical neurons cultured from E2-25K/Hip-2 knockout mice lack Aβ-induced ER stress responses, including accumulation of caspase-12, and are resistant to Aβ toxicity. E2-25K/Hip-2–deficient cortical neurons are resistant to Aβ toxicity and to the induction of ER stress and caspase-12 expression by Aβ. E2-25K/Hip-2 is thus an essential upstream regulator of the expression and activation of caspase-12 in ER stress–mediated Aβ neurotoxicity [184].

CONCLUDING REMARKS

As is the case for Aβ accumulation, whether ER stress and protein misfolding in AD are a cause or consequence of AD is still to be determined. However, it is not surprising that a variety of diseases are caused by dysfunction in the ER because of the vital role that the ER plays in the cell. ER dysfunction causes disturbances in the correct folding of proteins and the accumulation of misfolded or damaged proteins in the secretary pathway. Accumulation of these proteins leads to the generation of the enzymatic machinery that degrades these malfolded proteins, as well as an impairment of the related enzymes. As a result of these dysfunctions, an increased generation of oxidative stress and an induction of apoptosis ultimately cause the death of neurons. In cellular and animal models for sporadic AD, calcium dyshomeostasis appears to be an early event that leads to initiation of the ER stress response and dysregulation in the ER chaperones expression, thus increasing Aβ production and/or secretion. The accumulation of Aβ peptide in sporadic AD may rather result from retention of Aβ intracellularly, following the inhibition or reduction of enzymes that normally carry Aβ to be degraded. Longer periods are therefore needed for Aβ to accumulate extracellularly. Environmental, dietary, and pathological factors can generate oxidative stress and alter the correct folding of proteins that degrade Aβ, thus resulting in reduced clearance of Aβ. In both familial and sporadic AD forms, ER dysfunction may also affect or be affected by mitochondrial stress, thus triggering a multitude of signaling pathways that converge to cause neuronal damage.

Mounting evidence indicates that genetic and environmental factors trigger prolonged dysfunction and/or stress in the ER, causing misfolding and aggregation of proteins. Incompletely folded molecules and an abnormal load of aggregated proteins can threaten living cells. The UPR and the UPS enable cells to deal with accumulations of unfolded proteins by mechanisms including transcriptional induction, translational attenuation, and degradation. However, under certain circumstances, the UPR as well as the UPS become partially or fully non-functional, thus contributing to the accumulation of aggregated proteins that characterize conformational diseases. In addition to AD, Parkinson's disease (PD), amyotrophic lateral sclerosis (ALS), Huntington's disease, and prion disease are the most prominent of the conformational disorders. While the extracellular aggregation of Aβ peptide is suggested to be a causal factor in AD, deposition of α-synuclein in intracellular proteinaceous aggregates- Lewy bodies- is the hallmark of PD (see for review [188]). The role of misfolded proteins in PD is further supported by the identification of another protein, parkin. Prion diseases are associated with the incomplete folding and subsequent misfolding and aggregation of the prion protein (PrP) [189].

Whether protein misfolding represents a common etiology for conformational diseases is still a controversial matter. Accumulating evidence has demonstrated the predominant neurotoxic role of prefibrillar intermediate forms (soluble oligomers and protofibrils) in these diseases. Large fibrillar protein aggregates may rather be non-toxic, representing a defensive mechanism to sequester or inactivate oligomers and protofibrils, or merely be a consequence of conformational diseases.

ACKNOWLEDGEMENTS

The author gratefully acknowledges grants from the National Center for Research Resources (5P20RR017699, Centers of Biomedical Research Excellence) and the NIH (NIEHS, R01ES014826).

REFERENCES

1.   Glenner, G. G.; Wong, C. W. *Biochem.Biophys.Res.Commun.* **1984**, *122*, 1131-1135.
2.   Glenner, G. G.; Wong, C. W. *Biochem.Biophys.Res.Commun.* **1984**, *120*, 885-890.
3.   Busciglio, J.; Gabuzda, D. H.; Matsudaira, P.; Yankner, B. A. *Proc.Natl.Acad.Sci.U.S.A* **1993**, *90*, 2092-2096.
4.   Haass, C.; Selkoe, D. J. *Cell* **1993**, *75*, 1039-1042.
5.   Selkoe, D. J. *J.Alzheimers.Dis.* **2001**, *3*, 75-80.
6.   Kuo, Y. M.; Emmerling, M. R.; Vigo-Pelfrey, C.; Kasunic, T. C.; Kirkpatrick, J. B.; Murdoch, G. H.; Ball, M. J.; Roher, A. E. *J.Biol.Chem.* **1996**, *271*, 4077-4081.
7.   Hardy, J.; Selkoe, D. J. *Science* **2002**, *297*, 353-356.
8.   Scheuner, D.; Eckman, C.; Jensen, M.; Song, X.; Citron, M.; Suzuki, N.; Bird, T. D.; Hardy, J.; Hutton, M.; Kukull, W.; Larson, E.; Levy-Lahad, E.; Viitanen, M.; Peskind, E.; Poorkaj, P.; Schellenberg, G.; Tanzi, R.; Wasco, W.; Lannfelt, L.; Selkoe, D.; Younkin, S. *Nat.Med.* **1996**, *2*, 864-870.
9.   Saura, C. A.; Choi, S. Y.; Beglopoulos, V.; Malkani, S.; Zhang, D.; Shankaranarayana Rao, B. S.; Chattarji, S.; Kelleher, R. J., III; Kandel, E. R.; Duff, K.; Kirkwood, A.; Shen, J. *Neuron* **2004**, *42*, 23-36.
10. Santacruz, K.; Lewis, J.; Spires, T.; Paulson, J.; Kotilinek, L.; Ingelsson, M.; Guimaraes, A.; DeTure, M.; Ramsden, M.; McGowan, E.; Forster, C.; Yue, M.; Orne, J.; Janus, C.; Mariash, A.; Kuskowski, M.; Hyman, B.; Hutton, M.; Ashe, K. H. *Science* **2005**, *309*, 476-481.
11. Strittmatter, W. J.; Saunders, A. M.; Schmechel, D.; Pericak-Vance, M.; Enghild, J.; Salvesen, G. S.; Roses, A. D. *Proc.Natl.Acad.Sci.U.S.A* **1993**, *90*, 1977-1981.
12. Saunders, A. M.; Strittmatter, W. J.; Schmechel, D.; George-Hyslop, P. H.; Pericak-Vance, M. A.; Joo, S. H.; Rosi, B. L.; Gusella, J. F.; Crapper-MacLachlan, D. R.; Alberts, M. J.; . *Neurology* **1993**, *43*, 1467-1472.
13. Lendon, C. L.; Talbot, C. J.; Craddock, N. J.; Han, S. W.; Wragg, M.; Morris, J. C.; Goate, A. M. *Neurosci.Lett.* **1997**, *222*, 187-190.
14. Blacker, D.; Wilcox, M. A.; Laird, N. M.; Rodes, L.; Horvath, S. M.; Go, R. C.; Perry, R.; Watson, B., Jr.; Bassett, S. S.; McInnis, M. G.; Albert, M. S.; Hyman, B. T.; Tanzi, R. E. *Nat.Genet.* **1998**, *19*, 357-360.
15. Okuizumi, K.; Onodera, O.; Namba, Y.; Ikeda, K.; Yamamoto, T.; Seki, K.; Ueki, A.; Nanko, S.; Tanaka, H.; Takahashi, H.; Oyanagi, K.; Mizusawa, H.; Kanazawa, I.; Tsuji, S. *Nat.Genet.* **1995**, *11*, 207-209.
16. Kang, D. E.; Saitoh, T.; Chen, X.; Xia, Y.; Masliah, E.; Hansen, L. A.; Thomas, R. G.; Thal, L. J.; Katzman, R. *Neurology* **1997**, *49*, 56-61.
17. Hollenbach, E.; Ackermann, S.; Hyman, B. T.; Rebeck, G. W. *Neurology* **1998**, *50*, 1905-1907.
18. Chyung, A. S.; Greenberg, B. D.; Cook, D. G.; Doms, R. W.; Lee, V. M. *J.Cell Biol.* **1997**, *138*, 671-680.
19. Haass, C.; Lemere, C. A.; Capell, A.; Citron, M.; Seubert, P.; Schenk, D.; Lannfelt, L.; Selkoe, D. J. *Nat.Med.* **1995**, *1*, 1291-1296.
20. Hartmann, T.; Bieger, S. C.; Bruhl, B.; Tienari, P. J.; Ida, N.; Allsop, D.; Roberts, G. W.; Masters, C. L.; Dotti, C. G.; Unsicker, K.; Beyreuther, K. *Nat.Med.* **1997**, *3*, 1016-1020.
21. Fluhrer, R.; Capell, A.; Westmeyer, G.; Willem, M.; Hartung, B.; Condron, M. M.; Teplow, D. B.; Haass, C.; Walter, J. *J.Neurochem.* **2002**, *81*, 1011-1020.
22. Van, B. C.; Backhovens, H.; Cruts, M.; De, W. G.; Bruyland, M.; Cras, P.; Martin, J. J. *Nat.Genet.* **1992**, *2*, 335-339.
23. Hutton, M.; Hardy, J. *Hum.Mol.Genet.* **1997**, *6*, 1639-1646.
24. De, S. B.; Saftig, P.; Craessaerts, K.; Vanderstichele, H.; Guhde, G.; Annaert, W.; Von, F. K.; Van, L. F. *Nature* **1998**, *391*, 387-390.
25. Vassar, R. *J.Mol.Neurosci.* **2004**, *23*, 105-114.
26. Michalak, M.; Lynch, J.; Groenendyk, J.; Guo, L.; Robert Parker, J. M.; Opas, M. *Biochim.Biophys.Acta* **2002**, *1600*, 32-37.
27. Verkhratsky, A. *Cell Calcium* **2002**, *32*, 393-404.
28. Orrenius, S.; Zhivotovsky, B.; Nicotera, P. *Nat.Rev.Mol.Cell Biol.* **2003**, *4*, 552-565.
29. Khachaturian, Z. S. *Ann.N.Y.Acad.Sci.* **1994**, *747*, 1-11.
30. Smith, I. F.; Green, K. N.; LaFerla, F. M. *Cell Calcium* **2005**, *38*, 427-437.
31. Mattson, M. P.; LaFerla, F. M.; Chan, S. L.; Leissring, M. A.; Shepel, P. N.; Geiger, J. D. *Trends Neurosci.* **2000**, *23*, 222-229.
32. Sherrington, R.; Rogaev, E. I.; Liang, Y.; Rogaeva, E. A.; Levesque, G.; Ikeda, M.; Chi, H.; Lin, C.; Li, G.; Holman, K.; . *Nature* **1995**, *375*, 754-760.
33. Levy-Lahad, E.; Wasco, W.; Poorkaj, P.; Romano, D. M.; Oshima, J.; Pettingell, W. H.; Yu, C. E.; Jondro, P. D.; Schmidt, S. D.; Wang, K.; . *Science* **1995**, *269*, 973-977.

34.   Guo, Q.; Fu, W.; Sopher, B. L.; Miller, M. W.; Ware, C. B.; Martin, G. M.; Mattson, M. P. *Nat.Med.* **1999**, *5*, 101-106.

35.   Chan, S. L.; Mayne, M.; Holden, C. P.; Geiger, J. D.; Mattson, M. P. *J.Biol.Chem.* **2000**, *275*, 18195-18200.

36.   Stutzmann, G. E.; Caccamo, A.; LaFerla, F. M.; Parker, I. *J.Neurosci.* **2004**, *24*, 508-513.

37.   Herms, J.; Schneider, I.; Dewachter, I.; Caluwaerts, N.; Kretzschmar, H.; Van, L. F. *J.Biol.Chem.* **2003**, *278*, 2484-2489.

38.   Smith, I. F.; Hitt, B.; Green, K. N.; Oddo, S.; LaFerla, F. M. *J.Neurochem.* **2005**, *94*, 1711-1718.

39.   Querfurth, H. W.; Jiang, J.; Geiger, J. D.; Selkoe, D. J. *J.Neurochem.* **1997**, *69*, 1580-1591.

40.   Querfurth, H. W.; Haughey, N. J.; Greenway, S. C.; Yacono, P. W.; Golan, D. E.; Geiger, J. D. *Biochem.J.* **1998**, *334 (Pt 1)*, 79-86.

41.   McNulty, T. J.; Taylor, C. W. *Biochem.J.* **1993**, *291 (Pt 3)*, 799-801.

42.   Suga, K.; Saito, A.; Tomiyama, T.; Mori, H.; Akagawa, K. *J.Neurochem.* **2005**, *94*, 425-439.

43.   Suga, K.; Tomiyama, T.; Mori, H.; Akagawa, K. *Biochem.J.* **2004**, *381*, 619-628.

44.   Sai, X.; Kawamura, Y.; Kokame, K.; Yamaguchi, H.; Shiraishi, H.; Suzuki, R.; Suzuki, T.; Kawaichi, M.; Miyata, T.; Kitamura, T.; De, S. B.; Yanagisawa, K.; Komano, H. *J.Biol.Chem.* **2002**, *277*, 12915-12920.

45.   Xu, C.; Bailly-Maitre, B.; Reed, J. C. *J.Clin.Invest* **2005**, *115*, 2656-2664.

46.   Schroder, M.; Kaufman, R. J. *Mutat.Res.* **2005**, *569*, 29-63.

47.   Schroder, M. *Cell Mol.Life Sci.* **2008**, *65*, 862-894.

48.   Lee, A. H.; Iwakoshi, N. N.; Glimcher, L. H. *Mol.Cell Biol.* **2003**, *23*, 7448-7459.

49.   Lee, A. S. *Methods* **2005**, *35*, 373-381.

50.   Cudna, R. E.; Dickson, A. J. *Biotechnol.Bioeng.* **2003**, *81*, 56-65.

51.   Oyadomari, S.; Mori, M. *Cell Death.Differ.* **2004**, *11*, 381-389.

52.   Marciniak, S. J.; Yun, C. Y.; Oyadomari, S.; Novoa, I.; Zhang, Y.; Jungreis, R.; Nagata, K.; Harding, H. P.; Ron, D. *Genes Dev.* **2004**, *18*, 3066-3077.

53.   Kogel, D.; Schomburg, R.; Schurmann, T.; Reimertz, C.; Konig, H. G.; Poppe, M.; Eckert, A.; Muller, W. E.; Prehn, J. H. *J.Neurochem.* **2003**, *87*, 248-256.

54.   Yasuda, Y.; Kudo, T.; Katayama, T.; Imaizumi, K.; Yatera, M.; Okochi, M.; Yamamori, H.; Matsumoto, N.; Kida, T.; Fukumori, A.; Okumura, M.; Tohyama, M.; Takeda, M. *Biochem.Biophys.Res.Commun.* **2002**, *296*, 313-318.

55.   Terro, F.; Czech, C.; Esclaire, F.; Elyaman, W.; Yardin, C.; Baclet, M. C.; Touchet, N.; Tremp, G.; Pradier, L.; Hugon, J. *J.Neurosci.Res.* **2002**, *69*, 530-539.

56.   Milhavet, O.; Martindale, J. L.; Camandola, S.; Chan, S. L.; Gary, D. S.; Cheng, A.; Holbrook, N. J.; Mattson, M. P. *J.Neurochem.* **2002**, *83*, 673-681.

57.   Kudo, T.; Katayama, T.; Imaizumi, K.; Yasuda, Y.; Yatera, M.; Okochi, M.; Tohyama, M.; Takeda, M. *Ann.N.Y.Acad.Sci.* **2002**, *977*, 349-355.

58.   Niwa, M.; Sidrauski, C.; Kaufman, R. J.; Walter, P. *Cell* **1999**, *99*, 691-702.

59.   Hoozemans, J. J.; Veerhuis, R.; Van Haastert, E. S.; Rozemuller, J. M.; Baas, F.; Eikelenboom, P.; Scheper, W. *Acta Neuropathol.(Berl)* **2005**, *110*, 165-172.

60.   Wolozin, B. *Neuron* **2004**, *41*, 7-10.

61.   Wolozin, B.; Brown, J., III; Theisler, C.; Silberman, S. *CNS.Drug Rev.* **2004**, *10*, 127-146.

62.   Sparks, D. L.; Scheff, S. W.; Hunsaker, J. C., III; Liu, H.; Landers, T.; Gross, D. R. *Exp.Neurol.* **1994**, *126*, 88-94.

63.   Sparks, D. L.; Schreurs, B. G. *Proc.Natl.Acad.Sci.U.S.A* **2003**, *100*, 11065-11069.

64.   Sparks, D. L.; Kuo, Y. M.; Roher, A.; Martin, T.; Lukas, R. J. *Ann.N.Y.Acad.Sci.* **2000**, *903*, 335-344.

65.   Refolo, L. M.; Malester, B.; LaFrancois, J.; Bryant-Thomas, T.; Wang, R.; Tint, G. S.; Sambamurti, K.; Duff, K.; Pappolla, M. A. *Neurobiol.Dis.* **2000**, *7*, 321-331.

66.   Shie, F. S.; Jin, L. W.; Cook, D. G.; Leverenz, J. B.; LeBoeuf, R. C. *Neuroreport* **2002**, *13*, 455-459.

67.   Racchi, M.; Baetta, R.; Salvietti, N.; Ianna, P.; Franceschini, G.; Paoletti, R.; Fumagalli, R.; Govoni, S.; Trabucchi, M.; Soma, M. *Biochem.J.* **1997**, *322 (Pt 3)*, 893-898.

68.   Simons, M.; Keller, P.; De Strooper, B.; Beyreuther, K.; Dotti, C. G.; Simons, K. *Proc.Natl.Acad.Sci.U.S.A* **1998**, *95*, 6460-6464.

69.   Frears, E. R.; Stephens, D. J.; Walters, C. E.; Davies, H.; Austen, B. M. *Neuroreport* **1999**, *10*, 1699-1705.

70.   Austen, B. M.; Sidera, C.; Liu, C.; Frears, E. *J.Nutr.Health Aging* **2003**, *7*, 31-36.

71.   Galbete, J. L.; Martin, T. R.; Peressini, E.; Modena, P.; Bianchi, R.; Forloni, G. *Biochem.J.* **2000**, *348 Pt 2*, 307-313.

72.   Lange, Y.; Ye, J.; Rigney, M.; Steck, T. L. *J.Lipid Res.* **1999**, *40*, 2264-2270.

73.   Jurevics, H.; Morell, P. *J.Neurochem.* **1995**, *64*, 895-901.

74.   Saher, G.; Brugger, B.; Lappe-Siefke, C.; Mobius, W.; Tozawa, R.; Wehr, M. C.; Wieland, F.; Ishibashi, S.; Nave, K. A. *Nat.Neurosci.* **2005**, *8*, 468-475.

75.   Bjorkhem, I.; Meaney, S. *Arterioscler.Thromb.Vasc.Biol.* **2004**, *24*, 806-815.

76.   Bretscher, M. S.; Munro, S. *Science* **1993**, *261*, 1280-1281.

77.   Feng, B.; Yao, P. M.; Li, Y.; Devlin, C. M.; Zhang, D.; Harding, H. P.; Sweeney, M.; Rong, J. X.; Kuriakose, G.; Fisher, E. A.; Marks, A. R.; Ron, D.; Tabas, I. *Nat.Cell Biol.* **2003**, *5*, 781-792.

78.   Hutter-Paier, B.; Huttunen, H. J.; Puglielli, L.; Eckman, C. B.; Kim, D. Y.; Hofmeister, A.; Moir, R. D.; Domnitz, S. B.; Frosch, M. P.; Windisch, M.; Kovacs, D. M. *Neuron* **2004**, *44*, 227-238.

79.   Benjannet, S.; Elagoz, A.; Wickham, L.; Mamarbachi, M.; Munzer, J. S.; Basak, A.; Lazure, C.; Cromlish, J. A.; Sisodia, S.; Checler, F.; Chretien, M.; Seidah, N. G. *J.Biol.Chem.* **2001**, *276*, 10879-10887.

80.   Cordy, J. M.; Hussain, I.; Dingwall, C.; Hooper, N. M.; Turner, A. J. *Proc.Natl.Acad.Sci.U.S.A* **2003**, *100*, 11735-11740.

81.   Ghribi, O. *Curr.Mol.Med.* **2006**, *6*, 119-133.

82.   Zhang, Q.; Powers, E. T.; Nieva, J.; Huff, M. E.; Dendle, M. A.; Bieschke, J.; Glabe, C. G.; Eschenmoser, A.; Wentworth, P., Jr.; Lerner, R. A.; Kelly, J. W. *Proc.Natl.Acad.Sci.U.S.A* **2004**, *101*, 4752-4757.

83.   Sayre, L. M.; Zelasko, D. A.; Harris, P. L.; Perry, G.; Salomon, R. G.; Smith, M. A. *J.Neurochem.* **1997**, *68*, 2092-2097.

84.   Takeda, A.; Smith, M. A.; Avila, J.; Nunomura, A.; Siedlak, S. L.; Zhu, X.; Perry, G.; Sayre, L. M. *J.Neurochem.* **2000**, *75*, 1234-1241.

85.   Pocernich, C. B.; Butterfield, D. A. *Neurotox.Res.* **2003**, *5*, 515-520.

86.   Gomez-Ramos, A.; az-Nido, J.; Smith, M. A.; Perry, G.; Avila, J. *J.Neurosci.Res.* **2003**, *71*, 863-870.

87.   Woltjer, R. L.; Maezawa, I.; Ou, J. J.; Montine, K. S.; Montine, T. J. *J.Alzheimers.Dis.* **2003**, *5*, 467-476.
88.   Johnstone, E. M.; Chaney, M. O.; Norris, F. H.; Pascual, R.; Little, S. P. *Brain Res.Mol.Brain Res.* **1991**, *10*, 299-305.
89.   Graur, D.; Duret, L.; Gouy, M. *Nature* **1996**, *379*, 333-335.
90.   Lee, H. G.; Castellani, R. J.; Zhu, X.; Perry, G.; Smith, M. A. *Int.J.Exp.Pathol.* **2005**, *86*, 133-138.
91.   Li, F.; Calingasan, N. Y.; Yu, F.; Mauck, W. M.; Toidze, M.; Almeida, C. G.; Takahashi, R. H.; Carlson, G. A.; Flint, B. M.; Lin, M. T.; Gouras, G. K. *J.Neurochem.* **2004**, *89*, 1308-1312.
92.   Paschen, W.; Mengesdorf, T.; Althausen, S.; Hotop, S. *J.Neurochem.* **2001**, *76*, 1916-1924.
93.   Gibson, G. E.; Huang, H. M. *J.Bioenerg.Biomembr.* **2004**, *36*, 335-340.
94.   Huang, H. M.; Chen, H. L.; Xu, H.; Gibson, G. E. *Free Radic.Biol.Med.* **2005**, *39*, 979-989.
95.   Loeffler, D. A.; Connor, J. R.; Juneau, P. L.; Snyder, B. S.; Kanaley, L.; DeMaggio, A. J.; Nguyen, H.; Brickman, C. M.; LeWitt, P. A. *J.Neurochem.* **1995**, *65*, 710-724.
96.   Grundke-Iqbal, I.; Fleming, J.; Tung, Y. C.; Lassmann, H.; Iqbal, K.; Joshi, J. G. *Acta Neuropathol.(Berl)* **1990**, *81*, 105-110.
97.   Smith, M. A.; Harris, P. L.; Sayre, L. M.; Perry, G. *Proc.Natl.Acad.Sci.U.S.A* **1997**, *94*, 9866-9868.
98.   Bush, A. I.; Pettingell, W. H.; Multhaup, G.; Paradis, M.; Vonsattel, J. P.; Gusella, J. F.; Beyreuther, K.; Masters, C. L.; Tanzi, R. E. *Science* **1994**, *265*, 1464-1467.
99.   Rottkamp, C. A.; Raina, A. K.; Zhu, X.; Gaier, E.; Bush, A. I.; Atwood, C. S.; Chevion, M.; Perry, G.; Smith, M. A. *Free Radic.Biol.Med.* **2001**, *30*, 447-450.
100. Ong, W. Y.; Tan, B.; Pan, N.; Jenner, A.; Whiteman, M.; Ong, C. N.; Watt, F.; Halliwell, B. *Mech.Ageing Dev.* **2004**, *125*, 305-313.
101. Ghribi, O.; Herman, M. M.; DeWitt, D. A.; Forbes, M. S.; Savory, J. *Brain Res.Mol.Brain Res.* **2001**, *96*, 30-38.
102. Ghribi, O.; DeWitt, D. A.; Forbes, M. S.; Herman, M. M.; Savory, J. *Brain Res.* **2001**, *903*, 66-73.
103. Pratico, D.; Uryu, K.; Sung, S.; Tang, S.; Trojanowski, J. Q.; Lee, V. M. *FASEB J.* **2002**, *16*, 1138-1140.
104. Rodella, L. F.; Ricci, F.; Borsani, E.; Stacchiotti, A.; Foglio, E.; Favero, G.; Rezzani, R.; Mariani, C.; Bianchi, R. *Histol.Histopathol.* **2008**, *23*, 433-439.
105. Mainous, A. G., III; Eschenbach, S. L.; Wells, B. J.; Everett, C. J.; Gill, J. M. *Fam.Med.* **2005**, *37*, 36-42.
106. Craft, S. *Curr.Alzheimer Res.* **2007**, *4*, 147-152.
107. Frolich, L.; Blum-Degen, D.; Bernstein, H. G.; Engelsberger, S.; Humrich, J.; Laufer, S.; Muschner, D.; Thalheimer, A.; Turk, A.; Hoyer, S.; Zochling, R.; Boissl, K. W.; Jellinger, K.; Riederer, P. *J.Neural Transm.* **1998**, *105*, 423-438.
108. Hoyer, S. *Eur.J.Pharmacol.* **2004**, *490*, 115-125.
109. Gasparini, L.; Gouras, G. K.; Wang, R.; Gross, R. S.; Beal, M. F.; Greengard, P.; Xu, H. *J.Neurosci.* **2001**, *21*, 2561-2570.
110. Ron, D. *J.Clin.Invest* **2002**, *110*, 1383-1388.
111. Kaufman, R. J. *J.Clin.Invest* **2002**, *110*, 1389-1398.
112. Schechter, R.; Beju, D.; Miller, K. E. *Biochem.Biophys.Res.Commun.* **2005**, *334*, 979-986.
113. Misra, U. K.; Pizzo, S. V. *J.Leukoc.Biol.* **2005**, *78*, 187-194.
114. Kruglikov, I.; Gryshchenko, O.; Shutov, L.; Kostyuk, E.; Kostyuk, P.; Voitenko, N. *Pflugers Arch.* **2004**, *448*, 395-401.

115. Ozcan, U.; Cao, Q.; Yilmaz, E.; Lee, A. H.; Iwakoshi, N. N.; Ozdelen, E.; Tuncman, G.; Gorgun, C.; Glimcher, L. H.; Hotamisligil, G. S. *Science* **2004**, *306*, 457-461.
116. Srinivasan, S.; Ohsugi, M.; Liu, Z.; Fatrai, S.; Bernal-Mizrachi, E.; Permutt, M. A. *Diabetes* **2005**, *54*, 968-975.
117. Johnson, R. J.; Xiao, G.; Shanmugaratnam, J.; Fine, R. E. *Neurobiol.Aging* **2001**, *22*, 387-395.
118. Taguchi, J.; Fujii, A.; Fujino, Y.; Tsujioka, Y.; Takahashi, M.; Tsuboi, Y.; Wada, I.; Yamada, T. *Acta Neuropathol.(Berl)* **2000**, *100*, 153-160.
119. Greenfield, J. P.; Tsai, J.; Gouras, G. K.; Hai, B.; Thinakaran, G.; Checler, F.; Sisodia, S. S.; Greengard, P.; Xu, H. *Proc.Natl.Acad.Sci.U.S.A* **1999**, *96*, 742-747.
120. Erickson, R. R.; Dunning, L. M.; Olson, D. A.; Cohen, S. J.; Davis, A. T.; Wood, W. G.; Kratzke, R. A.; Holtzman, J. L. *Biochem.Biophys.Res.Commun.* **2005**, *332*, 50-57.
121. Hamos, J. E.; Oblas, B.; Pulaski-Salo, D.; Welch, W. J.; Bole, D. G.; Drachman, D. A. *Neurology* **1991**, *41*, 345-350.
122. Anthony, S. G.; Schipper, H. M.; Tavares, R.; Hovanesian, V.; Cortez, S. C.; Stopa, E. G.; Johanson, C. E. *J.Alzheimers.Dis.* **2003**, *5*, 171-177.
123. Guo, Z. H.; Mattson, M. P. *Exp.Neurol.* **2000**, *166*, 173-179.
124. Yang, M.; Omura, S.; Bonifacino, J. S.; Weissman, A. M. *J.Exp.Med.* **1998**, *187*, 835-846.
125. Kakimura, J.; Kitamura, Y.; Taniguchi, T.; Shimohama, S.; Gebicke-Haerter, P. J. *Biochem.Biophys.Res.Commun.* **2001**, *281*, 6-10.
126. Hoshino, T.; Nakaya, T.; Araki, W.; Suzuki, K.; Suzuki, T.; Mizushima, T. *Biochem.J* **2007**, *402*, 581-589.
127. Yoo, B. C.; Kim, S. H.; Cairns, N.; Fountoulakis, M.; Lubec, G. *Biochem.Biophys.Res.Commun.* **2001**, *280*, 249-258.
128. McCullough, K. D.; Martindale, J. L.; Klotz, L. O.; Aw, T. Y.; Holbrook, N. J. *Mol.Cell Biol.* **2001**, *21*, 1249-1259.
129. Tamagno, E.; Bardini, P.; Obbili, A.; Vitali, A.; Borghi, R.; Zaccheo, D.; Pronzato, M. A.; Danni, O.; Smith, M. A.; Perry, G.; Tabaton, M. *Neurobiol.Dis.* **2002**, *10*, 279-288.
130. Tamagno, E.; Guglielmotto, M.; Bardini, P.; Santoro, G.; Davit, A.; Di Simone, D.; Danni, O.; Tabaton, M. *Neurobiol.Dis.* **2003**, *14*, 291-301.
131. Kopito, R. R.; Sitia, R. *EMBO Rep.* **2000**, *1*, 225-231.
132. Hung, C. C.; Davison, E. J.; Robinson, P. A.; Ardley, H. C. *Biochem.Soc.Trans.* **2006**, *34*, 743-745.
133. Shcherbik, N.; Haines, D. S. *J.Cell Biochem.* **2004**, *93*, 11-19.
134. Kopito, R. R. *Cell* **1997**, *88*, 427-430.
135. Hochstrasser, M. *Curr.Opin.Cell Biol.* **1995**, *7*, 215-223.
136. Ardley, H. C.; Hung, C. C.; Robinson, P. A. *FEBS Lett.* **2005**, *579*, 571-576.
137. Bulteau, A. L.; Lundberg, K. C.; Humphries, K. M.; Sadek, H. A.; Szweda, P. A.; Friguet, B.; Szweda, L. I. *J.Biol.Chem.* **2001**, *276*, 30057-30063.
138. Imai, Y.; Soda, M.; Hatakeyama, S.; Akagi, T.; Hashikawa, T.; Nakayama, K. I.; Takahashi, R. *Mol.Cell* **2002**, *10*, 55-67.
139. Maraganore, D. M.; Lesnick, T. G.; Elbaz, A.; Chartier-Harlin, M. C.; Gasser, T.; Kruger, R.; Hattori, N.; Mellick, G. D.; Quattrone, A.; Satoh, J.; Toda, T.; Wang, J.; Ioannidis, J. P.; de Andrade, M.; Rocca, W. A.; Toda, T. *Ann.Neurol.* **2004**, *55*, 512-521.

140. Keck, S.; Nitsch, R.; Grune, T.; Ullrich, O. *J.Neurochem.* **2003**, *85*, 115-122.
141. Keller, J. N.; Hanni, K. B.; Markesbery, W. R. *J.Neurochem.* **2000**, *75*, 436-439.
142. Lopez, S. M.; Morelli, L.; Castano, E. M.; Soto, E. F.; Pasquini, J. M. *J.Neurosci.Res.* **2000**, *62*, 302-310.
143. Gao, X.; Hu, H. *Acta Biochim.Biophys.Sin.(Shanghai)* **2008**, *40*, 612-618.
144. Qing, H.; Zhou, W.; Christensen, M. A.; Sun, X.; Tong, Y.; Song, W. *FASEB J.* **2004**, *18*, 1571-1573.
145. Schmitz, A.; Schneider, A.; Kummer, M. P.; Herzog, V. *Traffic.* **2004**, *5*, 89-101.
146. Hammad, S. M.; Ranganathan, S.; Loukinova, E.; Twal, W. O.; Argraves, W. S. *J.Biol.Chem.* **1997**, *272*, 18644-18649.
147. Zerbinatti, C. V.; Bu, G. *Rev.Neurosci.* **2005**, *16*, 123-135.
148. Von Arnim, C. A.; Kinoshita, A.; Peltan, I. D.; Tangredi, M. M.; Herl, L.; Lee, B. M.; Spoelgen, R.; Hshieh, T. T.; Ranganathan, S.; Battey, F. D.; Liu, C. X.; Bacskai, B. J.; Sever, S.; Irizarry, M. C.; Strickland, D. K.; Hyman, B. T. *J.Biol.Chem.* **2005**, *280*, 17777-17785.
149. Misra, U. K.; Gonzalez-Gronow, M.; Gawdi, G.; Wang, F.; Pizzo, S. V. *Cell Signal.* **2004**, *16*, 929-938.
150. Misra, U. K.; Gonzalez-Gronow, M.; Gawdi, G.; Hart, J. P.; Johnson, C. E.; Pizzo, S. V. *J.Biol.Chem.* **2002**, *277*, 42082-42087.
151. Orlando, R. A. *Exp.Cell Res.* **2004**, *294*, 244-253.
152. Willnow, T. E.; Rohlmann, A.; Horton, J.; Otani, H.; Braun, J. R.; Hammer, R. E.; Herz, J. *EMBO J.* **1996**, *15*, 2632-2639.
153. Gervais, F. G.; Xu, D.; Robertson, G. S.; Vaillancourt, J. P.; Zhu, Y.; Huang, J.; LeBlanc, A.; Smith, D.; Rigby, M.; Shearman, M. S.; Clarke, E. E.; Zheng, H.; Van Der Ploeg, L. H.; Ruffolo, S. C.; Thornberry, N. A.; Xanthoudakis, S.; Zamboni, R. J.; Roy, S.; Nicholson, D. W. *Cell* **1999**, *97*, 395-406.
154. LeBlanc, A.; Liu, H.; Goodyer, C.; Bergeron, C.; Hammond, J. *J.Biol.Chem.* **1999**, *274*, 23426-23436.
155. Hacki, J.; Egger, L.; Monney, L.; Conus, S.; Rosse, T.; Fellay, I.; Borner, C. *Oncogene* **2000**, *19*, 2286-2295.
156. Wang, S.; El Deiry, W. S. *Cancer Biol.Ther.* **2004**, *3*, 44-46.
157. Boehning, D.; Patterson, R. L.; Sedaghat, L.; Glebova, N. O.; Kurosaki, T.; Snyder, S. H. *Nat.Cell Biol.* **2003**, *5*, 1051-1061.
158. Barnes, N. Y.; Li, L.; Yoshikawa, K.; Schwartz, L. M.; Oppenheim, R. W.; Milligan, C. E. *J.Neurosci.* **1998**, *18*, 5869-5880.
159. Soriano, S.; Lu, D. C.; Chandra, S.; Pietrzik, C. U.; Koo, E. H. *J.Biol.Chem.* **2001**, *276*, 29045-29050.
160. Tesco, G.; Koh, Y. H.; Tanzi, R. E. *J.Biol.Chem.* **2003**, *278*, 46074-46080.
161. Pellegrini, L.; Passer, B. J.; Tabaton, M.; Ganjei, J. K.; D'Adamio, L. *J.Biol.Chem.* **1999**, *274*, 21011-21016.
162. Weidemann, A.; Paliga, K.; Durrwang, U.; Reinhard, F. B.; Schuckert, O.; Evin, G.; Masters, C. L. *J.Biol.Chem.* **1999**, *274*, 5823-5829.
163. Lu, D. C.; Rabizadeh, S.; Chandra, S.; Shayya, R. F.; Ellerby, L. M.; Ye, X.; Salvesen, G. S.; Koo, E. H.; Bredesen, D. E. *Nat.Med.* **2000**, *6*, 397-404.
164. Nakagawa, T.; Zhu, H.; Morishima, N.; Li, E.; Xu, J.; Yankner, B. A.; Yuan, J. *Nature* **2000**, *403*, 98-103.

165. Fischer, H.; Koenig, U.; Eckhart, L.; Tschachler, E. *Biochem.Biophys.Res.Commun.* **2002**, *293*, 722-726.
166. Ghribi, O.; Prammonjago, P.; Herman, M. M.; Spaulding, N. K.; Savory, J. *Brain Res.Mol.Brain Res.* **2003**, *119*, 201-206.
167. Ghribi, O.; Herman, M. M.; Savory, J. *J.Neurosci.Res.* **2003**, *71*, 853-862.
168. Ghribi, O.; Herman, M. M.; Pramoonjago, P.; Spaulding, N. K.; Savory, J. *Neurobiol.Dis.* **2004**, *16*, 417-427.
169. Mark, R. J.; Hensley, K.; Butterfield, D. A.; Mattson, M. P. *J.Neurosci.* **1995**, *15*, 6239-6249.
170. Mattson, M. P.; Cheng, B.; Davis, D.; Bryant, K.; Lieberburg, I.; Rydel, R. E. *J.Neurosci.* **1992**, *12*, 376-389.
171. Ferreiro, E.; Oliveira, C. R.; Pereira, C. *J.Neurosci.Res.* **2004**, *76*, 872-880.
172. Suen, K. C.; Lin, K. F.; Elyaman, W.; So, K. F.; Chang, R. C.; Hugon, J. *J.Neurochem.* **2003**, *87*, 1413-1426.
173. McLaurin, J.; Chakrabartty, A. *J.Biol.Chem.* **1996**, *271*, 26482-26489.
174. Kayed, R.; Sokolov, Y.; Edmonds, B.; McIntire, T. M.; Milton, S. C.; Hall, J. E.; Glabe, C. G. *J.Biol.Chem.* **2004**, *279*, 46363-46366.
175. Kremer, J. J.; Sklansky, D. J.; Murphy, R. M. *Biochemistry* **2001**, *40*, 8563-8571.
176. Quist, A.; Doudevski, I.; Lin, H.; Azimova, R.; Ng, D.; Frangione, B.; Kagan, B.; Ghiso, J.; Lal, R. *Proc.Natl.Acad.Sci.U.S.A* **2005**, *102*, 10427-10432.
177. Alarcon, J. M.; Brito, J. A.; Hermosilla, T.; Atwater, I.; Mears, D.; Rojas, E. *Peptides* **2005**.
178. Arispe, N.; Pollard, H. B.; Rojas, E. *Ann.N.Y.Acad.Sci.* **1994**, *747*, 256-266.
179. Arispe, N.; Pollard, H. B.; Rojas, E. *Mol.Cell Biochem.* **1994**, *140*, 119-125.
180. Pollard, H. B.; Arispe, N.; Rojas, E. *Cell Mol.Neurobiol.* **1995**, *15*, 513-526.
181. Durell, S. R.; Guy, H. R.; Arispe, N.; Rojas, E.; Pollard, H. B. *Biophys.J.* **1994**, *67*, 2137-2145.
182. Resende, R.; Ferreiro, E.; Pereira, C.; Resende de, O. C. *Neuroscience* **2008**, *155*, 725-737.
183. Schapansky, J.; Olson, K.; Van Der, P. R.; Glazner, G. *Exp.Neurol.* **2007**, *208*, 169-176.
184. Song, S.; Kim, S. Y.; Hong, Y. M.; Jo, D. G.; Lee, J. Y.; Shim, S. M.; Chung, C. W.; Seo, S. J.; Yoo, Y. J.; Koh, J. Y.; Lee, M. C.; Yates, A. J.; Ichijo, H.; Jung, Y. K. *Mol.Cell* **2003**, *12*, 553-563.
185. Lam, Y. A.; Pickart, C. M.; Alban, A.; Landon, M.; Jamieson, C.; Ramage, R.; Mayer, R. J.; Layfield, R. *Proc.Natl.Acad.Sci.U.S.A* **2000**, *97*, 9902-9906.
186. de Pril, R.; Fischer, D. F.; Maat-Schieman, M. L.; Hobo, B.; de Vos, R. A.; Brunt, E. R.; Hol, E. M.; Roos, R. A.; van Leeuwen, F. W. *Hum.Mol.Genet.* **2004**, *13*, 1803-1813.
187. Fischer, D. F.; de Vos, R. A.; Van Dijk, R.; De Vrij, F. M.; Proper, E. A.; Sonnemans, M. A.; Verhage, M. C.; Sluijs, J. A.; Hobo, B.; Zouambia, M.; Steur, E. N.; Kamphorst, W.; Hol, E. M.; van Leeuwen, F. W. *FASEB J.* **2003**, *17*, 2014-2024.
188. Agorogiannis, E. I.; Agorogiannis, G. I.; Papadimitriou, A.; Hadjigeorgiou, G. M. *Neuropathol.Appl.Neurobiol.* **2004**, *30*, 215-224.
189. Demarco, M. L.; Daggett, V. *C.R.Biol.* **2005**, *328*, 847-862.

CHAPTER 10

Endoplasmic Reticulum Stress Response in Prion Diseases

Abhisek Mukherjee and Claudio Soto*

Protein Misfolding Disorders Laboratory, George and Cynthia Mitchell Center for Neurodegenerative Diseases, Dept of Neurology, University of Texas Medical School at Houston

To whom correspondence should be addressed at claudio.soto@uth.tmc.edu

Abstract: Prion diseases are infectious neurodegenerative diseases associated with the brain accumulation of the misfolded prion protein. Despite substantial knowledge of the mechanism of infection and disease transmission, little is known about the molecular pathways involved in neurodegeneration. Recent findings implicate endoplasmic reticulum (ER) stress as a key event in brain dysfunction. The available evidence indicates that accumulation of misfolded prion protein induces ER stress, followed by the activation of the unfolded protein response. Chronic stress produced by the sustained formation of misfolded proteins lead to neuronal apoptosis and synaptic alterations. In this article we discuss the role of ER stress in prion neurodegeneration and the signaling pathways implicated.

INTRODUCTION

Prion diseases or transmissible spongiform encephalopathies (TSEs) are lethal, infectious disorders affecting the mammalian nervous system. The family of TSEs includes scrapie in sheep, bovine spongiform encephalopathy (BSE) or ''mad cow disease'' in cattle, and several human neuropathies: Creutzfeld–Jacob disease (CJD), fatal familial insomnia (FFI), Gertsmann–Straussler–Scheinker (GSS) syndrome, and kuru. Although TSEs are relatively rare in human, the recent appearance of a new form of CJD, termed variant CJD (vCJD), and the experimental evidence that this phenotype is linked to the BSE agent [1] has raised concerns about a possible outbreak of a large epidemic in the human population. While around 10-15% of all the human cases, including all GSS and FFI, have been reported to be inherited in an autosomic dominant manner, most of the cases (85%) [2] are sporadic where the cause that triggers the disease remains to be explained. The intriguing feature that distinguishes TSEs from other neurodegenerative diseases associated to protein misfolding is the infectious nature of the disease. Surgical supplies, cornea transplant or human growth hormone from affected individuals have been described to transmit the disease to normal people [3]. Recent report of transmission of vCJD by blood transfusion [4] set up a red alert through out European blood banks.

The hallmark neuropathological features of TSEs are the spongiform degeneration of the brain,

extensive synaptic dysfunction, neuronal loss, astrogliosis, and cerebral accumulation of PrP^{Sc} aggregates. The relationship between different brain abnormalities in TSE is not clear. A number of studies indicate that a major portion of cell death is caused by apoptosis in TSE [5, 6], but it is likely that neuronal death is a late event in the pathogenesis. The conversion of the cellular form of prion protein (PrP^{C}) into an abnormally folded form (PrP^{Sc}) and accumulation of PrP^{Sc} in the nervous system has been shown to be the central event in TSE pathogenesis.

PRION PROTEIN

The Rogue Infectious Agent in TSEs

Prion protein is a type 1 membrane protein expressed in wide variety of tissues, but expression in brain is much higher. In mammals, the sequence of PrP is highly conserved. Human prion precursor protein consists of 253 amino acids. Irrespective of the species, it has an N-terminal signal sequence that directs it towards the endoplasmic reticulum (ER) and a C-terminal signal domain that determine its association to lipid rafts through glycophosphatidyl inositol (GPI) anchoring [7, 8]. PrP is glycosylated in two sites during ER-Golgi trafficking. The protein is found as a mixture of mono-, di- and un-glycosyalted forms. The fact that PrP^{C} glycosylation is conserved in mammals suggests an important role of the sugar moieties [7]. Prion protein also has a disulfide bridge which is very important for its structure. PrP is mostly attached to the exterior leaflet of the cell membrane [7, 9], but it can also retro-translocate from ER to cytoplasm resulting in cytosolic PrP (CyPrP) [10]. The mature human prion protein consists of 209 amino acids. The length varies slightly in different species.

Although several putative activities have been described for PrP^C, its physiological function is still poorly understood [11, 12]. Proposed functions include copper binding and protection against oxidative stress, a role in calcium metabolism, and binding to a variety of proteins and nucleic acids. Evidence also suggests that PrP can be neuroprotective and participate in signal transduction pathways [13, 14]. However, the fact that PrP null and conditional knockout animals do not show any gross phenotype suggests that all these proposed functions are not critical for viability [11, 15]. Therefore, the gain of toxic function, by the conversion of cellular prion protein in to a partially protease-resistant, detergent insoluble form (PrP^{Sc}) became the widely accepted theory to explain the pathogenesis in TSEs.

As the name suggests, TSEs are transmissible and the infectious agent belongs to a new class of unprecedented agents whose nature of pathogenesis is not yet fully known. Compelling evidences suggest that PrP^{Sc} is the sole component of the infectious agent [16]. It is proposed that prions replicates by interaction of the incoming

PrP^{Sc} with the host PrP^C leading to the transformation of the normal protein into the pathogenic form. Although, there is no change in primary structure, this conversion involves a conformational change where α-helical content decreases and β-sheet content increases [16]. The mechanism of interaction between PrP^C and PrP^{Sc} is unclear but two steps have been identified in cell free conversion systems: binding of the cellular form to the abnormally folded protein followed by misfolding, oligomerization and acquisition of partial protease resistance [17]. Irrespective of how the misfolding occurs, it plays a paramount role in mediating neurodegeneration and transmitting infectivity. However, despite massive investigation, little is known about cellular factors modulating the conversion and how the generation of PrP^{Sc} leads to brain damage.

ER STRESS IN PRION DISEASE

ER is an important organelle for the synthesis, folding, and transport of nascent proteins. Almost all secreted and membrane proteins, which are around 1/3 of the total cellular proteins, including PrP^C, attain their folded conformation in the ER. The correct folding of a protein inside the ER involves proper post-translational modification such as glycosylation and disulfide bond formation. Conditions such as a reducing environment, viral infection, glucose starvation, inhibition of glycosylation, perturbation of Ca^{2+}

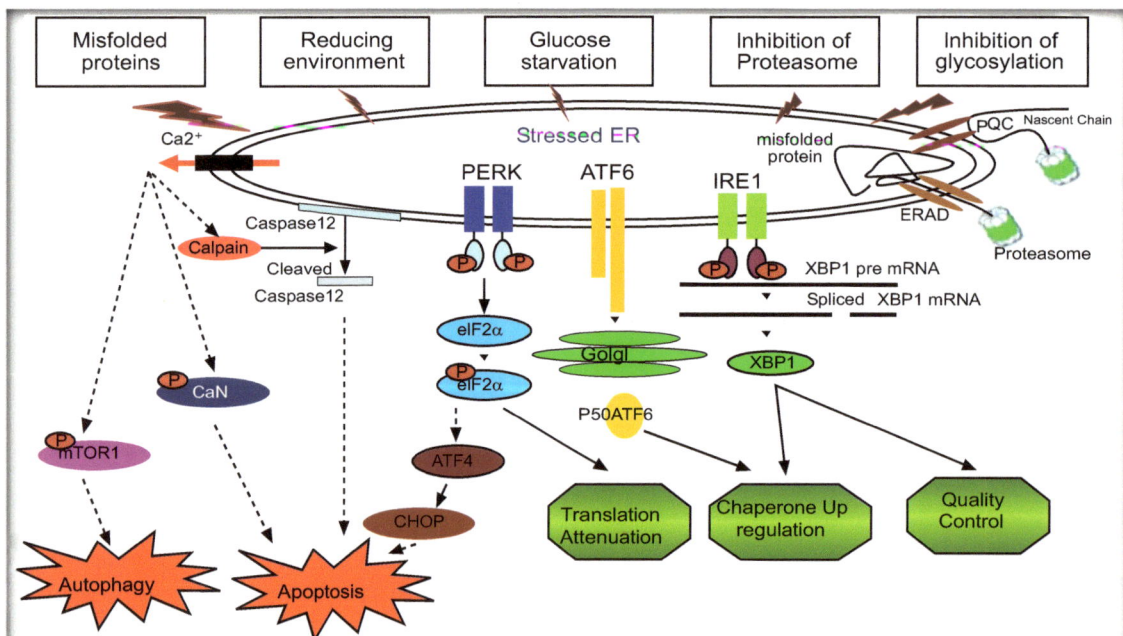

Fig. (1). Mechanism of activation of ER stress response pathways. Dotted line implies signaling events not shown in the diagram.

homeostasis, inhibition of proteosome disturbs the integrity of the ER, which finally results in a burden of misfolded proteins [18, 19]. Accumulation of misfolded proteins is sensed by the ER and it signals the nucleus to induce the genes required to combat against these misfolded proteins. This intracellular signaling event in response to ER stress is called Unfolded Protein Response (UPR) [18, 19]. UPR consist of activation of three different mechanisms Fig. (**1**): (1) translational attenuation to decrease load of misfolded proteins in the ER. (2) Transcriptional activation of different ER resident chaperones, including BiP/(glucose regulated protein) GrP78, Protein Disulfide Isomerase (PDI), GrP94 and GrP58, to combat against misfolding. (3) Activation of ER associated degradation (ERAD) of proteins by directing them back to the cytosol for 26S proteosome mediated clearance. Recent demonstration of activation of a Pre-Emptive Quality Control (pQC) pathway in presence of an acute ER stress provides one more way to direct ER bound proteins into proteosomic degradation in presence of an existing protein overload in the ER lumen [20]. It should be noted that pQC is mechanistically and spatially different from the ERAD pathway. While in ERAD the misfolded protein from ER is retro-translocated into the cytosol, the nascent ER bound protein never becomes able to enter the lumen of ER during activation of pQC.

We and others have previously shown that ER stress plays an important role on TSE pathogenesis [21-25]. The up-regulation of UPR responsive chaperones, such as GrP78/BiP, GrP94 and GrP58, was observed in the cortex of patients affected with variant and sporadic Creutzfeldt-Jacob disease, in mice infected with scrapie prions and in neuroblastoma cells treated with brain-derived PrP^{Sc} [21-23]. Moreover, the overexpression of the disulfide isomerase GrP58 was shown to be an early event in prion pathogenesis, closely following PrP^{Sc} formation [22]. The interaction between PrP and this chaperone modulates the neurotoxic activity of PrP^{Sc} [22]. The mechanisms described above combat to alleviate the cellular stress by either correcting the misfolding or clearing the misfolded proteins in a direct of indirect fashion [18, 19]. This comprises the protective part of the ER stress response. However, in presence of long sustained stressing conditions or chronic production of misfolded proteins, the protective mechanisms are not enough to relieve the cells. In these conditions, ER stress lead to a suicidal

response when the cell is no more able to handle the burden of misfolded and unfunctional proteins Fig. (**1**). In the next sections we will describe in more details the mechanism of the defense response and the cell death pathway produced as a consequence of ER stress.

THE ER STRESS DEFENSE PATHWAY

At the molecular level the protective response to ER stress, that is the UPR consist of activation of three different signaling pathways linked to ATF6 (activated transcription factor 6), PERK (double stranded RNA activated protein kinase–like ER kinase) and IRE1α (inositol-requiring transmembrane kinase and endonuclease) [18, 19] Fig. (**1**). Following, we will proceed with short description of each of these molecular effectors and their implication in prion protein misfolding.

ATF6

This is a type II transmembrane protein, which in presence of ER stress translocates from ER to Golgi. In Golgi apparatus ATF6 is transcriptionally activated through cleavage by the site 1 and 2 proteases [26, 27] near the transmembrane region. The activated N-terminal cytosolic region, termed p50ATF6, translocates to the nucleus and binds to the promoters containing an ER-Stress Response Element using its bZIP domain [26-27]. This binding result in transcription activation of ER resident chaperones (such as BiP) and another important transcript, related to ER stress, XBP1 [18, 19]. BiP is one of the most important chaperones present in the lumen of ER and it also plays a major role in UPR activation. This chaperon has been shown to be upregulated during late-stages in the mouse model of prion disease [21, 21, 28]. *In vitro* studies suggesting a direct interaction with PrP [28] indicate a possible role of BiP in correcting prion protein misfolding. However, more studies are required to confirm this hypothesis.

PERK –eIF2α

PERK is a type I transmembrane Ser/Thr protein kinase, which is activated in the presence of accumulated proteins inside the ER by oligomerization and *trans*-autophophorylation [29]. Under physiological conditions, BiP is attached to the luminal domain of PERK, preventing its oligomerization. However, in the presence of a misfolded protein overload, BiP shifts from PERK towards binding the misfolded proteins, allowing the PERK inter-molecular oligomerization. Activated PERK blocks the classical translational initiation pathway by phosphorylating the Ser51 residue of eukaryotic initiation factor α (*eIF2α*) [30]. Thus, activated PERK attenuates protein synthesis in order to decrease the net protein trafficking through the ER. PERK is also implicated in inducing some UPR elements by indirectly activating another transcription factor, ATF4 [31]. ATF4 mRNA is constitutively expressed in many cell lines and translated efficiently under condition of *eIF2α* phosphorylation [31]. The role of PERK signaling in TSEs pathogenesis has not yet been studied.

IRE1

This is also a type I transmembrane Ser/Thr protein kinase and endonuclease, which activates in the same fashion as does PERK. Several group of studies demonstrated that activated IRE1 alternatively splices an UPR element, XBP1 mRNA, and turns into an active transcription factor [32]. Active XBP1 binds to ER-stress Response Elements and UPR elements (UPRE) upregulating the expression of different ER chaperones required to prevent misfolding inside the ER lumen [18, 19]. IRE1 has also been shown to induce the ER resident type II trans-membrane protein EDEM, which is a central executor of ERAD. EDEM specifically binds to misfolded glycosylated proteins and facilitates their degradation [33]. PrP mutants associated to TSEs have been shown to be retained inside the ER [34]. Furthermore, accumulation of PrP in the cytoplasm in presence of a known ER stressor suggests an important role of ERAD pathway in TSE pathology. Being an N-Glycosylated protein PrP may be an important target for EDEM, however this possibility has not been explored yet. Thus, IRE1 plays an important role in the protective response to ER stress. Interestingly, recent work from Hetz *et.al* [35] has shown that inactivation of XPB1 by knocking out the gene does not change the course of TSE pathogenesis. The lack of effect of one of the key components of the ER stress response can be explained in two ways: ER stress associated neurodegeneration is a consequence of prion protein misfolding and does not play a direct role in the disease process. Alternatively, in absence of one of the important components of ER stress signaling, the other two may compensate activating the UPR pathway.

UPR AND CHAPERONES

One of the main components of the ER stress response is the activation of UPR which leads to the induction of ER chaperones such as the glucose regulated family. BiP/GrP78, PDI and GrP94 are the best characterized among the family. Although there is upregulation of these proteins in TSEs, it is not as early and pronounced as GrP58 [21, 22]. GrP58, also known as Erp-60, ER-60, ERp-58, ERp61 and Q2 [36], is a 504 amino acid protein, which shares a considerable sequence homology with protein disulfide isomerase (PDI). This protein has several activities but the most important in this context is its chaperone activity with specificity for N-glycosylated proteins [37]. GrP58 also resembles PDI in its activity of catalyzing disulfide bond formation [36]. This protein is mainly localized in the ER. Interestingly, it is one of the very few chaperones found active in the plasma membrane, especially in the lipid rafts where most of PrP is found [36]. It has been shown that Grp58 can be co-immunoprecipitated with anti-PrP antibodies [22]. Upregulation of GrP58 using pharmacological agents may become an important therapeutic strategy against prion disorders.

DEATH RESPONSE ASSOCIATED TO ER STRESS

Till now we have talked about the defensive response of ER stress with respect to protein misfolding in general, with special focus on prion misfolding. As discussed earlier sustained conditions producing ER stress, which cannot be rescued by the defensive mechanism, have been described to induce a death response. The later has been described in neurodegenerative disorders associated to protein misfolding and aggregation, including Alzheimer's disease (AD), Parkinson's disease (PD) or Huntington's disease (HD) [38]. As in TSEs, these diseases are characterized by the continuous cerebral accumulation of misfolded protein aggregates producing a sustained ER stress [39].

In the case of TSEs, due to the unique ability of PrP[Sc] to auto-catalytically induce misfolding to normally folded monomeric PrP[C], the misfolding and aggregation proceeds in an exponential way. This is expected to create even worst situation with respect to a sustained ER stress environment. The suicidal or death response from ER stress consists of mainly two different mechanisms [40]:

(1) Activation of ER stress mediated apoptosis. (2) Activation of autophagy Fig. (**1**). While ER stress mediated apoptosis is well documented in TSEs [21-22], recent findings also suggest an important role of autophagy in this process [41-43]. Following is a brief overview of suicidal signaling pathways related to ER stress during TSE pathogenesis.

APOPTOTIC SIGNALING

The apoptotic pathway induced by ER stress involves several elements, including CHOP, caspases and perturbation of calcium homeostasis [18, 19].

CHOP is a member of C/EBP family of bZIP transcription factors. CHOP (also known as GADD153), is one of the first molecules reported to be associated with ER stress mediated apoptosis [44]. There is a low-level expression of CHOP in the normal situation, which increase several folds in the presence of sustained ER stress. Over-expression of CHOP has been described to induce cell-cycle arrest and apoptosis. Post-translational modifications, such as phophorylation at residue Ser 78, were reported to increase its transcriptional activity on several genes, including the Bcl-2 family [45]. CHOP-/- mice are resistant to neuronal cell death [46], indicating an important role of CHOP cellular apoptosis. CHOP is one of the important targets of PERK and has been shown to be upregulated both *in vitro* and at the late stage of prion disease in mouse model [23].

Caspases are the central executor of apoptosis [47]. Activation of an initiator caspase triggers apoptosis. Stimulus either from cell surface (through caspase 8) or mitochondria (through caspase 9) can activate the initiator caspases. However, both pathways finally converge into the executor caspases 3 and/or 7 [47], leading to cell death. An analogous pathway has been suggested to exist at the ER, involving murine caspase 12 or human caspase 4 acting as an initiator caspase [47]. These molecules normally reside on the ER membrane. However, upon activation by ER stress it translocates to cytoplasm. Previous studies from our lab have shown upregulation of caspase12 in prion infected mouse brains [21]. Caspase 3 which is downstream of other caspases has also been shown to be activated in prion infected cultured cells [21]. Although caspase12 and 4 are likely to be involved in ER stress

mediated apoptosis, the upstream events leading to their activation are not clear.

Disruption of calcium homeostasis in the cell is probably the most adverse and immediate effect caused by ER stress [18, 19]. When it comes to neuron the effect becomes even more deleterious, because of the significant role of calcium waves in neuronal activity. Ca^{2+} plays an important role as a second messenger in different cellular signaling pathways, where the final outcome is controlled by cellular calcium concentration [48]. For this reason, maintaining a specific concentration of Ca^{2+} in the cytoplasm is critical for normal cellular biology. Cell utilizes different Ca^{2+} channels and ATP driven Ca^{2+} pumps to maintain a gradient of Ca^{2+} to stabilize the calcium homeostasis inside the cytoplasm [48]. ER functions as an intra-cellular Ca^{2+} storage. Ca2+ uptake in ER from cytoplasm is guided by sarcoplasmic/ER Ca2+ ATPase (SERCA) and released via inositol 1,4,5 –triphosphate receptor (IP3R) or Raynodine receptor (RyR) [49]. Several studies have suggested increase of cytoplasmic Ca^{2+} due to ER stress in presence of misfolded proteins [18, 19]. Previous works form our lab and others have shown the release of calcium from the ER to the cytoplasm when cells are exposed to misfolded prion protein [21]. Indeed, Ca^{2+} release appears to be one of the first adverse effects after prion infection in cells. However, it is not entirely clear whether the deleterious flow of Ca^{2+} in the cytoplasm is coming from the extracellular space or due to leakage from the ER through RyR. Recent evidences strongly suggest that at least a major source of elevated Ca2+ in the cytoplasm of prion infected cultured cortical neurons is leakage from the ER (Hetz and Soto, unpublished results). Whatever the cause of Ca^{2+} increase in cytoplasm, this event creates a hue and cry inside the cell by deregulating different down-stream targets. Calcineurin (CaN) a phosphatase of type 2B is one of the important targets of Ca^{2+} [50]. The activity of this enzyme is regulated by the Ca^{2+}-calmoudulin complex. Optimum activity of CaN is required to maintain the proper phosphorylation state of different important targets, like apoptosis inducer BAD or transcription factor CREB [50]. Hyper-activation of CaN due to chronic uprglation of $[Ca^{2+}]$ reduces the phosphorylation of Bad, which then disassociate from the scaffolding protein 14-3-3 and interacts with Bcl-Lx or other Bcl2 family protein located in the mitochondrial membrane [51]. As a result cytochrome C is released in the cytoplasm, leading to caspase activation and finally causing apoptosis. On the other hand dephosphorylated by hyper-activated CaN, CREB is not able to translocate into the nucleus to act as a transcription factor to regulate expression of different genes required for synaptic plasticity [52]. Current work from our lab suggests that blocking CaN activity in terminally sick prion infected mouse, decrease neuronal death and increase survival.

AUTOPHAGY

Massive neuronal loss in TSEs might not be explained by apoptosis only. Evidences suggesting the involvement of autophagy in prion pathology have been recently reported [41-43]. Autophagy is a mechanism by which intracellular materials are recycled [52]. The first step of autophagy is the envelopment of cytosol or organelles in a bilayered autophagosome. Autophagosome matures and fuses with endolysosomal vesicle creating an autolysosome where the cargo is degraded [52]. The initial nucleation and the assembly of the primary autophagosomal membrane require a kinase complex consisting of phosphatidylinositol 3–kinase (PI3K), p150 myristylated kinase and becilin 1 (or Atg6). The next elongation step requires conversion of a microtubule associated protein 1 light chain 3 (LC3-I, also known as Atg8) from free to a lipid conjugated form (LC3-II). LC3-II is used as a marker of autophagy. Although, autophagy is utilized as a pro-survival machinery to supply the cell with nutrient and energy, it can also be directed for non-apoptotic cell death [52]. Accumulating evidences indicate ER stress acts as a potent stimulus to induce autophagy [40]. PERK and IRE1 have been implicated as mediators of ER stress-induced autophagy [54]. Induction of autophagy has also been demonstrated in presence of ER stress caused by cytosolic accumulation of misfolded proteins [55]. As discussed earlier Ca^{2+} release from ER is one of the earliest pathogenic changes reported in *in vitro* and *in vivo* models of TSE. Elevated Ca^{2+} activates Ca^{2+}/calmodulin dependent-kinase kinase ß (CaMKK ß), which in turn activates AMPK that ultimately leads to inhibition of mammalian target of rapamycin complex1 (mTOR1) [56]. Expression and activity of several Atgs has been suggested to be inhibited by mTOR1. Thus, it will be very interesting to study if elevation of cytosolic calcium in prion pathogenesis can induce autophagy by inhibiting mTORC1.

ROLE OF ER STRESS IN PRION MISFOLDING

So far we have discussed mostly about the effect of prion protein misfolding on ER stress response, however recent works also suggested that ER stress itself can modulate prion protein misfolding. A recent study form our lab has shown that treatment with pharmacological agents known to cause ER stress leads to the formation of detergent insoluble PrP aggregates in N2A cells or primary cortical neurons, without changes in the total level of PrP [57]. Interestingly, PrP^C from cells treated in this manner are more prone to conversion into the PrP^{Sc} form, suggesting a direct role of ER stress on the prion protein conformational changes. Several other pieces of evidence also point to the involvement of ER stress response in prion replication. Indeed, treatment of cells with proteosome inhibitors, which in turn produces ER stress, leads to the formation of a protease-resistance PrP^{Sc}-like form that accumulates in the cytosol [58]. In this process, known as ERAD, ER overloaded with misfolded proteins delivers some of its burden to the cytosol for degradation by ubiqutin-proteosome machinery. ERAD is normally a protective response [18]. However, PrP accumulated in the cytosol has been shown to acquire a PrP^{Sc} like conformation and it is partially toxic to neuronal cells [59]. Misfolded PrP has also recently been shown to block the proteosome machinery causing a protein "traffic jam", which is probably one of the potential mechanisms by which cytosolic PrP^{Sc}-like is toxic [60]. Moreover, expression of several mutant PrP molecules associated with human hereditary TSEs resulted in the formation of cytotoxic PrP forms that were retained early in the secretory pathway [34, 61]. Stimulation of retrograde transport towards the ER increases the accumulation of PrP^{Sc} in prion-infected neuroblastoma cells [57]. We also showed that scrapie infection triggers changes on PrP^C glycosylation suggesting that the homeostasis of the ER and Golgi is altered by prion replication [62]. It has been hypothesized that the prion conversion process involves the generation of a folding intermediate, termed PrP*, which likely represents a partially unfolded form of PrP^C with exposed fragments to permit the interaction with PrP^{Sc} [16]. It is possible that ER stress may contribute to the formation of this putative intermediate, which is more prone to be converted into PrP^{Sc}. Imbalances of ER homeostasis are a frequent event in aging [63], which may provide a molecular explanation for the higher incidence of most forms of TSEs in elderly people. In addition, considering extensive data that PrP^{Sc} replication induces ER stress, it is possible to envision that the relationship between PrP^{Sc} and ER stress falls into a vicious cycle, in which the induction of ER stress by prion infection may promote conformational changes in PrP^C rendering the protein more susceptible to be converted into PrP^{Sc}. These cycles may result in an amplification loop leading to an exponential increase in PrP^{Sc} generation, neuronal dysfunction and disease. Therefore, ER-stress seems to play a central and crucial role in the development of prion diseases. In this scenario, compounds protecting ER homeostasis such as chemical chaperons or disrupting the connection between alterations in ER functioning and PrP misfolding may be able to delay prion replication and disease onset. Non-invasive manipulation of ER stress may, therefore, represent a novel therapeutic target against prion diseases.

Acknowledgments: This work was support in part by NIH grant R01 NS05349 to CS.

LIST OF ABBREVIATIONS

AD	=	Alzheimer's Disease
Atg	=	Autophagy related
AMPK	=	5' Adenosine Monophosphate-Activated Protein Kinase
ATF4	=	Activating Transcription Factor4
ATF6	=	Activating Transcription Factor 6
BSE	=	Bovine Spongiform Encephalopathy
CaN	=	Calcineurin
CJD	=	Creutzfeldt - Jakob disease
CREB	=	cAMP Response Element Binding
CyPrP	=	Cytosolic PrP
EDAM	=	ER Degradation-Enhancing α-Mannosidase
eIF2α	=	Eukaryotic Initiation Factor 2 α
ER	=	Endoplasmic Reticulum
ERAD	=	ER Associated Degradation
ERSE	=	ER stress Responsive Element
FFI	=	Fatal Familial Insomnia
GPI	=	Glycosylphosphatidylinositol
GrP	=	Glucose Regulated Protein
GSS	=	Gerstmann Sträussler Syndrome
HD	=	Huntington's Disease
IRE1α	=	Inositol-Requiring
LC	=	Light Chain
mRNA	=	Messenger-Ribonucleic Acid
mTOR1	=	Mammalian Target of Rapamycin Complex 1Enzyme 1α
PDI	=	Protein Disulfide Isomerase
PERK	=	PKR like ER Kinase
PI3K	=	Phosphatidylinositol 3–Kinase
PKR	=	Protein Kinase R
PD	=	Parkinson's Disease
PrP	=	Prion Protein
PrP^C	=	Cellular form of Prion Protein
PrP^{Sc}	=	Abnormally folded form of Prion Protein
pQC	=	Pre-emptive Quality Control
RyR	=	Raynodine Receptor
UPR	=	Unfolded Protein Response
TSEs	=	Transmissible Spongiform Encephalopathies
vCJD	=	Variant Creutzfeldt - Jakob disease
XBP1	=	X-box Binding Protein1

REFERENCES

[1] Bruce ME, Will RG, Ironside JW, McConnell I, Drummond D, Suttie A, McCardle L, Chree A, Hope J, Birkett C, Cousens S, Fraser H, Bostock CJ. Transmissions to mice indicate that 'new variant' CJD is caused by the BSE agent. Nature 1997; 389: 498-501.

[2] Johnson RT. Prion diseases. Lancet Neurol. 2005; 4: 635-642.

[3] Brown, P. Preece M, Brandel JP, Sato T, McShane L, Zerr I, Fletcher A, Will RG, Pocchiari M, Cashman NR, d'Aignaux JH, Cervenáková L, Fradkin J, Schonberger LB, Collins SJ. Iatrogenic Creutzfeldt-Jakob disease at the millennium. Neurology 2000; 55: 1075-1081.

[4] Llewelyn CA, Hewitt PE, Knight RS, Amar K, Cousens S, Mackenzie J, Will RG. Possible transmission of variant Creutzfeldt-Jakob disease by blood transfusion. Lancet. 2004; 363: 417-421.

[5] Jesionek-Kupnicka D, Buczyński J, Kordek R, Liberski PP. Neuronal loss and apoptosis in experimental Creutzfeldt-Jakob disease in mice. Folia Neuropathol. 1999; 37: 283-286.

[6] Jesionek-Kupnicka D, Buczyński J, Kordek R, Sobów T, Kłoszewska I, Papierz W, Liberski PP.

Programmed cell death (apoptosis) in Alzheimer's disease and Creutzfeldt-Jakob disease. Folia Neuropathol. 1997; 35: 233-235.

[7]   Harris DA. Trafficking, turnover and membrane topology of PrP. Br. Med. Bull. 2003; 66: 71-85.

[8]   Abid K, Soto C. The intriguing prion disorders. Cell Mol. Life Sci. 2006; 63: 2342-2351.

[9]   Vey M, Pilkuhn S, Wille H, Nixon R, DeArmond SJ, Smart EJ, Anderson RG, Taraboulos A, Prusiner SB. Subcellular colocalization of the cellular and scrapie prion proteins in caveolae-like membranous domains. Proc Natl Acad Sci USA. 1996; 93: 14945-14949.

[10] Ma J, Lindquist S.. Wild-type PrP and a mutant associated with prion disease are subject to retrograde transport and proteasome degradation. Proc Natl Acad Sci USA. 200; 98: 14955-14960.

[11] Hetz C, Maundrell K, Soto C. Is the loss of function of prion protein the cause of prion disorders? Trends Mol. Med. 2003; 9: 237-243.

[12] Lasmezas CI. Putative functions of PrP(C). British Med. Bull. 2003; 66: 61-70.

[13] Kuwahara C, Takeuchi AM, Nishimura T, Haraguchi K, Kubosaki A, Matsumoto Y, Saeki K, Matsumoto Y, Yokoyama T, Itohara S, Onodera T.. Prions prevent neuronal cell-line death. Nature 1999; 400: 225-226.

[14] Mouillet-Richard S. Ermonval M, Chebassier C,Laplanche JL, Lehmann S, Launay JM, Kellermann O. Signal transduction through prion protein. Science 2000 ; 289: 1925-1928.

[15] Moore RC, Lee IY, Silverman GL, Harrison PM, Strome R, Heinrich C, Karunaratne A, Pasternak SH, Chishti MA, Liang Y, Mastrangelo P, Wang K, Smit AF, Katamine S, Carlson GA, Cohen FE, Prusiner SB, Melton DW, Tremblay P, Hood LE, Westaway D. Ataxia in prion protein (PrP)-deficient mice is associated with upregulation of the novel PrP-like protein doppel. J Mol Biol. 1999; 292: 797-817.

[16] Prusiner SB. Prions. Proc Natl Acad Sci USA 1998; 95: 13363-13383.

[17] Horiuchi M, Priola SA, Chabry J, Caughey B. Interactions between heterologous forms of prion protein: binding, inhibition of conversion, and species barriers. Proc Natl Acad Sci USA. 2000; 97: 5836-5841.

[18] Schröder M, Kaufman RJ. ER stress and the unfolded protein response. Mutat Res. 2005; 569; 29-63.

[19] Lindholm D, Wootz H, Korhonen L. ER stress and neurodegenerative diseases. Cell Death Differ. 2006; 13: 385-392.

[20] Kang SW, Rane NS, Kim SJ, Garrison JL, Taunton J, Hegde RS. Substrate-specific translocational attenuation during ER stress defines a pre-emptive quality control pathway. Cell. 2006; 127: 999-1013.

[21] Hetz C, Russelakis-Carneiro M, Maundrell K, Castilla J, Soto C. Caspase-12 and endoplasmic reticulum stress mediate neurotoxicity of pathological prion protein. EMBO J. 2003; 22: 5435-5445

[22] Hetz C, Russelakis-Carneiro M, Wälchli S, Carboni S, Vial-Knecht E, Maundrell K, Castilla J, Soto C. The disulfide isomerase Grp58 is a protective factor against prion neurotoxicity. J Neurosci. 2005; 25: 2793-2802.

[23] Yoo BC, Krapfenbauer K, Cairns N, Belay G, Bajo M, Lubec G. Overexpressed protein disulfide isomerase in brains of patients with sporadic Creutzfeldt-Jakob disease. Neurosci Lett. 2002; 334: 196-200.

[24] Hetz CA, Soto C. Stressing out the ER: a role of the unfolded protein response in prion-related disorders. Curr Mol Med. 2006; 6: 37-43.

[25] Rane NS, Kang SW, Chakrabarti O, Feigenbaum L, Hegde RS. Reduced translocation of nascent prion protein during ER stress contributes to neurodegeneration. Dev Cell. 2008; 15: 359-370.

[26] Yoshida H, Haze K, Yanagi H, Yura T, Mori K. Identification of the cis-acting endoplasmic reticulum stress response element responsible for transcriptional induction of mammalian glucose-regulated proteins. Involvement of basic leucine zipper transcription factors. J Biol Chem. 1998; 273: 33741–33749.

[27] Yoshida H, Okada T, Haze K, Yanagi H, Yura T, Negishi M, Mori.. ATF6 activated by proteolysis binds in the presence of NF-Y (CBF) directly to the cis-acting element responsible for the mammalian unfolded protein response. Mol Cell Biol. 2000; 20: 6755-6767.

[28] Jin T, Gu Y, Zanusso G, Sy M, Kumar A, Cohen M, Gambetti P, Singh N. The chaperone protein BiP binds to a mutant prion protein and mediates its degradation by the proteasome. J Biol Chem. 2000; 275: 38699-38704.

[29] Bertolotti A, Zhang Y, Hendershot LM, Harding HP, Ron D. Dynamic interaction of BiP and ER stress transducers in the unfolded-protein response. Nat Cell Biol. 2000; 2: 326–332.

[30] Harding HP, Zhang Y, Ron D. Protein translation and folding are coupled by an endoplasmic-reticulum-resident kinase. Nature 1999; 397: 271–274.

[31] Harding HP, Zhang Y, Bertolotti A, Zeng H, Ron D. Perk is essential for translational regulation and cell survival during the unfolded protein response. Mol Cells. 2000; 5: 897–904.

[32] Lee K, Tirasophon W, Shen X, Michalak M, Prywes R, Okada T, Yoshida H, Mori K, Kaufman RJ. IRE1-mediated unconventional mRNA splicing and S2P-mediated ATF6 cleavage merge to regulate XBP1 in signaling the unfolded protein response. Genes Dev. 2002; 16: 452-466.

[33] Yoshida H, Matsui T, Hosokawa N, Kaufman RJ, Nagata K, Mori K. A time-dependent phase shift in the mammalian unfolded protein response. Dev Cell 2003; 4: 265–271.

[34] Drisaldi B, Stewart RS, Adles C, Stewart LR, Quaglio E, Biasini E, Fioriti L, Chiesa R, Harris DA. Mutant PrP is delayed in its exit from the endoplasmic reticulum, but neither wild-type nor mutant PrP undergoes retrotranslocation prior to proteasomal degradation. J Biol Chem. 2003; 278: 21732-21743.

[35] Hetz C, Lee AH, Gonzalez-Romero D, Thielen P, Castilla J, Soto C, Glimcher LH. Unfolded protein response transcription factor XBP-1 does not influence prion replication or pathogenesis. Proc Natl Acad Sci USA. 2008; 105: 757-762.

[36] Turano C, Coppari S, Altieri F, Ferraro A. Proteins of the PDI family: unpredicted non ER locations and functions. J Cell Physiol. 2002; 193: 154-163.

[37] Elliott JG, Oliver JD, High S.. The thiol-dependent reductase ERp57 interacts specifically with N-glycosylated integral membrane proteins. J Biol Chem. 1997; 272: 13849-13855.

[38] Matus S, Lisbona F, Torres M, León C, Thielen P, Hetz C. The stress rheostat: an interplay between the unfolded protein response (UPR) and autophagy in neurodegeneration. Curr Mol Med. 2008: 157-172.

[39] Soto C. Unfolding the role of Protein Misfolding in Neurodegenerative Diseases. Nature Rev Neurosci. 2003; 4: 49-60.

[40]   Heath-Engel HM, Chang NC, Shore GC. The endoplasmic reticulum in apoptosis and autophagy: role of the BCL-2 protein family. Oncogene. 2008; 27: 6419–6433.

[41]   Dron M, Bailly Y, Beringue V, Haeberlé AM, Griffond B, Risold PY, Tovey MG, Laude H, Dandoy-Dron F.. Scrg1 is induced in TSE and brain injuries, and associated with autophagy. Eur J Neurosci. 2005; 22: 133-146.

[42]   Sikorska B, Liberski PP, Giraud P, Kopp N, Brown P. Autophagy is a part of ultrastructural synaptic pathology in Creutzfeldt-Jakob disease: a brain biopsy study. Int J Biochem Cell Biol. 2004; 36: 2563-2573.

[43]   Liberski PP, Sikorska B, Bratosiewicz-Wasik J, Gajdusek DC, Brown P. Neuronal cell death in transmissible spongiform encephalopathies (prion diseases) revisited: from apoptosis to autophagy. Int J Biochem Cell Biol. 2004; 36: 2473-2490.

[44]   Wang XZ, Lawson B, Brewer JW, Zinszner H, Sanjay A, Mi LJ. Signals from the stressed endoplasmic reticulum induce C/EBP-homologous protein (CHOP/GADD153). Mol Cell Biol. 1996; 16: 4273–4280.

[45]   Wang XZ, Ron D. Stress-induced phosphorylation and activation of the transcription factor CHOP (GADD153) by p38 MAP Kinase. Science 1996; 272: 1347–1349.

[46]   Tajiri S, Oyadomari S, Yano S, Morioka M, Gotoh T, Hamada JI. Ischemia-induced neuronal cell death is mediated by the endoplasmic reticulum stress pathway involving CHOP. Cell Death Differ. 2004; 11: 403–415.

[47]   Li J, Yuan J. Caspases in apoptosis and beyond. Oncogene. 2008; 27: 6194-6206.

[48]   Pinton P, Giorgi C, Siviero R, Zecchini E, Rizzuto R. Calcium and apoptosis: ER-mitochondria Ca2+ transfer in the control of apoptosis. Oncogene. 2008; 27: 6407-6418

[49]   Zalk R, Lehnart SE, Marks AR.. Modulation of the ryanodine receptor and intracellular calcium. Annu Rev Biochem. 2007; 76: 367–385.

[50]   Crabtree GR. Calcium, calcineurin, and the control of transcription. J Biol Chem. 2001; 276: 2313-2316

[51]   Wang HG, Pathan N, Ethell IM, Krajewski S, Yamaguchi Y, Shibasaki F, McKeon F, Bobo T, Franke TF, Reed JC. Ca2+-induced apoptosis through calcineurin dephosphorylation of BAD. Science 1999; 284: 339-343.

[52]   Kingsbury TJ, Bambrick LL, Roby CD, Krueger BK. Calcineurin activity is required for depolarization-induced, CREB-dependent gene transcription in cortical neurons. J Neurochem. 2007; 103: 761-770.

[53]   Uchiyama Y, Shibata M, Koike M, Yoshimura K, Sasaki M. Autophagy-physiology and pathophysiology. Histochem. Cell Biol. 2008; 129: 407-420.

[54]   Kouroku Y, Fujita E, Tanida I, Ueno T, Isoai A, Kumagai H, Ogawa S, Kaufman RJ, Kominami E, Momoi T.. ER stress (PERK/eIF2alpha phosphorylation) mediates the polyglutamine-induced LC3 conversion, an essential step for autophagy formation. Cell Death Differ. 2007; 14: 230-239.

[55]   Field MC, Moran P, Li W, Keller GA, Caras IW.. Retention and degradation of proteins containing an uncleaved glycosyl phosphatidylinositol signal. J Biol Chem. 1994; 269: (14):10830-7

[56]   Høyer-Hansen M, Bastholm L, Szyniarowski P, Campanella M, Szabadkai G, Farkas T, Bianchi K, Fehrenbacher N, Elling F, Rizzuto R, Mathiasen IS, Jäättelä M.. Control of macroautophagy by calcium, calmodulin-dependent kinase kinase-beta, and Bcl-2. 2007; 25: 193-205.

[57]   Hetz C, Castilla J, Soto C. Perturbation of endoplasmic reticulum homeostasis facilitates prion replication. J Biol Chem. 2007; 282: 12725-12733.

[58]   Ma J, Lindquist S. Conversion of PrP to a self-perpetuating PrP^Sc-like conformation in the cytosol. Science 2002; 298: 1785-1788.

[59]   Ma J, Wollmann R, Lindquist S. Neurotoxicity and neurodegeneration when PrP accumulates in the cytosol. Science 2002; 298: 1781-1785.

[60]   Kristiansen M, Deriziotis P, Dimcheff DE, Jackson GS, Ovaa H, Naumann H, Clarke AR, van Leeuwen FW, Menéndez-Benito V, Dantuma NP, Portis JL, Collinge J, Tabrizi SJ. Disease-associated prion protein oligomers inhibit the 26S proteasome. Mol Cell. 2007; 26: 175-188.

[61]   Zanusso G, Petersen RB, Jin T, Jing Y, Kanoush R, Ferrari S, Gambetti P, Singh N.. Proteasomal degradation and N-terminal protease resistance of the codon 145 mutant prion protein. J Biol Chem. 1999; 274: 23396-23404.

[62]   Russelakis-Carneiro M, Saborio GP, Anderes L, Soto C.. Changes in the glycosylation pattern of prion protein in murine scrapie. Implications for the mechanism of neurodegeneration in prion diseases. J Biol Chem. 2002; 277: 36872-36877.

[63]   Naidoo N, Ferber M, Master M, Zhu Y, Pack AI.. Aging impairs the unfolded protein response to sleep deprivation and leads to proapoptotic signaling. J Neurosci. 2008; 28: 6539-6548.

CHAPTER 11

Autophagy and the Ubiquitin-Proteasome System – Protein Catabolism Comes Full Circle

Natalia B. Nedelsky and J. Paul Taylor*

Department of Developmental Neurobiology, St. Jude Children's Research Hospital, 262 Danny Thomas Place, Memphis, TN 38120 USA

Department of Developmental Neurobiology, St. Jude Children's Research Hospital, MS 343, D-4026, 262 Danny Thomas Place. Memphis, TN 38105-3678, USA; Tel: (901) 595-6047; Fax: (901) 595-2032; E-mail: jpaul.taylor@stjude.org

Abstract: All cells are endowed with two catabolic pathways for degrading protein: the ubiquitin-proteasome system (UPS) and autophagy. While these routes of protein degradation were long considered to be parallel and complementary systems, new evidence has revealed interaction between the UPS and autophagy, suggesting a coordinated relationship that becomes critical in times of cellular stress. Here we introduce the basics and parallels of the UPS and autophagy, review the evidence for cross-regulation of the two systems, and highlight their emerging coordinated relationship. Throughout, we review the evidence suggesting that impairment of autophagy could contribute to the initiation or progression of age-related neurodegeneration.

INTRODUCTION

In awarding the Nobel Prize in Chemistry to Aaron Ciechanover, Avram Hershko and Irwin Rose in 2004, the Royal Swedish Academy of Sciences praised these scientists as innovators. After decades of work focusing on how the cell produces proteins, these pioneers had broken with tradition and highlighted the equally important process of how the cell *degrades* proteins. Indeed, the idea that the proteome (a term yet to be invented) was dynamic, with proteins continually synthesized and degraded, was challenged well into the 1950s. What Ciechanover, Hershko, and Rose discovered in the mid-1980s was an exquisitely controlled and efficient system of selectively labeling and targeting proteins for degradation, now well known as the ubiquitin-proteasome system (UPS). According to Ciechanover, the identification of the UPS marked the end of a long search for a non-lysosomal proteolytic system [1]. Although the lysosome had been characterized as a catabolic organelle some 30 years before, several lines of evidence indicated that some portion of intracellular protein degradation could not be explained based on the known mechanisms of lysosomal activity. If the lysosome non-selectively degraded all proteins, one might predict that all proteins would be degraded at approximately the same rate. Yet, empirically, protein half-lives varied widely from a few minutes to as long as several days. Secondly, the discovery that the stability of only a subset of proteins was sensitive to physiological conditions (most notably nutrient availability) was difficult to reconcile with a single, bulk lysosome-based degradation system. A third line of evidence for a non-lysosomal proteolytic system was the differential sensitivity of particular proteins to lysosomal inhibitors, suggesting that distinct groups of proteins are degraded by distinct degradation pathways, only one of which is dependent on lysosomal proteases. Finally, the fact that degradation of some proteins was ATP-dependent suggested that lysosomal proteases (which degrade proteins in an exergonic manner) could not be the sole means of degradation. This delineation between lysosomal- and non-lysosomal-based degradation permitted these astute investigators to intuit an alternative degradation system, culminating in elucidation of the UPS as we understand it today.

The manner in which the UPS was discovered and initially characterized underscored the differences between the UPS and lysosome-mediated degradation. Indeed, for many years these two catabolic pathways were viewed as distinct catabolic pathways with no point of intersection. Recent years have seen renewed interest in that which the UPS specifically is *not* – that is, relatively non-selective bulk degradation of intracellular proteins that requires lysosomal proteases – a process broadly defined as *autophagy*. The recent heightened interest in autophagy, combined with the wealth of knowledge of the UPS, has highlighted the similar goals of the two catabolic pathways: first, their complementary role in recycling macromolecules, and second, their turnover of misfolded and/or damaged proteins. Further studies have begun to identify functional and physical interactions between the two systems, uncovering what may be a hierarchical relationship between the pathways. Thus the two systems that were identified based on their differences are presently being revealed to be surprisingly similar and intimately interrelated.

The UPS and Autophagy: A Division of Labor

The distinctions used by researchers in the 1980s to differentiate the UPS from autophagy remain the key characteristics of these systems as they are defined today. The UPS is a highly selective catabolic process which serves as the primary route of degradation for thousands of short-lived proteins, many of which serve regulatory functions in such key processes as cell cycle control, transcriptional regulation, and signal transduction. An important class of substrates for degradation by the UPS is misfolded and damaged proteins, since elimination of these proteins is important to prevent their accumulation in protein aggregates that are inherently toxic. UPS substrates are first marked for degradation by the covalent addition of a ubiquitin molecule to particular lysine(s) within the target protein; these ubiquitin molecules are added in an ATP-dependent manner through the sequential action of ubiquitin-activating (E1), -conjugating (E2), and -ligating (E3) enzymes. An additional ubiquitin moiety is added to a specific lysine residue in the preceding ubiquitin molecule, and this process is repeated to form a polyubiquitin chain on the substrate, sometimes involving the activity of a polyubiquitin (E4) ligase. Ubiquitin molecules have a total of seven lysine residues (at positions 6, 11, 27, 29, 33, 48, and 63), and the particular lysine residue used for conjugation of one ubiquitin monomer to another – defining distinct ubiquitin topologies – appears to have important functional consequences for the substrate. For example, K48-linked polyubiquitin chains are targeted to the proteasome, while K63-linked polyubiquitin chains are involved in other functions, as will be explored below [1, 2]. Those substrates targeted for UPS degradation are directed to the proteasome, where ubiquitin molecules are recycled and substrates are enzymatically degraded to oligopeptides. These oligopeptides are subsequently broken down into amino acids by non-specific peptidases, thereby

regenerating molecules essential to metabolic homeostasis.

In contrast, autophagy (literally "self-eating") describes a process in which cellular components such as organelles and longer-lived proteins are delivered to the lysosome for degradation. While autophagy serves a diverse array of functions (reviewed in [3]), this chapter will focus on its evolutionarily conserved function as the critical mediator of metabolic homeostasis in the face of changing nutrient availability [4] as well as its role in neuroprotection. Autophagy is generally considered to be a less selective degradative system than the UPS, and is typically described as a process in which large portions of cytoplasm are engulfed within membranes and delivered to the lysosome in bulk. This characterization describes the best-studied subtype of autophagy, known as macroautophagy. However, more several specialized forms of autophagy exist, including microautophagy and chaperone-mediated autophagy (CMA). These subsystems are distinguished by the identity of the substrates and the route by which these substrates reach the lysosomal compartment. Microautophagy consists of direct engulfment of small volumes of cytosol by lysosomes, while CMA involves selective, receptor-mediated translocation of proteins into the lysosomal lumen. In contrast, macroautophagy involves the *de novo* formation of an isolation membrane which expands to engulf a portion of the cytosol, eventually fusing to form a new vacuole termed an autophagosome. Autophagosomes undergo a series of maturation steps before fusing with lysosomes to deliver their cargo for degradation by lysosomal proteases. Breakdown products from the lysosome are translocated across the lysosomal membrane to the cytosol, where they are reused in metabolic processes. There appears to be capacity for selectivity within the process of macroautophagy, as some processes have been observed that appear to be specific for mitochondria (mitophagy), portions of the nucleus (*nucleophagy*), peroxisomes (*pexophagy*), endoplasmmic reticulum (*reticulophagy*), microorganisms (*xenophagy*), ribosomes *(ribophagy)* or protein aggregates (*aggrephagy*) (reviewed in [5]). Macroautophagy forms the basis of this chapter and will be referred to hereafter simply as "autophagy".

The UPS and Autophagy: Functional Parallels

Despite such gross differences between the UPS and autophagy at a mechanistic level, two key functional parallels have been well-established. First, both systems play important roles in maintaining cellular pool of free amino acids, particularly in the setting of limited nutrient availability. Protein catabolism mediated by the UPS and autophagy are crucial for recycling amino acids during acute and chronic starvation, respectively. Second, both systems play essential roles in protecting the integrity of the proteome which is continually threatened by non-native protein-protein interactions and can lead to the formation of insoluble aggregates. Even under normal conditions cells constitutively produce aberrant proteins, and the challenge to protein quality control can become even greater with proteotoxic insults such as protein oxidation, aberrant translation, or mutant gene products. To counteract protein aggregation and its consequences, cells are equipped with protective mechanisms that scrutinize the cell for non-native proteins and assist in their refolding or degradation. The UPS and autophagy are both important to this quality control system and deficiency of either system is associated with accumulation of defective proteins in insoluble aggregates with attendant cytotoxicity.

The importance of eliminating misfolded or defective proteins is perhaps most evident in the context of the nervous system. As post-mitotic, highly metabolically active cells, neurons are particularly vulnerable to the long-term accumulation of proteins that engage in aberrant interactions or acquire other toxic properties. Indeed, a broad array of neurodegenerative diseases are characterized by the accumulation of misfolded proteins in affected brain regions. These deposits are frequently immuno-positive for ubiquitin and other UPS components, suggesting a failure in the cell's capacity to clear proteins marked for degradation. In addition, accumulations of autophagic vacuoles in affected brain regions of patients with Alzheimer's disease, Parkinson's disease, Creutzfeldt-Jakob disease, and many of the polyglutamine diseases suggest that autophagy could play a role in the initiation or progression of disease [6-9].

The observation that these protein deposits in the setting of disease occur alongside (and despite) signs of both UPS and autophagic activity raises the question of which system has failed in its task of degrading these misfolded proteins. The answer may be both: the *in vitro* turnover of neurodegenerative disease-causing proteins such as polyglutamine-expanded proteins, polyalanine-

expanded proteins, and α-synuclein can be altered by manipulation of either the UPS or the autophagy-lysosomal system [10-17]. Such wide-ranging sensitivities indicate that more than one degradative route may be available to some proteins, and have led to the suggestion that the choice of route for a particular substrate may be influenced by which system is most capable of degrading it. For example, in the case of α-synuclein, it has been suggested that soluble forms of the protein can be efficiently degraded by the proteasome, while aggregated or oligomeric forms require the bulk degradation of the autophagic pathway [16]. Such a model further suggests that autophagy could provide an alternate, compensatory route of degradation when a particular substrate cannot be cleared efficiently by the proteasome, or when the UPS is more globally compromised.

While the clearance of disease proteins is likely to be cytoprotective in and of itself, degradation of intracellular proteins in general – whether misfolded, damaged, or simply no longer useful – has the advantage of recycling amino acids for further use by the cell. As mentioned above, the best-characterized and evolutionarily conserved role for autophagy lies in its response to chronic starvation. As such, autophagy is negatively regulated by the nutrition-dependent insulin/PI3K and TOR signaling pathways; when nutrients are removed, active PI3K inhibits TOR, allowing autophagy to reallocate nutrients from nonessential cytoplasmic components to vital cellular processes. The UPS has also been implicated in response to starvation, though its major role appears to be mobilization of nutrients in the context of acute starvation.

The UPS and Autophagy: Molecular Parallels

Apart from functional parallels between the UPS and autophagy with respect to recycling amino acids and implications of impaired function in the setting of neurodegenerative disease, a number of molecular parallels between autophagy and the UPS have emerged as the details of each system have been delineated. Of particular note is the striking similarity between the processes of autophagy induction and ubiquitin conjugation. Both processes utilize molecules that have come to be defined as UBLs (ubiquitin-like proteins): while the UPS uses the eponymous ubiquitin molecule, autophagy induction is regulated by post-translational modification by two UBL proteins, known as Atg8 and Atg12. Atg8 and Atg12 are also members of a family of evolutionarily conserved proteins known as the Atg (autophagy-related) proteins; these Atg proteins are the effectors and regulatory proteins that initiate and elongate the autophagosomal membrane (reviewed in [18]). UBLs share similar structural domains and are likely ancestrally related Fig. (**1**) [19]. Moreover, the UBL conjugation system is also highly conserved between the UPS and autophagy Fig. (**2**): in both cases, the carboxyl group of the C-terminal glycine of the UBL is activated and attacked by a thiol-group-containing E1-activating enzyme to generate an E1-UBL thiolester. The activated UBL is then transferred to an E2-conjugating enzyme, and finally ligated to the target. In the case of the UBL Atg8, this target is not a protein, but the membrane-bound phospholipid phosphotidylethanolamine (PE). As PE is a component of the autophagosomal membrane, this PE-Atg8 reaction results in the studding of the inner and outer membrane of the autophagosome with Atg8. A mammalian homolog of Atg8 known as MAP-LC3 (microtubule-associated protein light chain 3, typically abbreviated as LC3) associates with phagophores in an analogous manner, and is therefore used as a primary histological marker of autophagosomes. Pro-LC3 is cleaved cotranslationally to yield a protein known as "LC3-I." When LC3-I becomes conjugated to PE and covalently associates with the phagophore, it forms "LC3-II." Consequently, the generation and turnover of LC3-II is used as an index of autophagy induction and/or flux [20]. Because LC3-II remains on the inner membrane of autophagosomes until lysosomal enzymes degrade it, increased steady-state levels of LC3-II may be due to induction of autophagosome formation, a blockade in their maturation, or both. The striking similarities between the ubiquitination system that precedes proteasomal digestion and the autophagy induction system that culminates in lysosomal digestion have led to the suggestion that these two catabolic pathways may have evolved from a common, ancestral biological pathway.

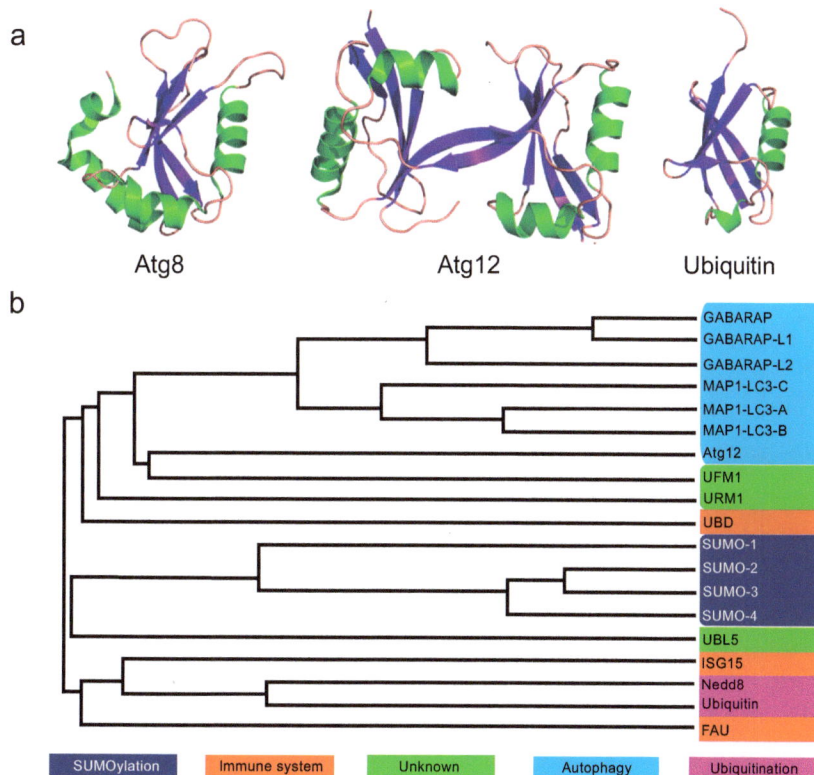

Fig (1). Ubiquitin-like (UBL) molecules share three-dimensional structures and common ancestry. (a) Ribbon diagrams of the UBL proteins Atg8, Atg12, and ubiquitin reveal a common ubiquitin fold. α-helices are shown in green, β-strands in purple, and unstructured loops in orange. Images were generated using PDB codes 1UBQ (ubiquitin), 1UGM (Atg8), and 1WZ3 (Atg12) and PYMOL. (b) Cladogram of human UBL proteins demonstrate the evolutionary relationships between UBL molecules and illustrate the ancestral relationship between ubiquitin and autophagy-related genes. Cladogram generated by multiple sequence alignment of human UBL proteins using Clustal W2.0.10.

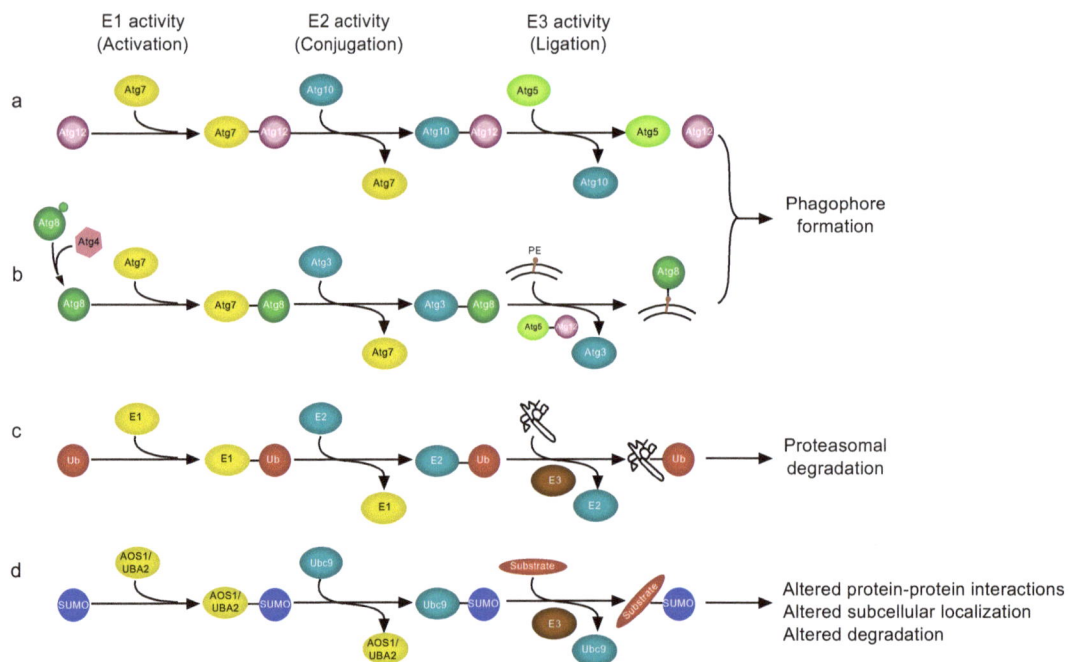

Fig. (2). Autophagy, the UPS, and SUMOylation use parallel conjugation systems of UBL modification. (a) In the autophagy pathway, the UBL Atg12 is activated by the E1-like molecule Atg7, transferred to the E2-like Atg10, and is subsequently conjugated to Atg5. No E3-like protein has been identified in this pathway. (b) Also in the autophagy pathway, the UBL Atg8 is activated by the E1-like molecule Atg7, transferred to the E2-like Atg3, and is conjugated to phosphotidylethanolamine (PE) via the E3-like activity of the Atg5-Atg12 complex. (c) In the UPS, the UBL protein ubiquitin is activated by an E1-activating enzyme, transferred to an E2-conjugating enzyme, and linked to its target substrate through the action of an E3-ligating enzyme. (d) In the SUMOylation pathway, SUMO is first activated via the E1-like complex formed by AOS1 and UBA2, transferred to the E2-conjugating enzyme Ubc9, and finally ligated to its substrate through an E3-ligating enzyme. Though each conjugation pathway is similar, each has significantly different downstream effects.

Points of Intersection Between the UPS and Autophagy: Cross-Regulation

As the list of similarities between the UPS and autophagy continued to grow, several groups began to realize that these shared characteristics did not simply reflect two parallel systems, but that these pathways could intersect in meaningful ways. This intersection was not predicted by the early researchers working to characterize the UPS, because of the apparently strict rule that agents that disrupt lysosomal function have no effect on the ATP-dependent turnover of short-lived and abnormal proteins [21].

The first solid evidence that the UPS intersected with autophagy emerged in the mid-1990s, when ubiquitin modification was identified as an essential signal in the endosomal-lysosomal system that permits lysosomal degradation of certain integral membrane proteins. Specifically, several groups showed that a subset of endocytosed proteins requires ubiquitin conjugation in order to achieve internalization from the plasma membrane [22, 23] and that monoubiquitination is sufficient as an endocytic internalization signal [24]. In addition, K63-linked ubiquitin topologies were found to stimulate endocytosis [25]. Ubiquitination was also found to serve as a sorting signal for endosomes, targeting endosomal cargo to multivesicular bodies (MVBs) in the lysosomal degradation pathway [26]. This pathway is also used in lysosome biogenesis, indicating that ubiquitination can influence the autophagy-lysosomal pathway at its most fundamental level. This latter observation was also the first of several observations suggesting a hierarchical relationship between these catabolic pathways, with autophagy under the control of the ubiquitin-proteasome system, as discussed below.

More recent evidence linking the UPS and autophagy comes from research into p53, a short-lived transcription factor whose steady-state levels are tightly controlled by the UPS. p53 plays multiple well-described roles in the regulation of the cell cycle and cell death, and several groups have now confirmed an additional function for p53 in the regulation of autophagy. Activation of p53 is believed to activate autophagy through both transcription-dependent and -independent mechanisms [27-32], while inhibition of p53 also appears to activate autophagy, though strictly in a transcription-independent manner [33]. The paradox in which autophagy may be induced by both activation and inhibition of p53 remains to be resolved, though it has been suggested that the different types of p53-dependent autophagy activation could potentially be dictated by the nature of the stress signal [34]. The notion that the UPS can dictate the steady-state levels of a key autophagy signaling molecule such as p53 suggests a model in which the UPS holds the reins of autophagy induction, acting upstream of autophagy to control the signals that induce or inhibit this degradative pathway.

Further intersection of the UPS and autophagy can be found in the specialized form of macroauto-phagy known as mitophagy (mitochondria-specific autophagy), a process vital to protecting cells from oxidative stress [35]. Parkin, a protein best known as a gene deleted in juvenile Parkinson's disease, is also an E3 ubiquitin ligase that was recently shown to be recruited to impaired mitochondria, where it mediates the engulfment of mitochondria by autophagosomes [36]. Though the ubiquitination activity of Parkin was not directly tested in this paper, it will be interesting to determine whether its ubiquitination signal involves mono- or poly-ubiquitination. Of particular interest is Parkin's ability to assemble K63-linked polyubiquitin chains, which form a ubiquitin chain topology that has been linked to autophagy and will be discussed more below [37].

Autophagy and the UPS: Coordinated Function

While these points of intersection highlighted regulatory crosstalk between the UPS and autophagy, there was until recently little evidence to show functional overlap between the two systems beyond their shared abilities to degrade disease-associated proteins. However, two papers published back-to-back in *Nature* in 2006 revealed a level of interaction that few would have predicted

[38, 39]. Both of these papers described conditional knockouts of individual Atg genes within the nervous system, and both reported that these mice showed neurodegeneration with extensive ubiquitin-positive pathology despite evidence of an intact UPS Fig. (**3**). These papers were significant in two respects. First, they revealed an essential role for basal autophagy (as opposed to nutritionally-induced autophagy) in the development and maintenance of the central nervous system, even in the absence of any disease-related mutant proteins. Second, the accumulation of ubiquitin conjugates despite an intact, functioning UPS was the first evidence that autophagy might play a role the degradation of ubiquitin-tagged substrates. Subsequent to the determination that a deficiency of autophagy leads to neurodegeneration with accumulation of ubiquitin conjugates, it was determined that induction of autophagy was able to suppress degeneration associated with UPS impairment and accelerate the clearance of misfolded protein in *Drosophila melanogaster*. These results demonstrated for the first time that not only does autophagy functionally complement the UPS, but is able to compensate for an impaired UPS [40]. In fact, impairment of the UPS is such a potent and consistent stimulus of autophagy that it has become a frequent method of experimentally inducing autophagy both *in vitro* and *in vivo* [41, 42].

Molecular Links between the UPS and Autophagy

The UPS and autophagy clearly share roles in maintaining metabolic homeostasis and degrading abnormal proteins, while ubiquitin modification evidently can lead substrates into the autophagic system. What signals might mediate this coordination between the UPS and autophagy? Several clues have come to light from *in vitro* studies in which cells are challenged by either high-level expression of misfolded protein or direct impairment of the UPS. In such contexts, many cells actively transport ubiquitinated, misfolded proteins to juxtanuclear bodies termed aggresomes [43]. Aggresomes are thought to be cytoprotective, acting as a mechanism to sequester potentially toxic proteins and facilitate their clearance by autophagy [11]. While controversy surrounds the question of whether aggresomes are formed *in vivo*, they have provided significant insight into the molecular machinery that protects cells from misfolded stress. In particular, several proteins involved in aggresome formation have subsequently been shown to play roles in managing

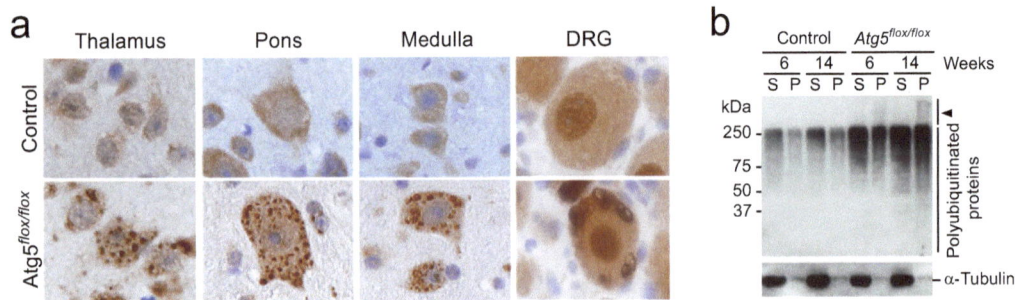

Fig. (3). Conditional knockout of Atg5 in the mouse nervous system results in ubiquitin-positive inclusions and accumulation of polyubiquitinated proteins. (a) Immunohistochemistry of brain sections from control and Atg5 conditional knockout mice at six weeks of age. Ubiquitin staining (1B3) reveals ubiquitin-positive inclusion bodies in the cytoplasm of large neurons in the thalamus, pons, medulla, and dorsal root ganglion (DRG). Genotypes shown: control (Atg5$^{flox/+}$; nestin-Cre) and Atg5 knockout (Atg5$^{flox/flox}$; nestin-Cre). Scale bar 10□m. (b) Triton-X-100-soluble polyubiquitinated proteins accumulate in Atg5$^{flox/flox}$; nestin-Cre brains. Brain homogenate was prepared at indicated times and separated into Triton-X-100-soluble (S) and −insoluble (P) fractions and immunoblotted with anti-ubiquitin antibodies. Arrowhead indicates the stacking gel. Reprinted from [39] with permission.

toxic proteins *in vivo,* including Parkin, histone deacetylase 6 (HDAC6) and p62. The common threads linking HDAC6 and p62 to aggresomes are K63-linked polyubiquitin chains, which are thought to target proteins to aggresomes, among other functions. The E3 ubiquitin ligase Parkin is capable of generating such K63 linkages [37], and overexpression of Parkin leads to aggresome formation [44]. HDAC6 is a cytoplasmic deacetylase whose targets include α-tubulin, Hsp90, and cortactin. HDAC6 interacts with polyubiquitinated proteins through a Zn-finger ubiquitin-binding domain, and also interacts with dynein motors, suggesting that it may provide a link between ubiquitinated proteins and transport machinery [42, 45, 46]. Indeed, HDAC6 was recently demonstrated to operate as an adaptor between Parkin-mediated K63-linked polyubiquitinated substrates and the dynein motor complex, effectively coordinating delivery of substrates to autophagic machinery [47, 48]. In *Drosophila,* HDAC6 overexpression was found to suppress degeneration associated with UPS impairment as well as degeneration caused by toxic polyglutamine expression; this suppression was autophagy-dependent, supporting a role for HDAC6 in linking the UPS with compensatory autophagy [40]. p62 is a second aggresome-related cytosolic protein that is thought to operate as an adaptor between ubiquitinated proteins and autophagic machinery, as it harbors both a ubiquitin-associated domain and an LC3-interacting region [49-51]. p62 has been observed in ubiquitin-positive inclusions in a variety of neurodegenerative disease brains [52-54], and converging evidence from experimental studies suggest that p62 protects against misfolded stress

by facilitating a connection between ubiquitinated substrates and autophagic machinery [51, 55-59]. In a model similar to that described for HDAC6, p62 has been proposed to partner specifically with K63-linked polyubiquitin to promote the clearance of protein inclusions by autophagy [60].

Autophagy is Cytoprotective (Except When it Isn't)

Whereas the neurodegeneration with ubiquitin-pathology observed in autophagy-deficient mice was unexpected, it was consistent with prior observations that genetic alteration of lysosomal activity has dramatic impact on the central nervous system. For example, knockout of cathepsin D, a lysosomal protease enriched in neuronal tissues, resulted in neurodegeneration and accumulation of autophagosomes and lysosomes in both mice and *Drosophila* [61-63]. On the basis of these observations one might predict that impairment of autophagy could contribute to neurodegenerative disease in humans. Indeed, primary lysosomal dysfunction in inherited congenital "lysosomal storage disorders" has long been recognized to cause severe neurodegenerative phenotypes characterized pathologically by accumulations of lysosomes and autophagic vacuoles [64]. For example, the neuronal ceroid lipofuscinoses (NCLs) are a heterogeneous group of inherited, neurodegenerative disorders with onset ranging from infancy to late adulthood that are caused by a variety of defects in lysosomal function. Furthermore, a growing list of adult-onset, familial neurological diseases have been linked to mutations expected to have an impact on autophagy-lysosomal function (reviewed in [64]), including Parkinson's disease (mutations in the lysosomal protein ATP13A2 are linked to early-onset PD) [65], Charcot- Marie-Tooth type 2B (a dominantly inherited form of peripheral neuropathy caused by mutations in the endosomal-lysosomal trafficking protein Rab7) [66], and distal-spinobulbar muscular atrophy (a form of motor neuron disease caused by mutations in the lysosomal trafficking protein dynactin) [67]. These latter two diseases are caused by mutations in components of the vesicular transport machinery, implicating impaired trafficking of autophagic components as important to pathogenesis. Indeed, microtubule-based vesicular trafficking is essential to the delivery of autophagosomes to lysosomes [68], and the relatively long axons of the sensory and motor neurons affected in these diseases may impart particular vulnerability.

How might autophagy be cytoprotective? One possibility, given the evidence that autophagy can degrade disease-causing proteins, is that autophagy's protective action is mediated through accelerated turnover of misfolded proteins. This idea is supported by experimental evidence in models of neurodegenerative disease. In these studies, genetic inhibition of autophagy enhanced degeneration in spinobulbar muscular atrophy (SBMA) and Alzheimer's disease models [40, 69] and was associated with higher levels of disease-related proteins, suggesting that augmenting autophagic clearance of these cytotoxic proteins could provide benefit. Indeed, pharmacological activation of TOR using rapamycin suppressed toxicity in *in vitro* and *in vivo* models of SBMA and Huntington's disease [10, 40, 70, 71].

Such a model, however, may be too simplistic. Accelerated turnover of mutant disease-causing proteins would be predicted to be cytoprotective, but such a mechanism does not explain how autophagy can suppress degeneration in models of proteasome impairment. It seems unlikely that autophagy upregulation can normalize the turnover of short-lived proteins that are normally degraded by the UPS, effectively replacing the UPS function with respect to regulatory networks. Instead, it seems reasonable to invoke another shared function of the UPS and autophagy – that of maintaining metabolic balance. Perhaps, through induction of autophagy, the metabolic balance that is disrupted with UPS impairment can be restored, replenishing the cellular pool of nutrients and allowing the cell to regain essential functions.

However, the role for autophagy in neurodegeneration may not always be so straightforward. In the case of Alzheimer's disease, a complex picture is emerging in which impaired autophagosome-lysosome fusion, combined with decreasing efficiency of the lysosomal system, causes accumulation of autophagic vacuoles [72]. These vacuoles may contribute to pathology by interfering with normal cellular functions such as intracellular trafficking and metabolic turnover of nutrients. In addition, recent studies have suggested that the toxic amyloid-β species may be generated by autophagic degradation of the amyloid beta precursor protein [73]. These findings support a model of Alzheimer's disease pathogenesis in which autophagy induction produces toxic species, while defective clearance of autophagic vacuoles lead to exacerbation of disease [72].

Final Thoughts

The complex relationship between autophagy and neurodegeneration, as illustrated by the example of Alzheimer's disease, highlights several unresolved questions. As mentioned above, many neurodegenerative diseases show accumulations of autophagic vacuoles; in addition, autophagosomes are frequently found in dying neurons. However, these morphological studies cannot determine whether the increased frequency of autophagic vacuoles in disease brain is due to induced autophagy or impaired autophagic flux. Furthermore, these studies cannot distinguish between the role of autophagy in cytoprotection or in cell death. Finally, if the increased autophagic vacuoles reflect endogenous upregulation of autophagy, it is unclear why this induction is insufficient to protect against proteotoxicity.

Further questions concern the details of the interrelatedness of the UPS and autophagy. Several questions in particular concern the compensatory function of autophagy in the context of UPS impairment. For example, it is not known whether this compensatory relationship is reciprocal – that is, whether induction of the UPS is able to compensate for impaired autophagy. Few reagents exist to upregulate the UPS, though one study found that upregulation of the UPS may afford neuroprotection from toxicity caused by disease proteins [74]. However, the authors did not examine the effects of UPS upregulation in autophagy-deficient cells. In addition, the molecular players that might transduce signals to induce compensatory autophagy remain unknown. Also, how is the decision made between

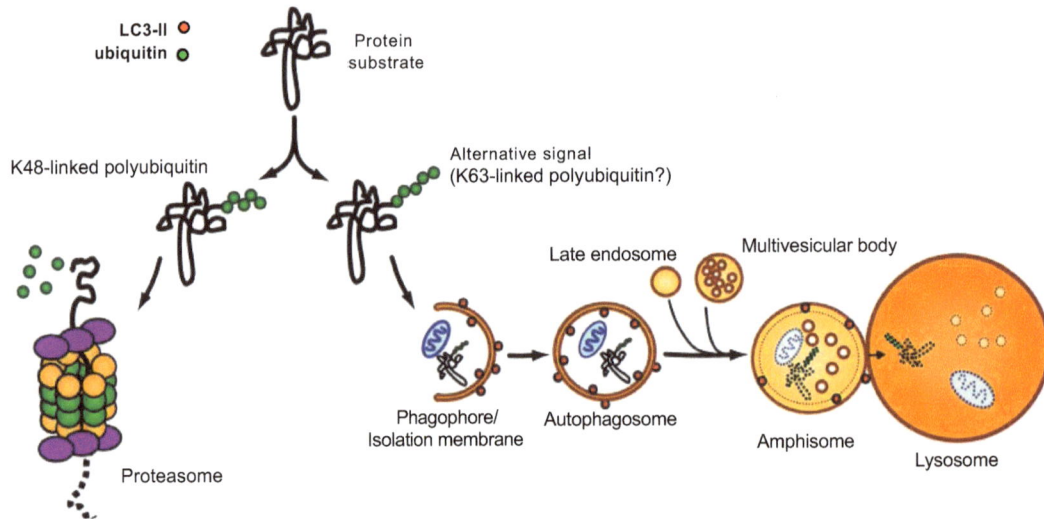

Fig. (4). Protein degradation can be accomplished by two major intracellular pathways: the UPS and autophagy. In the UPS pathway, misfolded protein substrates are tagged with K48-linked polyubiquitin chains and targeted to the proteasome for degradation. The signal for degradation by macroautophagy is not known, but *in vitro* evidence suggests that K63-linked polyubiquitination leads to aggresome formation and subsequent degradation of misfolded proteins by autophagy. The process of macroautophagy involves the expansion of a phagophore or isolation membrane that surrounds a portion of the cytoplasm. The phagophore seals and matures to form an autophagosome, which in mammals joins with late endosomes and multivesicular bodies (MVBs) to form a new structure termed an amphisome. Amphisomes then fuse with lysosomes to deliver their cargo for lysosomal degradation.

degradative pathways for any particular protein substrate when more than one route is available? HDAC6 and p62 have both been implicated in directing ubiquitinated proteins for autophagic degradation, but the mechanisms whereby these proteins identify their targets and influence their degradation are still unknown. Some evidence suggests that different ubiquitin topologies might identify different classes of substrates, with K48-linked chains being degraded by the UPS, while K63-linked chains are recognized by HDAC6 and p62 and possibly degraded by autophagy Fig. (**4**). However, experimental limitations in distinguishing the effects of K48- and K63-ubiquitin chains must be overcome in order these questions, and *in vivo* evidence for a link between K63-linked chains and autophagy is still lacking.It is further evidence of the irony of nature that the molecule that Ciechanover, Hershko, and Rose discovered at the heart of their search for a non-lysosomal proteolytic pathway appears to be intimately linked to lysosomal proteolysis. At the very least, their decision to name the molecule "ubiquitin" turns out to have been made with remarkable foresight.

ACKNOWLEDGEMENTS

JPT is supported by a grants from the Dana Foundation, the Muscular Dystrophy Association and NIH grants NS053825 and AG031587.

REFERENCES

1. V. Chau, J.W. Tobias, A. Bachmair, D. Marriott, D.J. Ecker, D.K. Gonda, A. Varshavsky, A multiubiquitin chain is confined to specific lysine in a targeted short-lived protein, Science 243 (1989) 1576-1583.
2. T. Arnason, M.J. Ellison, Stress resistance in Saccharomyces cerevisiae is strongly correlated with assembly of a novel type of multiubiquitin chain, Mol Cell Biol 14 (1994) 7876-7883.
3. N. Mizushima, The pleiotropic role of autophagy: from protein metabolism to bactericide, Cell Death Differ 12 Suppl 2 (2005) 1535-1541.
4. H. Abeliovich, D.J. Klionsky, Autophagy in yeast: mechanistic insights and physiological function, Microbiol Mol Biol Rev 65 (2001) 463-479, table of contents.
5. M. Kundu, C.B. Thompson, Autophagy: basic principles and relevance to disease, Annu Rev Pathol 3 (2008) 427-455.
6. R.A. Nixon, J. Wegiel, A. Kumar, W.H. Yu, C. Peterhoff, A. Cataldo, A.M. Cuervo, Extensive involvement of autophagy in Alzheimer disease: an immuno-electron microscopy study, J Neuropathol Exp Neurol 64 (2005) 113-122.
7. P. Anglade, S. Vyas, F. Javoy-Agid, M.T. Herrero, P.P. Michel, J. Marquez, A. Mouatt-Prigent, M. Ruberg, E.C. Hirsch, Y. Agid, Apoptosis and autophagy in nigral neurons of patients with Parkinson's disease, Histol Histopathol 12 (1997) 25-31.
8. B. Sikorska, P.P. Liberski, P. Giraud, N. Kopp, P. Brown, Autophagy is a part of ultrastructural synaptic pathology in Creutzfeldt-Jakob disease: a brain biopsy study, Int J Biochem Cell Biol 36 (2004) 2563-2573.
9. E. Sapp, C. Schwarz, K. Chase, P.G. Bhide, A.B. Young, J. Penney, J.P. Vonsattel, N. Aronin, M. DiFiglia, Huntingtin localization in brains of normal

and Huntington's disease patients, Ann Neurol 42 (1997) 604-612.

10. B. Ravikumar, R. Duden, D.C. Rubinsztein, Aggregate-prone proteins with polyglutamine and polyalanine expansions are degraded by autophagy, Hum Mol Genet 11 (2002) 1107-1117.

11. J.P. Taylor, F. Tanaka, J. Robitschek, C.M. Sandoval, A. Taye, S. Markovic-Plese, K.H. Fischbeck, Aggresomes protect cells by enhancing the degradation of toxic polyglutamine-containing protein, Hum Mol Genet 12 (2003) 749-757.

12. K.B. Kegel, M. Kim, E. Sapp, C. McIntyre, J.G. Castano, N. Aronin, M. DiFiglia, Huntingtin expression stimulates endosomal-lysosomal activity, endosome tubulation, and autophagy, J Neurosci 20 (2000) 7268-7278.

13. E. Martin-Aparicio, A. Yamamoto, F. Hernandez, R. Hen, J. Avila, J.J. Lucas, Proteasomal-dependent aggregate reversal and absence of cell death in a conditional mouse model of Huntington's disease, J Neurosci 21 (2001) 8772-8781.

14. C.J. Cummings, E. Reinstein, Y. Sun, B. Antalffy, Y. Jiang, A. Ciechanover, H.T. Orr, A.L. Beaudet, H.Y. Zoghbi, Mutation of the E6-AP ubiquitin ligase reduces nuclear inclusion frequency while accelerating polyglutamine-induced pathology in SCA1 mice, Neuron 24 (1999) 879-892.

15. J.E. Davies, S. Sarkar, D.C. Rubinsztein, Trehalose reduces aggregate formation and delays pathology in a transgenic mouse model of oculopharyngeal muscular dystrophy, Hum Mol Genet 15 (2006) 23-31.

16. J.L. Webb, B. Ravikumar, J. Atkins, J.N. Skepper, D.C. Rubinsztein, Alpha-Synuclein is degraded by both autophagy and the proteasome, J Biol Chem 278 (2003) 25009-25013.

17. M.C. Bennett, J.F. Bishop, Y. Leng, P.B. Chock, T.N. Chase, M.M. Mouradian, Degradation of alpha-synuclein by proteasome, J Biol Chem 274 (1999) 33855-33858.

18. Z. Xie, D.J. Klionsky, Autophagosome formation: core machinery and adaptations, Nat Cell Biol 9 (2007) 1102-1109.

19. K.R. Love, A. Catic, C. Schlieker, H.L. Ploegh, Mechanisms, biology and inhibitors of deubiquitinating enzymes, Nat Chem Biol 3 (2007) 697-705.

20. D.J. Klionsky, H. Abeliovich, P. Agostinis, D.K. Agrawal, G. Aliev, D.S. Askew, M. Baba, E.H. Baehrecke, B.A. Bahr, A. Ballabio, B.A. Bamber, D.C. Bassham, E. Bergamini, X. Bi, M. Biard-Piechaczyk, J.S. Blum, D.E. Bredesen, J.L. Brodsky, J.H. Brumell, U.T. Brunk, W. Bursch, N. Camougrand, E. Cebollero, F. Cecconi, Y. Chen, L.S. Chin, A. Choi, C.T. Chu, J. Chung, P.G. Clarke, R.S. Clark, S.G. Clarke, C. Clave, J.L. Cleveland, P. Codogno, M.I. Colombo, A. Coto-Montes, J.M. Cregg, A.M. Cuervo, J. Debnath, F. Demarchi, P.B. Dennis, P.A. Dennis, V. Deretic, R.J. Devenish, F. Di Sano, J.F. Dice, M. Difiglia, S. Dinesh-Kumar, C.W. Distelhorst, M. Djavaheri-Mergny, F.C. Dorsey, W. Droge, M. Dron, W.A. Dunn, Jr., M. Duszenko, N.T. Eissa, Z. Elazar, A. Esclatine, E.L. Eskelinen, L. Fesus, K.D. Finley, J.M. Fuentes, J. Fueyo, K. Fujisaki, B. Galliot, F.B. Gao, D.A. Gewirtz, S.B. Gibson, A. Gohla, A.L. Goldberg, R. Gonzalez, C. Gonzalez-Estevez, S. Gorski, R.A. Gottlieb, D. Haussinger, Y.W. He, K. Heidenreich, J.A. Hill, M. Hoyer-Hansen, X. Hu, W.P. Huang, A. Iwasaki, M. Jaattela, W.T. Jackson, X. Jiang, S. Jin, T. Johansen, J.U. Jung, M. Kadowaki, C. Kang, A. Kelekar, D.H. Kessel, J.A. Kiel, H.P. Kim, A. Kimchi, T.J. Kinsella, K. Kiselyov, K. Kitamoto, E. Knecht, M.

Komatsu, E. Kominami, S. Kondo, A.L. Kovacs, G. Kroemer, C.Y. Kuan, R. Kumar, M. Kundu, J. Landry, M. Laporte, W. Le, H.Y. Lei, M.J. Lenardo, B. Levine, A. Lieberman, K.L. Lim, F.C. Lin, W. Liou, L.F. Liu, G. Lopez-Berestein, C. Lopez-Otin, B. Lu, K.F. Macleod, W. Malorni, W. Martinet, K. Matsuoka, J. Mautner, A.J. Meijer, A. Melendez, P. Michels, G. Miotto, W.P. Mistiaen, N. Mizushima, B. Mograbi, I. Monastyrska, M.N. Moore, P.I. Moreira, Y. Moriyasu, T. Motyl, C. Munz, L.O. Murphy, N.I. Naqvi, T.P. Neufeld, I. Nishino, R.A. Nixon, T. Noda, B. Nurnberg, M. Ogawa, N.L. Oleinick, L.J. Olsen, B. Ozpolat, S. Paglin, G.E. Palmer, I. Papassideri, M. Parkes, D.H. Perlmutter, G. Perry, M. Piacentini, R. Pinkas-Kramarski, M. Prescott, T. Proikas-Cezanne, N. Raben, A. Rami, F. Reggiori, B. Rohrer, D.C. Rubinsztein, K.M. Ryan, J. Sadoshima, H. Sakagami, Y. Sakai, M. Sandri, C. Sasakawa, M. Sass, C. Schneider, P.O. Seglen, O. Seleverstov, J. Settleman, J.J. Shacka, I.M. Shapiro, A. Sibirny, E.C. Silva-Zacarin, H.U. Simon, C. Simone, A. Simonsen, M.A. Smith, K. Spanel-Borowski, V. Srinivas, M. Steeves, H. Stenmark, P.E. Stromhaug, C.S. Subauste, S. Sugimoto, D. Sulzer, T. Suzuki, M.S. Swanson, I. Tabas, F. Takeshita, N.J. Talbot, Z. Talloczy, K. Tanaka, K. Tanaka, I. Tanida, G.S. Taylor, J.P. Taylor, A. Terman, G. Tettamanti, C.B. Thompson, M. Thumm, A.M. Tolkovsky, S.A. Tooze, R. Truant, L.V. Tumanovska, Y. Uchiyama, T. Ueno, N.L. Uzcategui, I. van der Klei, E.C. Vaquero, T. Vellai, M.W. Vogel, H.G. Wang, P. Webster, J.W. Wiley, Z. Xi, G. Xiao, J. Yahalom, J.M. Yang, G. Yap, X.M. Yin, T. Yoshimori, L. Yu, Z. Yue, M. Yuzaki, O. Zabirnyk, X. Zheng, X. Zhu, R.L. Deter, Guidelines for the use and interpretation of assays for monitoring autophagy in higher eukaryotes, Autophagy 4 (2008) 151-175.

21. C.M. Pickart, Back to the future with ubiquitin, Cell 116 (2004) 181-190.

22. L. Hicke, H. Riezman, Ubiquitination of a yeast plasma membrane receptor signals its ligand-stimulated endocytosis, Cell 84 (1996) 277-287.

23. R. Kolling, C.P. Hollenberg, The ABC-transporter Ste6 accumulates in the plasma membrane in a ubiquitinated form in endocytosis mutants, EMBO J 13 (1994) 3261-3271.

24. J. Terrell, S. Shih, R. Dunn, L. Hicke, A function for monoubiquitination in the internalization of a G protein-coupled receptor, Mol Cell 1 (1998) 193-202.

25. J.M. Galan, R. Haguenauer-Tsapis, Ubiquitin lys63 is involved in ubiquitination of a yeast plasma membrane protein, EMBO J 16 (1997) 5847-5854.

26. M. Komada, N. Kitamura, The Hrs/STAM complex in the downregulation of receptor tyrosine kinases, J Biochem 137 (2005) 1-8.

27. Z. Feng, H. Zhang, A.J. Levine, S. Jin, The coordinate regulation of the p53 and mTOR pathways in cells, Proc Natl Acad Sci U S A 102 (2005) 8204-8209.

28. X. Zeng, T. Yan, J.E. Schupp, Y. Seo, T.J. Kinsella, DNA mismatch repair initiates 6-thioguanine--induced autophagy through p53 activation in human tumor cells, Clin Cancer Res 13 (2007) 1315-1321.

29. W.M. Abida, W. Gu, p53-Dependent and p53-independent activation of autophagy by ARF, Cancer Res 68 (2008) 352-357.

30. D. Crighton, S. Wilkinson, J. O'Prey, N. Syed, P. Smith, P.R. Harrison, M. Gasco, O. Garrone, T. Crook, K.M. Ryan, DRAM, a p53-induced modulator of autophagy, is critical for apoptosis, Cell 126 (2006) 121-134.

31.   R.K. Amaravadi, D. Yu, J.J. Lum, T. Bui, M.A. Christophorou, G.I. Evan, A. Thomas-Tikhonenko, C.B. Thompson, Autophagy inhibition enhances therapy-induced apoptosis in a Myc-induced model of lymphoma, J Clin Invest 117 (2007) 326-336.

32.   K.H. Maclean, F.C. Dorsey, J.L. Cleveland, M.B. Kastan, Targeting lysosomal degradation induces p53-dependent cell death and prevents cancer in mouse models of lymphomagenesis, J Clin Invest 118 (2008) 79-88.

33.   E. Tasdemir, M.C. Maiuri, L. Galluzzi, I. Vitale, M. Djavaheri-Mergny, M. D'Amelio, A. Criollo, E. Morselli, C. Zhu, F. Harper, U. Nannmark, C. Samara, P. Pinton, J.M. Vicencio, R. Carnuccio, U.M. Moll, F. Madeo, P. Paterlini-Brechot, R. Rizzuto, G. Szabadkai, G. Pierron, K. Blomgren, N. Tavernarakis, P. Codogno, F. Cecconi, G. Kroemer, Regulation of autophagy by cytoplasmic p53, Nat Cell Biol 10 (2008) 676-687.

34.   B. Levine, J. Abrams, p53: The Janus of autophagy?, Nat Cell Biol 10 (2008) 637-639.

35.   I. Kim, S. Rodriguez-Enriquez, J.J. Lemasters, Selective degradation of mitochondria by mitophagy, Arch Biochem Biophys 462 (2007) 245-253.

36.   D. Narendra, A. Tanaka, D.F. Suen, R.J. Youle, Parkin is recruited selectively to impaired mitochondria and promotes their autophagy, J Cell Biol 183 (2008) 795-803.

37.   K.L. Lim, K.C. Chew, J.M. Tan, C. Wang, K.K. Chung, Y. Zhang, Y. Tanaka, W. Smith, S. Engelender, C.A. Ross, V.L. Dawson, T.M. Dawson, Parkin mediates nonclassical, proteasomal-independent ubiquitination of synphilin-1: implications for Lewy body formation, J Neurosci 25 (2005) 2002-2009.

38.   M. Komatsu, S. Waguri, T. Chiba, S. Murata, J. Iwata, I. Tanida, T. Ueno, M. Koike, Y. Uchiyama, E. Kominami, K. Tanaka, Loss of autophagy in the central nervous system causes neurodegeneration in mice, Nature 441 (2006) 880-884.

39.   T. Hara, K. Nakamura, M. Matsui, A. Yamamoto, Y. Nakahara, R. Suzuki-Migishima, M. Yokoyama, K. Mishima, I. Saito, H. Okano, N. Mizushima, Suppression of basal autophagy in neural cells causes neurodegenerative disease in mice, Nature 441 (2006) 885-889.

40.   U.B. Pandey, Z. Nie, Y. Batlevi, B.A. McCray, G.P. Ritson, N.B. Nedelsky, S.L. Schwartz, N.A. DiProspero, M.A. Knight, O. Schuldiner, R. Padmanabhan, M. Hild, D.L. Berry, D. Garza, C.C. Hubbert, T.P. Yao, E.H. Baehrecke, J.P. Taylor, HDAC6 rescues neurodegeneration and provides an essential link between autophagy and the UPS, Nature 447 (2007) 859-863.

41.   H.J. Rideout, I. Lang-Rollin, L. Stefanis, Involvement of macroautophagy in the dissolution of neuronal inclusions, Int J Biochem Cell Biol 36 (2004) 2551-2562.

42.   A. Iwata, B.E. Riley, J.A. Johnston, R.R. Kopito, HDAC6 and microtubules are required for autophagic degradation of aggregated huntingtin, J Biol Chem 280 (2005) 40282-40292.

43.   J.A. Johnston, C.L. Ward, R.R. Kopito, Aggresomes: a cellular response to misfolded proteins, J Cell Biol 143 (1998) 1883-1898.

44.   E. Junn, S.S. Lee, U.T. Suhr, M.M. Mouradian, Parkin accumulation in aggresomes due to proteasome impairment, J Biol Chem 277 (2002) 47870-47877.

45.   Y. Kawaguchi, J.J. Kovacs, A. McLaurin, J.M. Vance, A. Ito, T.P. Yao, The deacetylase HDAC6 regulates aggresome formation and cell viability in response to misfolded protein stress, Cell 115 (2003) 727-738.

46.   R.R. Kopito, The missing linker: an unexpected role for a histone deacetylase, Mol Cell 12 (2003) 1349-1351.

47.   J.A. Olzmann, L. Li, M.V. Chudaev, J. Chen, F.A. Perez, R.D. Palmiter, L.S. Chin, Parkin-mediated K63-linked polyubiquitination targets misfolded DJ-1 to aggresomes via binding to HDAC6, J Cell Biol 178 (2007) 1025-1038.

48.   J.A. Olzmann, L.S. Chin, Parkin-mediated K63-linked polyubiquitination: a signal for targeting misfolded proteins to the aggresome-autophagy pathway, Autophagy 4 (2008) 85-87.

49.   T. Geetha, M.W. Wooten, Structure and functional properties of the ubiquitin binding protein p62, FEBS Lett 512 (2002) 19-24.

50.   M.L. Seibenhener, J.R. Babu, T. Geetha, H.C. Wong, N.R. Krishna, M.W. Wooten, Sequestosome 1/p62 is a polyubiquitin chain binding protein involved in ubiquitin proteasome degradation, Mol Cell Biol 24 (2004) 8055-8068.

51.   S. Pankiv, T.H. Clausen, T. Lamark, A. Brech, J.A. Bruun, H. Outzen, A. Overvatn, G. Bjorkoy, T. Johansen, p62/SQSTM1 binds directly to Atg8/LC3 to facilitate degradation of ubiquitinated protein aggregates by autophagy, J Biol Chem 282 (2007) 24131-24145.

52.   E. Kuusisto, A. Salminen, I. Alafuzoff, Ubiquitin-binding protein p62 is present in neuronal and glial inclusions in human tauopathies and synucleinopathies, Neuroreport 12 (2001) 2085-2090.

53.   K. Zatloukal, C. Stumptner, A. Fuchsbichler, H. Heid, M. Schnoelzer, L. Kenner, R. Kleinert, M. Prinz, A. Aguzzi, H. Denk, p62 Is a common component of cytoplasmic inclusions in protein aggregation diseases, Am J Pathol 160 (2002) 255-263.

54.   E. Kuusisto, A. Salminen, I. Alafuzoff, Early accumulation of p62 in neurofibrillary tangles in Alzheimer's disease: possible role in tangle formation, Neuropathol Appl Neurobiol 28 (2002) 228-237.

55.   G. Bjorkoy, T. Lamark, A. Brech, H. Outzen, M. Perander, A. Overvatn, H. Stenmark, T. Johansen, p62/SQSTM1 forms protein aggregates degraded by autophagy and has a protective effect on huntingtin-induced cell death, J Cell Biol 171 (2005) 603-614.

56.   M. Komatsu, S. Waguri, M. Koike, Y.S. Sou, T. Ueno, T. Hara, N. Mizushima, J. Iwata, J. Ezaki, S. Murata, J. Hamazaki, Y. Nishito, S. Iemura, T. Natsume, T. Yanagawa, J. Uwayama, E. Warabi, H. Yoshida, T. Ishii, A. Kobayashi, M. Yamamoto, Z. Yue, Y. Uchiyama, E. Kominami, K. Tanaka, Homeostatic levels of p62 control cytoplasmic inclusion body formation in autophagy-deficient mice, Cell 131 (2007) 1149-1163.

57.   J. Ramesh Babu, M. Lamar Seibenhener, J. Peng, A.L. Strom, R. Kemppainen, N. Cox, H. Zhu, M.C. Wooten, M.T. Diaz-Meco, J. Moscat, M.W. Wooten, Genetic inactivation of p62 leads to accumulation of hyperphosphorylated tau and neurodegeneration, J Neurochem 106 (2008) 107-120.

58.   I.P. Nezis, A. Simonsen, A.P. Sagona, K. Finley, S. Gaumer, D. Contamine, T.E. Rusten, H. Stenmark, A. Brech, Ref(2)P, the Drosophila melanogaster homologue of mammalian p62, is required for the formation of protein aggregates in adult brain, J Cell Biol 180 (2008) 1065-1071.

59.   Y. Ichimura, T. Kumanomidou, Y.S. Sou, T. Mizushima, J. Ezaki, T. Ueno, E. Kominami, T. Yamane, K. Tanaka, M. Komatsu, Structural basis for

sorting mechanism of p62 in selective autophagy, J Biol Chem 283 (2008) 22847-22857.

60. J.M. Tan, E.S. Wong, V.L. Dawson, T.M. Dawson, K.L. Lim, Lysine 63-linked polyubiquitin potentially partners with p62 to promote the clearance of protein inclusions by autophagy, Autophagy 4 (2007) 251-253.

61. M. Koike, H. Nakanishi, P. Saftig, J. Ezaki, K. Isahara, Y. Ohsawa, W. Schulz-Schaeffer, T. Watanabe, S. Waguri, S. Kametaka, M. Shibata, K. Yamamoto, E. Kominami, C. Peters, K. von Figura, Y. Uchiyama, Cathepsin D deficiency induces lysosomal storage with ceroid lipofuscin in mouse CNS neurons, J Neurosci 20 (2000) 6898-6906.

62. J.J. Shacka, B.J. Klocke, C. Young, M. Shibata, J.W. Olney, Y. Uchiyama, P. Saftig, K.A. Roth, Cathepsin D deficiency induces persistent neurodegeneration in the absence of Bax-dependent apoptosis, J Neurosci 27 (2007) 2081-2090.

63. L. Myllykangas, J. Tyynela, A. Page-McCaw, G.M. Rubin, M.J. Haltia, M.B. Feany, Cathepsin D-deficient Drosophila recapitulate the key features of neuronal ceroid lipofuscinoses, Neurobiol Dis 19 (2005) 194-199.

64. R.A. Nixon, D.S. Yang, J.H. Lee, Neurodegenerative lysosomal disorders: a continuum from development to late age, Autophagy 4 (2008) 590-599.

65. Y.P. Ning, K. Kanai, H. Tomiyama, Y. Li, M. Funayama, H. Yoshino, S. Sato, M. Asahina, S. Kuwabara, A. Takeda, T. Hattori, Y. Mizuno, N. Hattori, PARK9-linked parkinsonism in eastern Asia: mutation detection in ATP13A2 and clinical phenotype, Neurology 70 (2008) 1491-1493.

66. K. Verhoeven, P. De Jonghe, K. Coen, N. Verpoorten, M. Auer-Grumbach, J.M. Kwon, D. FitzPatrick, E. Schmedding, E. De Vriendt, A. Jacobs, V. Van Gerwen, K. Wagner, H.P. Hartung, V. Timmerman, Mutations in the small GTP-ase late endosomal protein RAB7 cause Charcot-Marie-Tooth type 2B neuropathy, Am J Hum Genet 72 (2003) 722-727.

67. I. Puls, S.J. Oh, C.J. Sumner, K.E. Wallace, M.K. Floeter, E.A. Mann, W.R. Kennedy, G. Wendelschafer-Crabb, A. Vortmeyer, R. Powers, K. Finnegan, E.L. Holzbaur, K.H. Fischbeck, C.L. Ludlow, Distal spinal and bulbar muscular atrophy caused by dynactin mutation, Ann Neurol 57 (2005) 687-694.

68. S. Kimura, T. Noda, T. Yoshimori, Dynein-dependent Movement of Autophagosomes Mediates Efficient Encounters with Lysosomes, Cell Struct Funct 33 (2008) 109-122.

69. F. Pickford, E. Masliah, M. Britschgi, K. Lucin, R. Narasimhan, P.A. Jaeger, S. Small, B. Spencer, E. Rockenstein, B. Levine, T. Wyss-Coray, The autophagy-related protein beclin 1 shows reduced expression in early Alzheimer disease and regulates amyloid beta accumulation in mice, J Clin Invest 118 (2008) 2190-2199.

70. B. Ravikumar, C. Vacher, Z. Berger, J.E. Davies, S. Luo, L.G. Oroz, F. Scaravilli, D.F. Easton, R. Duden, C.J. O'Kane, D.C. Rubinsztein, Inhibition of mTOR induces autophagy and reduces toxicity of polyglutamine expansions in fly and mouse models of Huntington disease, Nat Genet 36 (2004) 585-595.

71. Z. Berger, B. Ravikumar, F.M. Menzies, L.G. Oroz, B.R. Underwood, M.N. Pangalos, I. Schmitt, U. Wullner, B.O. Evert, C.J. O'Kane, D.C. Rubinsztein, Rapamycin alleviates toxicity of different aggregate-prone proteins, Hum Mol Genet 15 (2006) 433-442.

72. R.A. Nixon, Autophagy, amyloidogenesis and Alzheimer disease, J Cell Sci 120 (2007) 4081-4091.

73. W.H. Yu, A.M. Cuervo, A. Kumar, C.M. Peterhoff, S.D. Schmidt, J.H. Lee, P.S. Mohan, M. Mercken, M.R. Farmery, L.O. Tjernberg, Y. Jiang, K. Duff, Y. Uchiyama, J. Naslund, P.M. Mathews, A.M. Cataldo, R.A. Nixon, Macroautophagy--a novel Beta-amyloid peptide-generating pathway activated in Alzheimer's disease, J Cell Biol 171 (2005) 87-98.

74. H. Seo, K.C. Sonntag, W. Kim, E. Cattaneo, O. Isacson, Proteasome activator enhances survival of huntington's disease neuronal model cells, PLoS ONE 2 (2007) e238.

www.ingramcontent.com/pod-product-compliance
Lightning Source LLC
Chambersburg PA
CBHW041712210326
41598CB00007B/620